Dr. Sebi

Take Control of Your Health with Dr. Sebi Alkaline Diet, Herbs and Cure for Herpes. 200+ Mouth Watering Recipes to Effectively Cleanse Your Liver and Naturally Detox the Body. 3 Manuscripts in 1 Book

Neal Graham

© Copyright 2020 - All rights reserved.

The content contained within this book may not be reproduced, duplicated or transmitted without direct written permission from the author or the publisher.

Under no circumstances will any blame or legal responsibility be held against the publisher, or author, for any damages, reparation, or monetary loss due to the information contained within this book. Either directly or indirectly.

Legal Notice:

This book is copyright protected. This book is only for personal use. You cannot amend, distribute, sell, use, quote or paraphrase any part, or the content within this book, without the consent of the author or publisher.

Disclaimer Notice:

Please note the information contained within this document is for educational and entertainment purposes only. All effort has been executed to present accurate, up to date, and reliable, complete information. No warranties of any kind are declared or implied. Readers acknowledge that the author is not engaging in the rendering of legal, financial, medical or professional advice. The content within this book has been derived from various sources. Please consult a licensed professional before attempting any techniques outlined in this book.

By reading this document, the reader agrees that under no circumstances is the author responsible for any losses, direct or indirect, which are incurred as a result of the use of information contained within this document, including, but not limited to, — errors, omissions, or inaccuracies.

The Doctor Sebi Diet

Table of Contents

INTRODUCTION 7

CHAPTER 1: WHAT IS THE DOCTOR SEBI DIET 9
    Who Is Dr. Sebi? 9
    What Is the Dr. Sebi Diet? 9
    How to Follow the Dr. Sebi Diet? 9
    Can It Help You Lose Weight? 10

CHAPTER 2: FOOD PRINCIPLES 11

CHAPTER 3: DOCTOR SEBI'S DIET AND WEIGHT LOSS 14
    Dr. Sebi Alkaline Diet for Health and Weight Loss 14

CHAPTER 4: BENEFITS AND DOWNSIDES 18
    Benefits of the Dr. Sebi Food Regimen 18
    Downsides of the Dr. Sebi Food Regimen 19

CHAPTER 5: DOCTOR SEBI'S SUPPLEMENTS 21
    What Are the Supplements Made of? 21

CHAPTER 6: THE BENEFIT OF FASTING AS RECOMMENDED BY DR. SEBI 24
    Preparing for a Fast 24
    Why Should You Fast? 24

CHAPTER 7: REVERSE DISEASE 28
    Types of Diabetes 28
    Lifestyle Changes for Diabetes 30
    Dr. Sebi's Diabetes Cure 31

CHAPTER 8: DIFFERENCE BETWEEN PHLEGM AND MUCUS 32
    Phlegm Carries Disease 32
    Mucus Disease 32
    Mucus Is The Cause Of Every Disease 32
    Mucus and Phlegm Cause Disease 32
    Phlegm After Eating 34
    Symptoms of Constant Mucus in the Throat 34

CHAPTER 9: DETOXING THE LIVER 35
    The Seven Day Liver Detox Diet Plan 35
    The Most Effective Method to Cleanse Your Liver 35
    Outside Toxins and the Effect They Have on the Liver 38

CHAPTER 10: DECONSTRUCTING THE PLANT-BASED DIET 40
    Hybridization and Genetic Manipulation 40
    Hereditarily Modified Organisms 41
    Prepared Foods 42
    In Part Hydrogenated Oils 43

CHAPTER 11: CLASSIFICATION OF FOODS 44

HYBRIDIZED FOODS 44
RAW FOODS 44
LIVE FOODS 45
GENETICALLY MODIFIED FOODS (GMO) 45
DRUGS 45
DEAD FOODS 46
THE IMPORTANCE OF DR. SEBI'S NUTRITIONAL DIETS 46
HOW TO EMBRACE DR. SEBI'S DIET 46

CHAPTER 12: HERBS 47

IRISH SEA MOSS 47
BLADDERWRACK 48
CASCARA SAGRADA 50
BLUE VERVAIN 51
BURDOCK ROOT 52

CHAPTER 13: DR. SEBI'S MUCUS DIETS 53

DR. SEBI'S 14 DAYS FAST DETOXIFICATION HERBS TO REMOVE EXCESS MUCUS, AND REMOVE ACID 53

CHAPTER 14: DR. SEBI'S ALKALINE DIET TIPS AND TRICKS 56

THE ALKALINE DIET: A LITTLE-KNOWN AND POWERFUL WEIGHT-LOSS PLAN 56
WHAT'S WRONG WITH THE WAY YOU'RE EATING NOW? 56
PERHAPS YOU WONDER, "WHY DO THE PH BALANCE AND ALKALINITY MEAN TO ME?" 57
WHAT'S THE ALKALINE DIET LIKE, AND WHAT WOULD YOU EXPECT? 58
WHAT WOULD YOU FIND AN ALTERNATE STRATEGY, INCLUDING AN ALKALINE DIET FOR OTHER EATING
PLANS? 58
TIPS FOR SUCCESSFULLY FOLLOWING THE ALKALINE DIET 58

CHAPTER 15: RISKS AND CONCERNS 60

SYMPTOMS OF ALKALOSIS 60
HYPOKALEMIA 60
ARRHYTHMIAS 60
COMA 60
MISTAKES BEGINNERS STARTING ALKALINE DIET OFTEN MAKE 61
YOU NEED TO THINK IN ADVANCE 62

CHAPTER 16: BEFORE YOU BEGIN 63

DIETARY CHANGES 65
GET YOUR MIND READY 66

CHAPTER 17: ALKALINE-PLANT-BASED DIET 68

THE HEALTH BENEFITS OF ALKALINE PLANT-BASED DIET 68
WHY CHOOSE A PLANT-BASED DIET? 68
THE BENEFIT OF SOY IN AN ALKALINE DIET 70
ALTERNATIVES TO SOY FOR A PLANT-BASED DIET 70
ALKALINE FRUITS 71
Which Fruits are high in Alkaline? 72

CHAPTER 18: EATING NATURALLY WITH DR. SEBI'S TEACHINGS 73

CHAPTER 19: HOW THE ALKALINE DIET CAN HELP YOU 75

ANTI-AGING EFFECT 75

- Increased Vitality and Energy..75
- Prepares Your Body for Weight Loss 75
- Decreased Bloating and Constipation 76
- Better Brain Function and Mood.. 76
- A Shield against Diseases and Allergies 76
- Stronger Bones 77
- Enhanced Fertility..77
- Possible Symptoms or Illnesses Which Can Be Prevented by Using This Type of Diet 77
- Hypertension, Stroke and Heart Disease 77
- Kidney Stones 77
- Muscle Mass.. 78
- Type 2 Diabetes 78

CHAPTER 20: THE IDEAL 30-DAY MEAL PLAN FOR AN ALKALINE DIET 79
- Week 1... 80
- Week 2..81
- Week 3... 82
- Week 4... 83
- Breakfast 84
- Snacks 84

CONCLUSION 85

Introduction

Following Dr. Sebi's diet leads to numerous health benefits as it encourages the consumption of fruits and vegetables, unprocessed fresh products, and discourages the use of alcohol and other potentially harmful substances. It also makes you drink lots of water.

This diet results in steady weight loss, decrease the risks of many diseases and lowers the chances of developing them. Kidney stones and kidney diseases are less frequent. Bones and muscles get stronger. It results in higher functioning of the heart and brain, also lowering the chances of their deterioration. You are less likely to develop some type 2 diabetes as it is related to obesity, and this diet helps remove obesity by effective weight loss.

People who believe in Dr. Sebi's diet say that it reduces the built-up acidity in our body. If we stop eating alkaline foods, the acid will start to accumulate, and our body will attract many types of diseases. Eating a constant influx of alkaline foods helps to reduce diseases and acidity.

Almost anyone looking to better their life can follow this diet. Unhealthy eating has become prominent all over the world. People of all ages prefer to run away from vegetables and fruits these days practically. Apart from some popular ingredients, people don't know about the large variety of foods that are available at their disposal. Because of laziness and ignorance, people choose not to look at all of the options that might greatly benefit them and settle for the most natural thing they can get on the plate. Dieting, especially Dr. Sebi's dieting, which is mainly focused on vegetables and fruits, is a crucial step in improving people's health.

More people are obese than ever before. Heart disease and diabetes are the major causes of death. All these aspects are related to bad eating and can be improved if we switch to a healthy and nutritious eating routine, just like this diet.

The people that can benefit the most are obese people looking for a way to shed some pounds so that they don't invite diseases into their bodies. The diet effectively makes a person lose weight and reach their weight goals, so obese and overweight people can improve their lives significantly. Also, it can help people suffering from heart disease and diabetes. Still, before patients should opt for the diet, it is advised that they seek the guidance of a health professional before adopting such a restrictive and low caloric diet.

Many people have tried and commented on their diet. The people who started the diet were mostly people looking for an effective weight-loss method. The dieting plan ranges for about four weeks for some people with probably a cheat day or two. A complete strict adaptation of the diet for your whole life, just as you are starting, is a near-impossible thing to do even if you have high motivation.

People switching to the diet for the first time — whose meals consist of meat, rice, and bread, with occasional snacking — found the diet to be complicated during the first week, their daily routine was affected as they felt a loss in energy, and they sensed weakness for the first few days. Dieters who took supplements and planned their meals to be rich in calories found that they gained some of their energy back, but it was still not enough. After weeks three and four, the diet became more comfortable to follow. In the end, dieters on average saw a considerable reduction in their weight —approximately two to four pounds per day, after five or six weeks of dieting was completed.

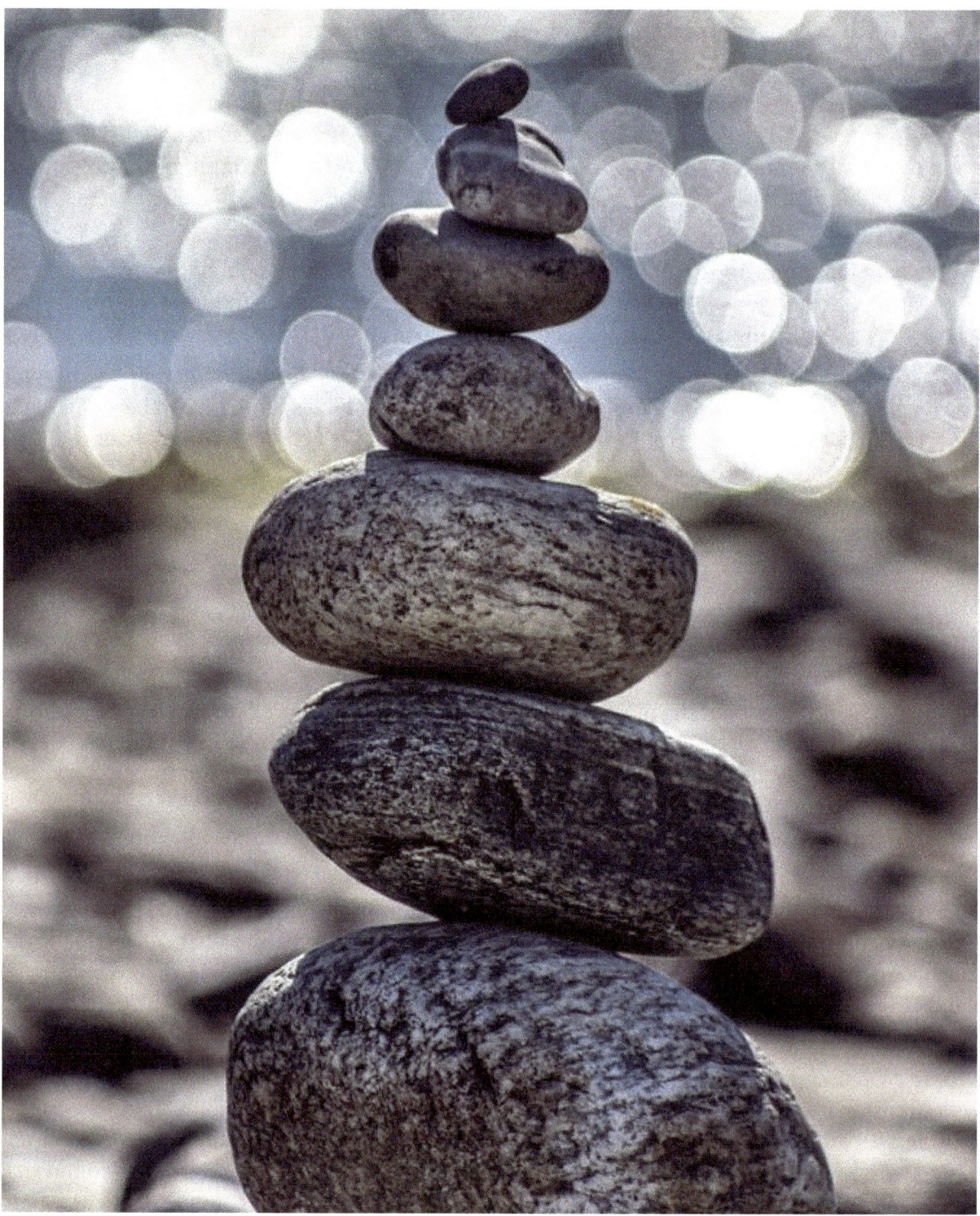

Chapter 1: What Is the Doctor Sebi Diet

Who Is Dr. Sebi?

This eating regimen was developed by the self-taught by an herbalist Alfredo Darrington Bowman – better known as Dr. Sebi. Despite his name, Dr. Sebi was not a medical specialist and did not hold a PH. D. The African bio-mineral balance theory was his basis.

An obituary describes about his controversial health claims, such as curing aids and leukemia. These and similar assertions resulted in a 1993 lawsuit that ended with the court ordering Dr. Sebi's organization to stop making these claims Dr. Sebi reportedly died in 2016 in police custody.

What Is the Dr. Sebi Diet?

Dr. Sebi believed the western approach to disease to be ineffective. He held that mucus and acidity – preferably bacteria and viruses, for example – caused disease. A central theory behind the diet is that disease can only survive in acidic environments. The diet aims to achieve an alkaline state in the body to prevent or eradicate the disease. The diet's main and official website sells botanical remedies that it claims will detoxify the body. Some of the remedies – called African bio-mineral balance supplements – retails at $1,500 per package. The site links to none research that would support its claims about health benefits. It does not mean that the food and drug administration (FDA) has not evaluated the statements. Those behind the site acknowledged that they are not medical doctors and do not intend the site's content to replace medical advice.

He designed this diet for anybody who wishes to naturally fix or prevent infection and improve their general health without relying on conventional western medicine. According to Dr. Sebi, sickness is a result of bodily fluid develops in an area of your body. For model, a build-up of mucus in the lungs is pneumonia, while overabundance mucus in the pancreas is diabetes. He debates that diseases cannot exist in an alkaline environment and start to occur when your body becomes too acidic. We need to strictly follow his diet and using his proprietary, costly supplements body. Formerly, Dr. Sebi claimed that his diet could cure conditions like aids, sickle cell anemia, leukemia, and lupus. Be that as it may, after a 1993 claim, he was requested to end making such claims. The diet contains a specific list of endorsed vegetables, natural products, grains, nuts, seeds, oils, and spices. As animal products are not allowable, the Dr. Sebi diet is considered a veggie lover diet. Sebi claimed that for your body to heal itself, you must follow all the eating routine consistently for the rest of your life. Finally, while numerous people insist that the program has healed them, no scientific studies support these cases.

How to Follow the Dr. Sebi Diet?

According to Dr. Sebi's nutritive guide, you must follow these essential rules:

- **Rule No. 1:** You must eat foods listed in the nutritional guide.

- **Rule No. 2:** Drink 1 gallon (3.8 liters) of water every day.
- **Rule No. 3:** Take Dr. Sebi's supplements an hour before medications.
- **Rule No. 4:** No animal products are permitted.
- **Rule No. 5:** No alcohol is allowed.
- **Rule No. 6:** Avoid wheat products and only consume the "natural-growing grains" listed in the guide.
- **Rule No. 7:** Avoid using a microwave to prevent killing your food.
- **Rule No. 8:** Avoid canned or seedless fruits.

There are no exact nutrient guidelines. However, this diet is low in protein, as it prohibits beans, lentils, and animal and soy foods. Protein is an essential nutrient needed for healthy muscles, skin, and joints. Additionally, you're also expected to purchase Dr. Sebi's cell food products, which are supplements that promise to cleanse your body and nurture your cells. It's suggested to buy the "all-inclusive" package, which encompasses 20 different products that are claimed to cleanse and restore your entire body at the fastest rate possible. Besides this, no specific enhancement recommendations are provided. Instead, you're predictable to order any supplement that matches your health concerns. For example, the "bio ferry" capsules claim to treat liver issues, cleanse your blood, boost immunity, promote weight loss, digestive aid issues, and increase overall well-being.

Furthermore, the enhancements don't contain a complete list of nutrients or their quantities, making it difficult to know whether they will meet your daily needs.

Can It Help You Lose Weight?

The diet depresses eating a western diet, which is high in ultra-processed foods and loaded with salt, sugar fat, and calories. Instead, it promotes an unprocessed, plant-based diet. Compared with the western diet, these who follow a plant-based diet tend to have lower rates of obesity and heart disease. A 12-month study in 65 people set up that those who followed an unlimited whole-food, low-fat, plant-based diet lost significantly more weight than people who did not follow the diet.

At the 6-month mark, those on a diet had lost an average of 26.6 pounds (12.1 kg), compared with 3.5 pounds (1.6 kg) in the regulator group. Furthermore, most foods on this diet are low in calories, except for nuts, seeds, avocados, and oils. Therefore, even if you ate a large volume of permitted foods, it's unlikely that it would result in a surplus of calories and lead to weight gain. However, very-low-calorie diets usually cannot be sustained long term. Most people who follow these diets regain the mass once they resume a regular eating outline. Since this diet does not identify quantities and portions, it's difficult to say whether it will provide enough calories for sustainable weight loss.

Chapter 2: Food Principles

The adequacy of the alkaline diet is highly reliant on the food you eat and how you combine them. If you want to achieve your weight misfortune goals, and get superior health, be knowledgeable about maintaining an acid-alkaline balance. With this, there is an appropriate food combination rule that you can follow to have the option to deliver many healthy and functional body cells. We coordinate these standards towards the anticipation of heartburn and acidosis, which are two significant obstructions to a successful alkaline diet. There are food combinations that interfere with your assimilation. If such food hampers the procedure of assimilation, your stomach won't have the option to flexibly vitamins and minerals to the different body organs and systems. On-going investigations have revealed that the foods that make up our usual meal cannot be processed appropriately. It is because of the inappropriate combination of the foods, making it difficult for the digestive enzymes to finish their work. As an impact, the level of acids and alkaline in the body becomes unstable. Doing the best food joining standards underneath won't just assist you with thinking of great alkaline food plans, but will also give you better processing. You may allude to the alkaline diet food chart as you read along.

1. Try not to eat carbohydrates and acid foods in combination; do not consume foods wealthy in carbohydrates, for example, potatoes, bread, bananas, beans, and dates with acid foods like limes, grapefruits, oranges, tomatoes, and pineapples with acidic foods. Ptyalin, an enzyme, is just activated by an alkaline medium, and by mellow acid, it's destroyed. Acidic fruits both forestall the assimilation of carbohydrates and bolster their fermentation. The acids found in these fruits, for example, oxalic acid, counter the action of ptyalin. In like manner, we must not eat tomatoes in combination with any starchy foods. Instead, eat them with green leafy vegetables and fatty foods. The acidic mixes present in tomatoes, such as malic, oxalic, and citrus extracts, contrast the way toward breaking down the starch in the mouth and the stomach. When there is hyperacidity in the stomach, starches become challenging to process. This brings distress as inappropriately processed starches become toxic substances to the body.

2. Try not to consume concentrated carbohydrates and concentrated protein inside the same meal. Concentrated carbohydrates incorporate bread, potatoes, cereals, cakes, and sweet fruits. Meanwhile, examples of concentrated protein are nuts, eggs, meat, and cheddar. The most widely recognized protein-carbohydrate food combinations are sandwiches and burgers. However, they are delicious; these food combinations are terrible for assimilation. Carbohydrate assimilation is altogether different from that of protein. When they are blended inside the stomach, they upset the processing of each other. We consider the absorption of protein as an acid procedure of gastric assimilation, while the processing of carbohydrates is a salivary absorption. Our system cannot carry these two sorts of processing for an extended

period because the stomach's increased acidity gradually thwarts the breakdown of carbohydrates. The exceptional gastric juices that are engaged with the assimilation of proteins hinder starch assimilation.

3. Similarly, sugar frustrates the release of these gastric squeezes and hinders the processing of protein. Because of this, the combination of starch and protein damages stomach activities. In an on-going report, we discovered that undigested carbs in enormous amounts absorb the enzyme pepsin. This blocks the acid from consolidating with proteins. In particular, beans are a combination of carbs and protein. They contain 25% protein and around half carbohydrates or starch. This is the reason the digestive system thinks it's taxing to process them. The carb substance of the beans stays in the stomach while it processes its protein segment and, later, produces toxins and gas. An excellent recommendation is to eliminate beans from your diet. Green beans, however, are a particular case because they contain a small amount of starch. Then again, dried or matured beans age rapidly and generate excessive amounts of gas.

4. Consume just one concentrated protein at a meal; you must separately take two concentrated proteins. For instance, don't consume nuts with meat, or meat with eggs, or nuts with cheddar, or eggs and cheddar at a single meal. The proteins in these foods have various syntheses and varying characters. It activates the uncommon inactive digestive squeezes. Because of this, the standard is supposed to be each rich in protein, and this ought to be handled carefully.

5. One must not devour protein and fat in one meal; this food joining rule includes not using butter, cream, or oil together with eggs, nuts, cheddar, and meat. The science behind this is that fat weakens the gastric glands and blocks the emission of correct gastric juices for the absorption of proteins. At the point when blended in with various foods, fats can hinder the activation of appetite juice, and decrease its quality. Fats in the stomach can smother the emission of chemical juices. Besides this, they diminish the level of pepsin and hydrochloric acid in the gastrointestinal tract. They cut down the activities of the digestive system to half lower. Oil, then again, when presented in the rectal area, decreases the number of gastric juices.

6. Never eat proteins with acidic fruits; oranges, pineapples, and tomatoes are suitable for consumption, together with eggs and meat (except for cheddar and nuts, which are protein fats). Studies have revealed the adverse effects of the combination of acids in fruits and the shaped acids after protein processing. Organic product acids block the progression of the gastric juices. Protein assimilation requires an unrestricted stream to avoid putrefaction. Just fresh cheese and nuts are protein sources that are not immediately festered.

7. One must not eat starches and sugars together; jams, nectar, molasses, syrups, jams, and organic product butter, when eaten with cake, bread, potatoes, and cereals, facilitates fermentation. In like manner, nectar glazed or syrup-secured

hotcakes are major no. The habit of devouring starches, camouflaged by sugar, isn't an ideal way of taking carbohydrates. Upon the intake of sugar, we indirectly loaded our mouth with instant saliva, but the enzyme ptyalin, which is essential in starch assimilation, is absent. When sugar covers a starch, syrups, jams, jams, etc., it deludes the taste buds in this manner, and cannot determine a way toward processing the carbs. The unhealthy combination of sugar and starch leads to fermentation. As an impact, the level of acidity in the stomach increases and brings inconvenience. Although nectar is a natural sugar and is beneficial to health, this food rule also applies. Here, nectar isn't any different from syrup, when put on cakes, hotcakes, and cereals. All these lead to fermentation and a sharp stomach. Similarly, sugar and molasses of all sorts when eaten with starches also spell fermentation. '

8. Never have concentrated starches and sugars at a single meal; take sugars and starches separately because combining them in one meal could cause the fermentation of some sugars originating from these food categories. The primary reason behind this fermentation is the time expected to break down these foods into sugar substances acceptable by the body. For instance, acid-natural product sugars that usually takes about an hour of processing will require two additional hours (making it three hours altogether) when joined with sweet organic product sugars like dates, fruits, grapes, and figs. The sugar part of the acid-fruits continues to wait for three hours or past before it gets processed. And because it was not well-processed inside the allotted timeframe, it would age. Also, starchy foods cause two hours or more to transform into sugar that the body cells will accept as supplements. Similarly, sugars from acid-fruits remain there for over two hours before processing. The acid originating from these fruits will damage the starch enzymes in this manner; this will delay the absorption of starch.

9. Eat melons alone; always eat melons (muskmelon, watermelon, honeydew melon, casaba melon, pie melon, and cantaloupe) alone with no other combination. There is no idea about the physiological basis of this standard. However, there are many reports about the ease of processing melon when one eats it alone. At the point when taken with another food, melons bring some distress.

10. Milk is best devoured alone; during the initial scarcity, milk is the leading natural food of infants, but it can give the essential supplements, vitamins, and minerals. When in doubt, infants ought not to get milk bombarded with various foods. This applies even to adults. Milk is a gastric insulator. It means that it discourages the creation of gastric squeezes after eating it. Organs in the stomach do not process milk. Instead, it left into the duodenum. This makes it difficult for the digestive system to accomplish its work when we consume milk along with various foods. As introduced above, food combinations mainly affect our intestinal processing.

Chapter 3: Doctor Sebi's Diet and Weight Loss

Numerous individuals endeavor prevailing fashion diets or those which guarantee snappy outcomes trying to get in shape. These diets may bring about the present moment, yet after some time, this can be an exceptionally unhealthy approach to get thinner. Also, numerous individuals recover the weight when they go off their exacting diet. At the point when an acid diet is utilized for weight loss and control, it is all the more a way of life change. The outcomes may not occur without any forethought. However, the weight won't be recovered.

An alkaline diet is wealthy in nourishments, which are generally low in calories, for example, most vegetables and natural products. A significant number of the nourishments that are high in fat and calories are likewise acidifying, so when these nourishments are expelled from the diet, a characteristic and healthy weight loss will happen. These nourishments incorporate red meat, greasy food sources, and high-fat dairy items, for example, whole milk and cheddar, sugar, pop, and liquor. When you quit eating these nourishments, your body will be a lot healthier, less acid, and you'll additionally get more fit all the while. Since the diet is healthy, you can stay with it long haul. Numerous individuals who start an alkaline diet exclusively to get in shape find countless different advantages. An expanded energy level, protection from an ailment, and a general improvement in health and prosperity are among the numerous benefits you can understand on an alkaline diet.

Dr. Sebi Alkaline Diet for Health and Weight Loss

There are a ton of insane diets available that guarantee to assist you with shedding pounds. Shockingly, on the off chance that you take a gander at the healthy benefit of a portion of these diets, they are regularly seriously deficient. If you have to get thinner, you ought to do it while eating food that is useful for your body, with the goal that you will get healthier rather than merely more slender. An alkaline diet is a healthy way to deal with weight loss that will keep you stimulated, healthy, and inspired to drop the pounds.

An alkaline diet is not the same as different diets since it centers mostly around the impact that nourishments have on the acidity or the alkalinity of the body. At the point when nourishments are processed and used by the body, they produce what is usually alluded to as an "alkaline debris" or "acid debris." the first pH of the nourishment doesn't factor into this decisive impact inside the body. The absolute most acidic nourishments, for example, organic citrus products, really produce an alkaline effect when eaten. At the point when increasingly alkaline nourishments are eaten instead of acid nourishments, the pH of the body can be acclimated to an ideal degree of roughly 7.3. While this isn't incredibly alkaline, it is sufficient to receive numerous healthful rewards.

Alkaline Diet Can Save Your Life

Most vegetables and organic products contain a higher measure of essential shaping components than different nourishments. The more noteworthy the ratio of green nourishments devoured in the diet, the more prominent the health benefits are accomplished. These plant nourishments are purifying and alkalizing to the body, while the refined and handled nourishments can increment unhealthy degrees of acidity and poisons. Be that as it may, know that an excess of alkaline can likewise hurt you. You should have the best possible information on adjusting alkaline and acidic nourishments in your diet. After ingestion, essential nourishment and water are very quickly killed by hydrochloric acid present in the stomach. The harmony among alkaline and acidic nourishments must be kept up all together for your organs to perform well.

A healthy and adjusted diet is more alkaline than acid. Given your blood classification, the menu ought to be comprised of 60 to 80% alkaline nourishments and 20 to 40% acidic food sources. Typically, the A and AB blood classifications require the most alkaline diet, while the o and b blood classifications require creature items increasingly in their diet. In any case, remember, in case you're in torment, you're acidic. Progressing to an alkaline diet requires a move in one's mentality about nourishment. It is useful to investigate new tastes and surfaces while rolling out little improvements and improving old propensities.

The Perks of the Alkaline Diet Program

Society today is assaulted by such a significant number of various diet programs that it very well may be overpowering. A few diets place limitations on what nourishments can be eaten due to what's in them. In contrast, others are progressively indulgent with nourishment determination, however stringent on when you can eat. The reason for diets differs too; and some are intended to get more fit, and others are for improving health. The alkaline diet can be grouped into the last mentioned, as it comprises of expending healthy nourishments yet can at the previous outcome in weight loss too.

The pH level of the human body should be around 7.35, which is somewhat alkaline and implies that the body requires alkaline. Trackers and gatherers, a long-time prior, experienced no difficulty addressing this need as the vast majority of the nourishments they are wealthy in alkaline, for example, vegetables, nuts, and seeds.

These days notwithstanding, the cutting-edge diet isn't exceptionally alkaline, comprising mainly of handled nourishments and creature protein. At the point when these nourishments and different things, for example, espresso, beans, and fish, are expended, they discharge acids that happen to debilitate our bones.

The alkaline diet is engaging because it advances quality during the bones and joints. Acid debilitates the bones, so expending a diet high in alkaline will balance the impacts that acids have on our bodies. That is the reason this diet contains nourishments, for example, natural products, seeds, nuts, green tea, tomatoes, etc. Because they have low degrees of acid. However, more grounded joints and bones aren't the main advantages of the alkaline diet.

Extra advantages of the alkaline diet incorporate expanded energy levels and hindering an abundance of mucous generation. It can likewise enable the individuals to experience the ill effects of this season's flu virus, colds, and nasal clog as often as possible. Also, the individuals who have different indications, for example, polycystic ovaries, ovarian pimples, and kind-hearted bosom growths, can improve by changing to an alkaline-based diet. At last, it can decrease sentiments of crabbiness, uneasiness, and tension.

Dr. Sebi's diet plan is a carefully veggie lover dietary system centered on the entire nourishment plant-based eating routine. It underlines nourishments that Dr. Sebi recorded as an antacid. This implies you are not permitted to eat all plant-based nourishment (see beneath). Significantly, all the nourishments you expend while following this eating regimen plan are on the endorsed food sources list.

Here is Dr. Sebi nourishment list with what you can eat on Dr. Sebi's eating routine arrangement:

- **Vegetables**

  Permitted vegetables incorporate asparagus, chime peppers, lettuce (aside from iceberg), cucumbers, kale, chickpeas, Mexican squash, onions, tomatoes, squash, okra, zucchini, wild arugula, amaranth greens, olives, dandelion greens, amaranth, chayote.

  Mushrooms (except for shitake) are permitted on Dr. Sebi slim down as long as they are non-GMO or prepared in any capacity. You can hope to eat a lot of mushrooms on this dietary arrangement.

- **Natural products**

  You can eat numerous sorts of the natural product on this eating regimen: apples, bananas, oranges, fruits, melon, cherries, papayas, mango, limes, figs, seeded grapes, seeded melons, plums, pears, peaches, prickly plant organic product, seeded raisins, prunes, and pears.

- **Nuts**

  There are sure nuts permitted on this eating regimen plan: pecans, crude sesame seeds, Brazil nuts, and hemp seed.

- **Herbs**

  A few herbs are additionally permitted on the Dr. Sebi's diet, for example, basil, dill, oregano, cloves, cayenne, habanero, sage, thyme.

- **Oils**

  Permitted oils incorporate olive oil, coconut oil, avocado oil, hemp seed oil, and grape seed oil.

- **Grains**

  This eating routine arrangement permits just basic grains on your eating regimen. These are fonio rye, kamut, quinoa, amaranth, wild rice, spelt.

- **Salt**

You can expend pure ocean salt on this eating regimen.

- **Sugars**

    Soluble sugars. Sugar isn't permitted on this eating routine; however, certain antacid sugars are. You can eat date sugar (from dried dates) and pure agave syrup from the prickly plant.

- **Non – GMO foods**

    You should concentrate on plant-based nourishments that are crude or insignificantly prepared. It is likewise significant that the nourishments you devour are non-GMO.

It is ideal for eating natural nourishments however much as could reasonably be expected, to dodge pesticides and different synthetic concoctions included non-natural food sources. For whatever length of time that the nourishments of decision fit the above criteria, the odds are that they are permitted on Dr. Sebi's diet.

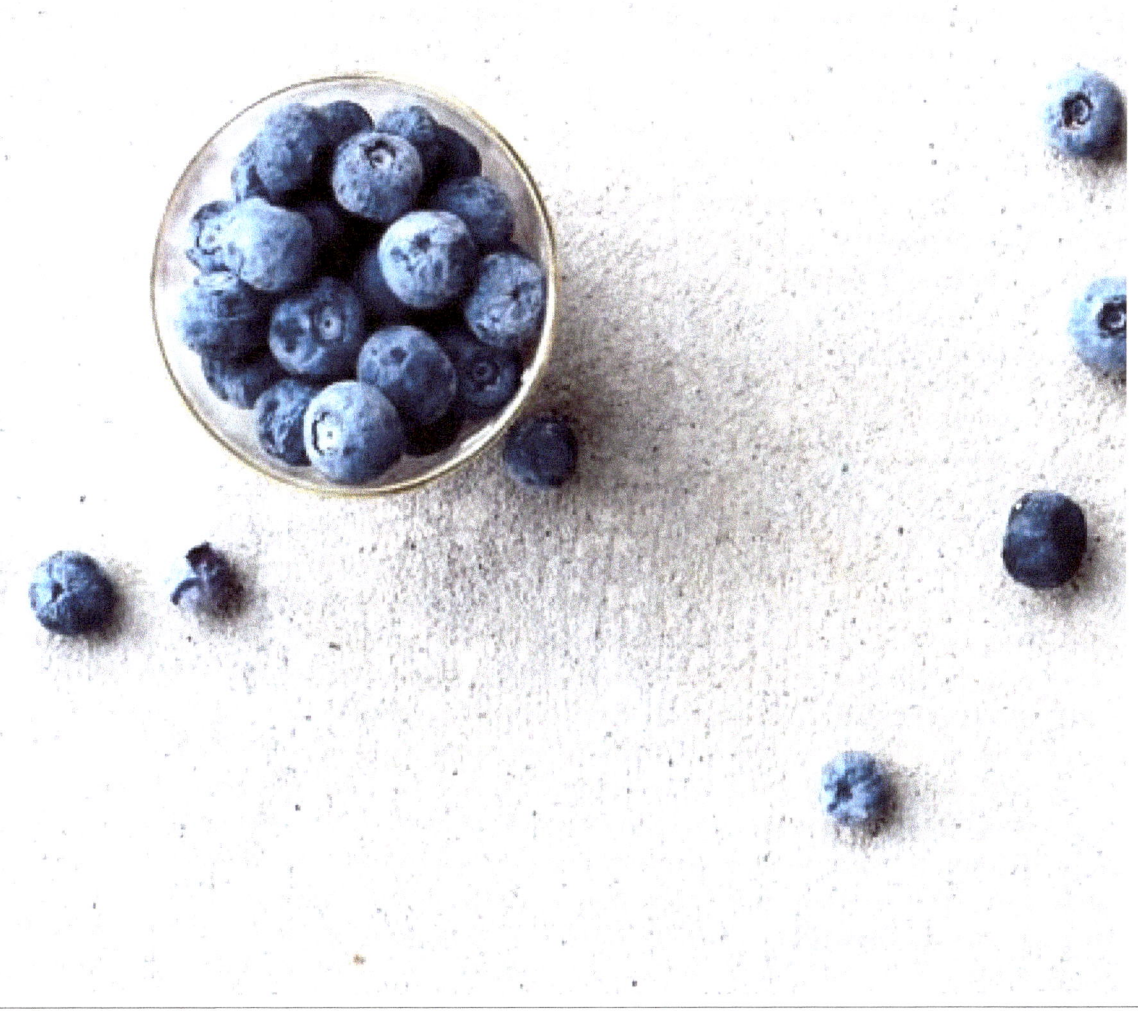

Chapter 4: Benefits and Downsides

Benefits of the Dr. Sebi Food Regimen

One benefit of Dr. Sebi's food regimen is its strong emphasis on plant-based ingredients.

The diet promotes eating a wide range of vegetables and fruit, which are excessive in fiber, vitamins, minerals, and plant compounds.

Diets wealthy in greens and fruit have been associated with decreased infection and oxidative pressure, similarly to safety in opposition to many sicknesses.

A take a look at 226 people, folks that ate 7 or more servings of veggies and fruit in line with day had a 25% and 31% lower occurrence of most cancers and coronary heart disorder, respectively.

Moreover, the majority aren't eating enough produce. In a 2017 file, 9.3% and 12.2% of people met the recommendations for vegetables and fruit, respectively.

Furthermore, Dr. Sebi diet promotes ingesting fiber-wealthy entire grains and wholesome fats, which includes nuts, seeds, and plant oils. That food had been linked to a decrease chance of coronary heart disease.

Sooner or later, diets that restriction extraordinarily-processed food are associated with a higher common weight-reduction plan fine.

Weight Loss

Despite that Dr. Sebi's alkaline diet is solely not focused on losing weight, strictly following the diet can aid weight loss and prevent obesity. The eating of alkaline food and limiting the intake of acidic foods can make it easy to lose weight. The alkaline diet reduces inflammation and leptin levels that affect fat-burning ability and hunger.

Consuming an alkaline diet, which is an anti-inflammatory food, helps the body achieve primal leptin levels, and helps you feel full from eating a few calories or the amount your body requires.

Reduced Risks of Diseases

The plant-based meals reduced the risk of diabetes, developing metabolic syndrome, improved cardiovascular health, reduced the risk of kidney stones, the risk of coronary heart disease, and memory loss. Dr. Sebi's diet advocates for a meatless diet that is low in calories but high in fiber.

The alkaline diet contains anti-aging effects that decrease inflammation and increase the production of growth hormone.

Lowers Chronic Pain and Inflammation

Chronic acidosis causes headaches, menstrual symptoms, back pains, joint pains, and inflammations. People with chronic pains are treated with daily alkaline supplements for 4 weeks. The alkaline diet is seen to lower the chronic pains significantly

Boost Vitamin Absorption

Many people in the world suffer from magnesium deficiency. Magnesium is increasingly required in many body processes and in the functioning of many enzyme systems in the body. Lack of magnesium causes muscle pains, sleep problems, heart complications, and headaches.

Eating an alkaline diet that is rich in magnesium prevents vitamin d deficiency by activating it. Vitamin d is responsible for the overall immune system and functioning of endocrine.

Protect the Bone Density and Muscle Mass

An alkaline diet involves mainly the intake of fruits and vegetables, which are rich in minerals. Eating more mineral-rich foods gives you better protection sarcopenia, which is muscle wasting and decreased bone strength.

Helps Improve Immune Function and Protect from Cancer

Body cells require minerals to fully oxygenate the body and dispose of waste products from the body. Lack of enough minerals compromise vitamin absorption and helps pathogens and toxins accumulate in the body. This highly weakens the immune system. Alkaline diet sees to it that your body is well packed with minerals, thus boosting your immune system; moreover, alkalinity in the body helps reduce inflammation and the risk of cancer. Alkaline diet highly benefits chemotherapeutic agents who require high ph to work effectively.

Appetite Control

Eating peas and beans found in the alkaline diet are more fillings than eating animal products like meat. Therefore, eating less of alkaline meals can help regulate the amount of food you eat, thus controlling your appetite. This may aid weight loss and overall body health.

Downsides of the Dr. Sebi Food Regimen

Keep up in mind that there are numerous drawbacks to this weight-reduction plan.

Incredibly restrictive

A crucial disadvantage of Dr. Sebi's food plan is that it restricts massive agencies of food, in conjunction with all products of animal eat, beans, lentils, and masses of forms of veggies and fruit.

In reality, it's so strict that it simplest lets in precise varieties of fruit. As an example, you're allowed to devour cherry or plum tomatoes, but now not other varieties like beefsteak or Roma tomatoes.

Moreover, following the sort of restrictive weight loss program isn't thrilling and might motive a poor dating with food, mainly whilst you don't forget that this food plan vilifies substances that are not listed inside the nutrients guide.

In the end, this food regimen encourages one-of-a-kind terrible behaviors, which encompass the usage of supplements to benefit fullness. Given that supplements aren't an excellent source of strength; this claim further drives risky eating styles.

Some dieters remember the Dr. Sebi's meals listing to be too proscribing for his or her liking. But, dedicated fans of the eating regimen experience that there are sufficient meals on the listing to allow for range. A general meal with the Dr. Sebi's weight loss program could likely look something like vegetables sautéed in avocado oil on a bed of untamed rice, or a large green salad with olive oil dressing even though it is able to take some getting used to, the Dr. Sebi's meals listing can be clean to stick to and useful to one's health.

May Lead to Vitamin b-12 Deficiency

Vitamin b-12 is a vitaol element in the body and is responsible for making DNA, healthy nerves, and healthy body cells. Dr. Sebi's diet excludes animal products in the foods to eat, which are major sources of vitamin b-12. Vitamin b-12 deficiency causes depression, tiredness, tingling hands and feet, and risk of pernicious anemia. People following Dr. Sebi's diet should, therefore, take vitamin-12 supplements.

May Lead to Protein deficiency

As we all know, proteins are bodybuilding foods and play an important role in our bodies. They support the health of bones, muscles, hormones, DNA, and above all, the brain. Dr. Sebi permits eating some food with proteins such as hemp seeds or walnuts. However, the food has low protein content, and one may be required to eat large amounts of these foods to meet the daily protein requirement. It's important to eat a very wide range of protein foods so that the body can absorb enough amino acids, which are proteins building blocks.

Deficiency of Omega-3 fatty Acids

Omega-3 fatty acids are significant elements in cell membranes. The fatty acids support the immune system, health of the heart, eyes, and brain and body energy. Some Dr. Sebi foods such as walnuts and hemp seed contain amino acids, but the body effectively absorbs them from animal products. If following Dr. Sebi's diet, you may be required to take omega-3 fatty acids supplements.

The body regulates its own ph the human body is created such that it can strictly regulate its own ph and keep it between 7.36 and 7.44, which is the kidney's major job. Sometimes due to medical conditions such as ketoacidosis in diabetes patients, the ph may go out of range. Some scientists, therefore, do not concur with the fact that a diet can alter the body ph.

Chapter 5: Doctor Sebi's Supplements

Along with the restrictive diet, you have to buy Dr. Sebi's original blend of supplements for effective disease curing therapy and weight loss. You can buy the supplements from Dr. Sebi's food cell website. Although the curing properties of these compounds were debunked a long time ago, the compounds' effectiveness in weight loss has still not been proven. There is no scientific study that has given definitive evidence that these chemicals/products do what they claim. Regardless, many of Dr. Sebi's clients and followers still believe that they are very beneficial and are irreplaceable.

What Are the Supplements Made of?

They are made by all organic and natural ingredients and blended with the knowledge of Dr. Sebi. They mostly contain seaweed and different types of herbs and algae. It mostly dispenses in the form of capsules and needs to be consumed daily by the practitioner of the diet. Some of Dr. Sebi's mixtures or products can contain exotic flowers and other pieces of plants. They can be a diverse mixture or consist of a single ingredient entirely. However, it is important to say that when you order a set of the products, many bottles are labeled that they contain some undisclosed ingredient not mentioned previously. This can be a serious hazard if you find yourself allergic to different substances or get sensitive reactions easily.

Are Supplements enough?

The diet has no nutritional or individual nutrient-based guidance. It doesn't tell us how to maintain normal levels of all the basic nutrients, which include proteins, fats, and other components of a balanced diet. One of the major concerns in any plant-based diet is malnutrition development from protein deficiency. Unlike vegetarian or vegan dieting, this diet restricts not only the meat of any animal-source but also some seeds, nuts, grains, and soy products. These ingredients are plant-based alternative foods to replenish protein supply. To get good amounts of protein and also other components this diet limits, you need to opt for protein supplements or any other kind of supplements that you may think is needed other than the ones provided by Dr. Sebi's food cell.

Are They Worth The Expense?

Some products are available in Dr. Sebi's food cell is too expensive for it to be a part of a daily regiment for most people. Getting a bottle of their products can cost up to $30 per bottle, and it is instructed that you have to take a pill each day. There have been no proven studies showing that the products even work, and on top of that, they sell the products with strict rules and great fare. Buying vegetables and whole foods are already very pricey as it is in this day and age for it to be capped by more expenses. For an effective weight-loss routine, you don't need these pills to help you reach your weight-loss goals. The diet itself is low enough in calories that you will see weight loss regardless.

Essential Dr. Sebi's Health Supplements

Proprietary supplements that the program expects you to consume to experience the full health benefits of the diet.

The recommended bundle would be the "all-inclusive package" that pretty much covers everything that would need to fully replenish the health of your body in the minimum amount of time.

Just so that you don't completely stay in the dark, let me talk about the major supplements found in the package to give you an idea of what to expect.

Keep in mind that you also have the option to purchase individual supplements as well. A great a certain type of health benefits from the program.

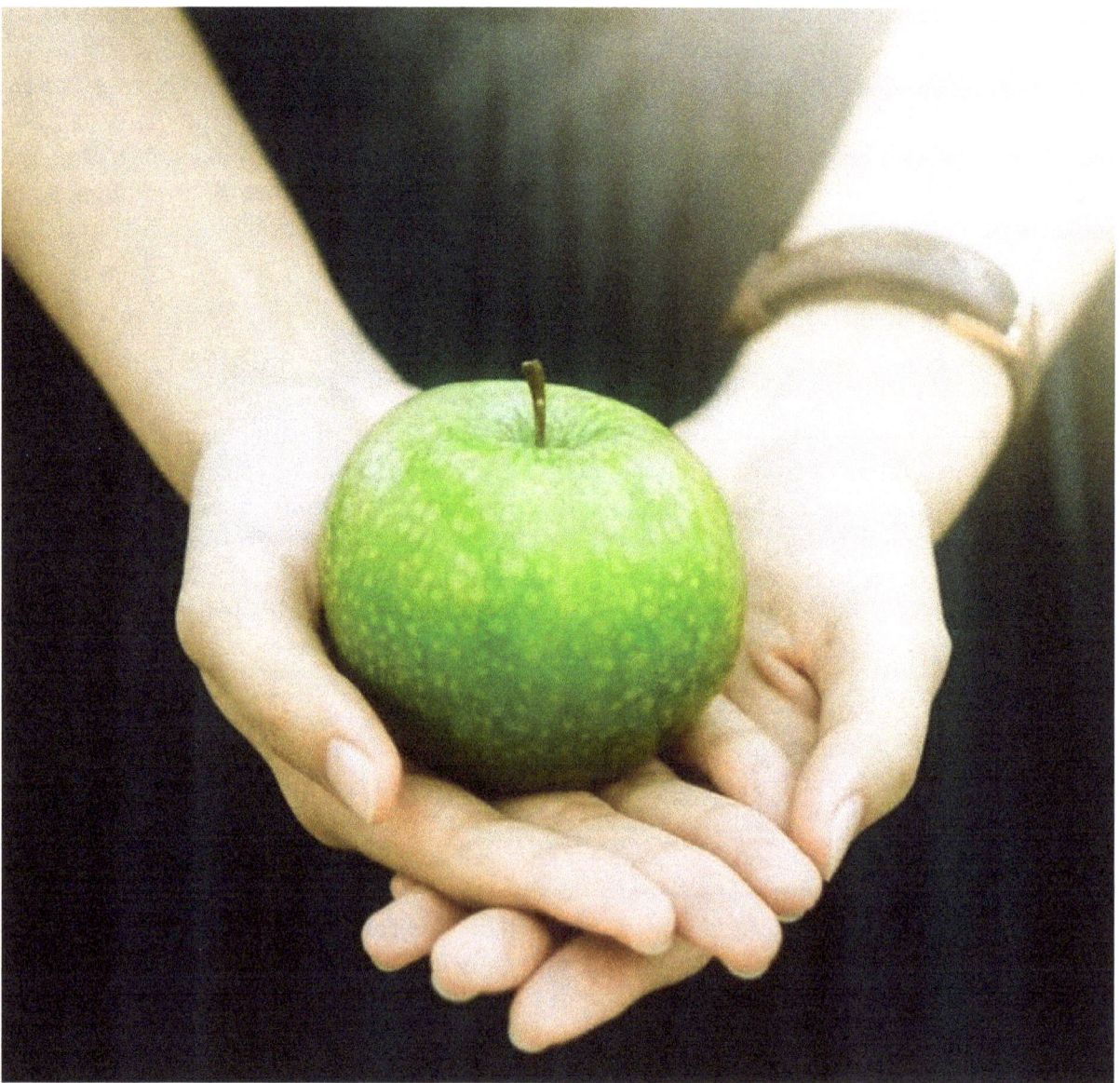

- **Green food plus:** This is a supplement that contains several different minerals that are collected from herbs that are rich in a compound known as chlorophyll. It helps to promote the healthy development of vital organs such as the nervous system, brain, heart, and so on.
- **Viento:** This is a cleanser and an energizer that will help to cleanse your body, revitalize your organs, and increase oxygen flow to your brain and blood. It is rich in iron and helps in the formation of red blood cells as well.
- **Sea moss/seaweed**: This is a nutritious plant that is rich in calcium, iron, magnesium alongside 92 other essential minerals and vitamins. This is an extremely versatile supplement and helps to improve the condition of your body. You may incorporate it into baking, blend into smoothies, or just consume it raw if you prefer. The factors and the ability to improve the effectiveness of the mucous membrane.
- **Testo:** This focuses on the endocrine system and helps to improve your hormonal balance libido. It also helps to improve sex drive in men by increasing blow flow to the male genitalia.
- **Tooth powder:** This one helps to cleanse your gum and prevent dental diseases. This powder is applied to a wet toothbrush and used.
- **Uterine wash and oil:** This is a wash that helps to improve and restore the health of your vaginal canal.
- **Estro:** This is a product that helps to increase libido and fertility in women and improves their sex drive. The dosage is 4 capsules per day.
- **Hair follicle fortifier:** This one is for the strengthening and growth of your hair follicles. It comes in paste form, and the instruction is to apply it to your scalp every day.
- **Banjul:** This supplement helps to deal with conditions with the nervous system that may lead to stress, irritability, and pain. Keep in mind that this is also found in a tonic version for children who are suffering from add or ADHD. The recommended dosage is 2 tablespoons twice a day.

Apart from those, other supplements that might interest you include:

- Hair food oil for scalp and hair nourishment
- Iron plus for fighting inflammation
- Eyewash for cleansing the eyes
- Bio Ferro capsules for blood purification
- Eva salve for skin nourishment
- Bromide plus powder

Chapter 6: The Benefit of Fasting as Recommended by Dr. Sebi

To learn how to fast with properly. The Dr. Sebi's diet for maximum results you must first understand how to prepare for a fast, why you do it and how it affects our bodies. So, let's dive into a bit more about fasting.

Preparing for a Fast

Your fasting should begin with purifying. Utilize distinctive common spices for 3 to 5 days before beginning your quick, be it a juice, a vegetable, or water quick. Take spices first to evacuate a portion of the poison and body squander. A great many people have poisons that have been in their bodies since they were children, so spices are significant before fasting. For instance, on the first occasion when I took a stab at fasting, on the 21st day, I was unable to get up rapidly enough to go to the washroom since I had a ton of poisons coming out of me. I am happy because what keeps us alive is purging.

Fasting comes in two stages to purify your body adequately. Right off the bat, you need to scrub your body with characteristic spices for at any rate five days before setting out on the genuine fasting.

To know when you are prepared for the quick, your body will give a sign of that, and the sign you will get is during the purifying with spices stage. At the point when you begin feeling hungry while purifying is the point at which you are prepared to start your quick. You should never quick when your body isn't prepared, on the off chance that you feel hungry during a quick, you ought to eat.

Why Should You Fast?

Realize how to address your body's inconveniences, fasting will fix your body and keep you more youthful. The best technique for fasting is to clean the body until there is no more yearning. When there is no appetite, you can quick as long as you like. Quickly until you're craving returns since it will vanish. The tongue will get white and delicate; quick until the tongue turns red once more, and quick until your breath and your body become sweet. The body will deliver its smell because of the evacuation of all the harmful material in the body.

Dr. Sebi's fasting technique advances glucose control. By reducing insulin resistance, which infers your body is dynamically feasible at moving glucose from your course framework to your phones, fasting improves glucose control. This bit of leeway is even more undeniably found in transient spasmodic fasting; for example, staying away from sustenance for 18 hours out of every day, and eating in a six-hour window.

Dr. Sebi's fasting technique battles irritation. The disturbance is a response of eating up an unreasonable number of acidic-molding sustenance, harms, or by being around a dangerous circumstance. Disturbance is moreover drawn in with the improvement of onerous conditions, for instance, coronary ailment, infection, various sclerosis, and rheumatoid joint agony. By fasting for only 12 hours consistently, it is possible to lessen disturbance, which helps in treating the afflictions.

Dr. Sebi's fasting strategy upgrades heart wellbeing. Coronary sickness is known as one of the principal wellsprings of death around the world. By clearing a path of life changes, for instance, following Dr. Sebi's healthful guide, and combining fasting into your day by day practice, it is possible to reduce hypertension, fatty oils, and cholesterol, all of which can provoke coronary ailment.

Dr. Sebi's fasting strategy supports mind work. Fasting does helpful things for the cerebrum, and this is clear by the whole of the valuable neurochemical changes that happen in the psyche when we snappy. It moreover improves the theoretical limit, increases neurotrophic factors and stress restriction, and diminishes irritation. You can help the cerebrum focal points of fasting by eating up banju while you are speedy. Dr. Sebi's banju quickens the psyche and assistants in the treatment of ailments related to the central tactile framework, for instance, distress, apprehension, fractiousness, and a resting issue.

Dr. Sebi's fasting strategy can defer maturing and increment life span. Wanting to live more? Try combining fasting technique as proposed by Dr. Sebi into your day by day plan, as it's shown to defer developing and addition life length to the people who practice it close by other strong lifestyle choices.

How Fasting Your Body & overall Health

You will look younger, feel younger, skin rejuvenated, and your hair and nails will be revitalized. Fasting will do all these things in your body. If you fast, your body will remain flexible, full of energy, and shine with vitality. This is what we all want, and nothing will do that well than cleansing and fasting. Fasting is the best way to heal, develop, and relieve our body of waste and toxins.

What Is Water Fasting & Is it different from a regular Fast?

Fasting with water is better because it will clean the body of toxic waste; heal the body of old dead cells that have been there for a long time. The best way to do this is to cleanse the body and then start the water fast. When you fast, you will find that your skin becomes resonant, young, and beautiful.

Your hair, your eyes, and every gland in your body will respond to fasting. This is what they all need, the intense cleansing that occurs from fasting. If you fast, your friends or people you know can say that you are killing yourself. But 1 did not listen to them; even during biblical days, people fasted for 21, 30, or 40 days, and no one died of fasting. The prophets, Jesus and the women of the bible, fasted, and no one died for it. Queen Esther fasted and saved the children of Israel from extinction. Fasting is a way of life.

How Long Should You Fast?

After cleaning the body with herbs, fast for 21 or 30 days until you no longer have a "coated" tongue, you no longer feel tired, weak, or nervous and you feel young again. The people around you are going to ask you what you are doing; you will look more youthful. Then, break the fast and begin again; if you cleanse the body quickly and adequately, you do not need to take drugs to do what you want. Male or female, your sex drive will continue to work well, and your hormones will work if they are cleansed and quickly.

Fasting with the Dr. Sebi's Diet to Cleanse Toxins

You will come to the realization that food does not keep humans alive. Rather clearing our bodies of waste and toxins revitalizes our bodies more than consuming food. When we begin to eat natural foods to cleanse our body instead of for fulfillment, our body and mind will change.

Our ancestors do not have prostate glands problems like the young men of nowadays. Our grandmothers as well did not lose their youthful factor as it is in today's world. In actuality, my great grandmother had twin babies at the age of 49, but this is unheard of in the 21st century despite all the medical discoveries. When we eat according to what nature has in store for us, we will stay healthy, live longer, and every pain in the body will vanish. Good health will ultimately triumph when we cleanse our body and stick to the right diet.

How to Properly Break a Fast

You are to break a fast exactly the way you started. By this, I mean, get a juice, warm it up and take that for 5 consecutive days. You will have more energy than you need. You won't feel hungry. If you jump right into taking steaks after an extensive fasting period, you will get sick.

That food will make you fall ill. You have to totally stop all those kinds of food as they cause body pains and ache. There are so many ways to fast. The aim of this guide and information therein is to know the correct way for you to fast. In the end, this is all about choosing a fasting method that works well for you.

Foods during Fasting

Dr. Sebi has recommended foods that are easy to digest and ones that will push the body's performance to its peak.

Basically, fasting is abstinence from food, and this act greatly improves the elimination of waste materials from the body. Pollution, environmental toxins, synthetic medication, electrical radiation are all forms of things we take that can diminish our overall health. Fasting is a mechanism that speedily removes toxins like mucus, fecal waste, parasites, and phlegm from the body.

Dr. Sebi's Fasting Foods Checklist

Here are the benefits of Dr. Sebi's fasting food; these are the benefits to your body when you eat the recommended fasting foods. Natural foods all contain 92 minerals found in the soil of the earth, 27 of which are found and play an important role in the human body to restore good health. These foods contain the following benefits that are essential for the optimal and proper functioning of the body.

Fasting foods provide:

- Alkalinity
- Iron, calcium, magnesium, copper, zinc, and many other minerals
- Expel mucus
- Easy to digest, assimilate and used by the body
- They flush out the body and detox harmful wastes
- Neutralize the body's ph balance
- Restore the body overall good health
- Get rid of toxins

Fasting Foods to Eat

Fruits:

- seeded melons
- mangoes
- all types of berries
- papaya and many more

Vegetables to Eat during Fasting?

If you have to eat during your fast for medical reasons or any other situation you are in.

These vegetables are ideal for consumption because of their ability to help the body expel mucus or toxins due to their high mineral content:

- Dandelion leaves
- Green leafy vegetables
- Kale
- Broth of burdock leaf, or root vegetable juices.

Dr. Sebi used these foods to remove mucus and other body wastes from his body system.

Chapter 7: Reverse Disease

Diabetes happens when your blood glucose turns out to be excessively high. Blood glucose is the thing that your body utilizes as vitality and is made from whatever you eat. Insulin, which is a hormone that your pancreas makes, enables the glucose to move into your cells with the goal that it very well may be utilized as vitality. There are times when the body doesn't make enough, or any, insulin. The body doesn't utilize insulin effectively. This makes the glucose stay in your blood, and it won't arrive at your cells.

The longer that this goes on, the excess glucose in the blood can end up creating severe health problems. Luckily, there is a way to reverse diabetes, and modern medicine also has medicine that can help manage diabetes if a person chooses not to make drastic dietary changes.

People can also be diagnosed with pre-diabetes. At this stage, it is easier to reverse things and prevent diabetes from developing at all. But that does not mean pre-diabetes is any less important than full-blown diabetes.

While type 1 and type 2 diabetes have different causes, there are still two factors that work in both. A person inherits some predisposition to this particular disease, and then something in your environment triggers the onset. Genes by themselves are not enough. A good example of this is with identical twins. For identical twins they have identical genes, but when one of them develops type 1 diabetes, the other one will only develop the disease, at most, half the time. If one of the develops type 2 diabetes, the odds of the other one developing it to is three in four.

Types of Diabetes

There isn't just one type of diabetes that a person can be diagnosed with. There are actually several different types.

This can be avoided and is normally found in childhood and is often referred to as juvenile diabetes. It is a type of auto-immune disease. In this case, your body doesn't make enough insulin. The immune system will also attack and destroy the pancreatic cells that create insulin. Most people with type 1 diabetes will have to take insulin every single day.

About five percent of people with diabetes have type 1 diabetes. Type 1 diabetes is considered incurable, but there are a lot of management tools out there.

- Weight loss without an apparent reason
- Fatigue and tiredness
- Unclear or blurred vision and problems with sight
- Frequent urination
- Increased thirst and hunger

Once a person is diagnosed with type 1 diabetes, they enter the honeymoon phase. During this time, the cells that are responsible for secreting insulin could continue to make the hormone for a bit before stopping altogether. At this stage, they won't need as many insulin shots to keep their glucose levels.

People with type 1 diabetes are faced with having to take insulin for the rest of their life. You will work with your doctor to figure out the best schedule for your insulin doses. There are now continuous blood sugar monitors and insulin pumps. This hybrid machine can act as artificial pancreas and remove the need for remembering when to take insulin. They will still need to manually check their blood sugar levels to make sure things are still okay.

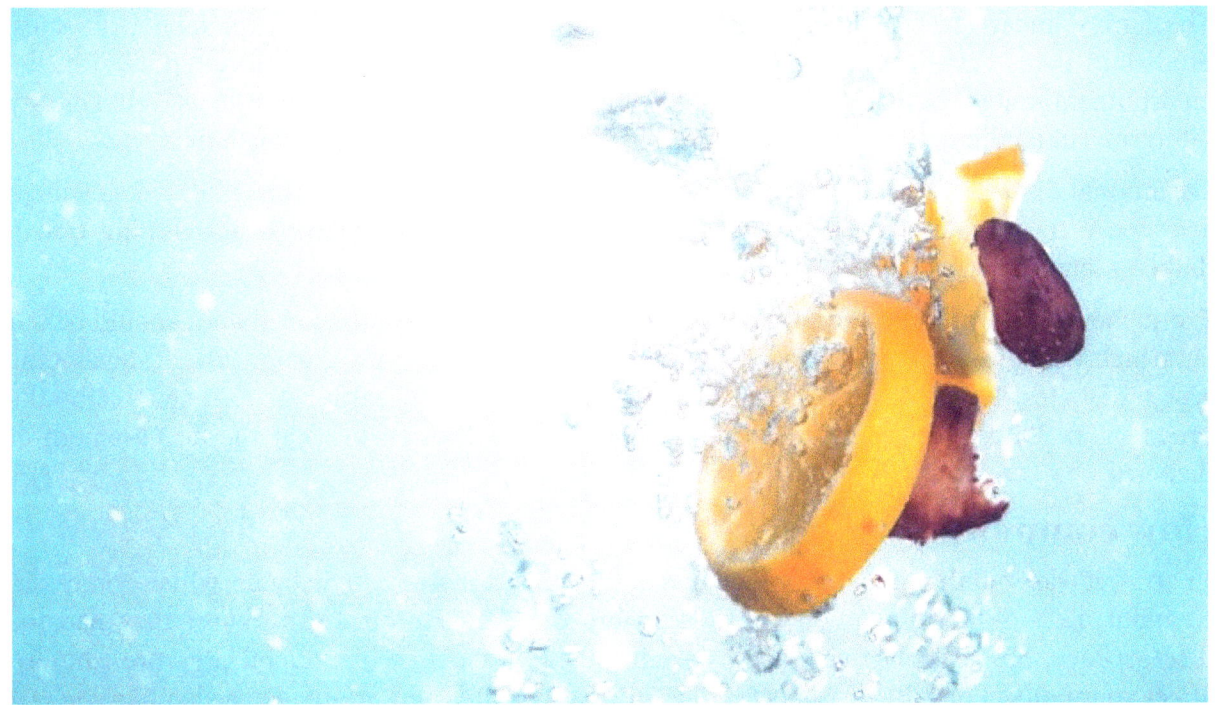

Diet as an infant may also play a role. Type 1 diabetes isn't as common in those who breastfed and in those who started eating solid foods at a later age. For most people, developing type 1 diabetes tends to take several years.

A man with type 1 diabetes has a 1 in 17 chance of having a child who develops it as well. A woman with type 2 diabetes, and gives birth before the age of 25, there is a 1 in 25 risks that your child will develop it. If you give birth after the age of 25, the odds go down to 1 in 100.

Type 2 diabetes is acquired during life because of poor dietary choices, and sometimes genetics. This can be developed at any age, and even as a child. However, it is more common for middle-aged and older adults to be diagnosed. This is known as the most common form of diabetes. They can include:

- Leading a sedentary life
- Being older than 45
- Being of Asian-pacific islander, Latin American, Native American, or African American descent

- History of PCOS
- Give birth to a child that weighed more than nine pounds, or having gestational diabetes
- History of high blood pressure
- Having an HDL cholesterol level that is less than 40 or 50 mg/dl
- Family history of diabetes
- Being overweight

The family lineage factor for type 2 diabetes is a lot stronger than it is for type 1 diabetes. Studies in twins have found that genetics plays a very big role in developing type 2. Yet, the environment still plays a big role as well. Lifestyle tends to play a very big role as well. Obesity often runs in families, and families will often have similar exercise and eating habits.

Gestational diabetes only affects women during pregnancy. For the most part, diabetes will go away once the woman gives birth. The mother is also at a higher risk of developing type 2 diabetes later in life.

Pre-diabetes simply means that you have a blood sugar level that is higher than it should be but isn't high enough to be considered diabetes. It does place you at a greater risk of developing type 2 diabetes. They will suggest that the person start making healthy life changes to stop the progression. Eating healthier foods and losing weight will often prevent the development of diabetes.

How common?

In 2015, it was said that 30.3 million people in the United States had diabetes, which comes out to about 9.4% of the population. Of those, more than one in four didn't know they had the disease Race, physical inactivity, some certain health issues like high blood pressure can also affect your odds of developing diabetes. Gestational diabetes and pre-diabetes also put you at a higher risk of developing type 2 diabetes.

Lifestyle Changes for Diabetes

At first, the doctor will tell a person with diabetes is to make some lifestyle changes to help support a healthy life and weight loss. Doctors may send you to a special nutritionist who can help you to manage the condition. Some of the most common changes diabetics are told make include:

- Recognize the signs for low blood sugar when they are exercising, which includes profuse sweating, weakness, confusion, and dizziness.
- Take part in at least 30 minutes of exercise each day, five days a week. Some of the best exercises for diabetics include swimming, biking, aerobics, and walking.
- Abstaining from drinking alcohol, or cutting back to one glass a day for women and two for men.
- Staying away from high-sugar foods that only provide you with empty calories or calories that won't provide you with any nutritional benefits, like sweets, fried foods, and sodas.

- Eating a diet that is high in healthful and fresh foods, like whole grains, healthy fats, vegetables, and fruits.

Lowering your BMI is also a great way to manage type 2 diabetes without the need for medications. Making your weight loss slow and steady will help you to retain the benefits.

Dr. Sebi's Diabetes Cure

Although there is a lot of upright advice for people with diabetes that doctors will share, such as lifestyle changes, there is also a lot of medication that you could end up being prescribed. And let's not get started on how scary it must be to learn how to give you insulin injections.

Dr. Sebi's diabetes cure is a super simple plan, and it doesn't cost that much. Very few people wanted to try his plan at first because it required fasting. Most would rather cut off their feet than not eat. Dr. Sebi was able to cure his diabetes with a 27 day fast.

There are a lot of other people who have reported similar results as well. You can find a lot of videos on YouTube, where people talk about having cured their diabetes with Dr. Sebi's plan.

Like with the STD treatments, the goal is to rid the body of excess mucus. For people with diabetes, excess mucus is found in the pancreatic duct. Dr. Sebi's own mother started fasting to help her diabetes, and after 57 days, she was cured.

During your fast, you should drink water, and you can also have herbal tea. A great herbal tea to drink is a combination of burdock, black walnut leaf, red raspberry, and elderberry. Practice a tablespoon of each and mix them into one and a half liters of spring water. Carry this to a boil and let it steep for 15 minutes. Take this off the heat and mix in another half-litter of water. Strain out the herbs and place them to the side to use the next day. Store the tea in the fridge and drink as much as you want during the day.

A lot of people, when they overhear the word fast, assume that means they can't take anything by mouth. But that's not Dr. Sebi's fast. See, when Dr. Sebi fasted to cure his diabetes, he would take three green plus tablets each day and drink sea moss tea, spring water, and tamarind juice. You don't have to drink tamarind juice, though. Any juice that is on the approved list of foods is okay. It must be fresh juice, though. You don't want pre-made juice with a bunch of added sugars.

Once you have fasted for a while, and your body will let you know when you have had enough, you will then need to start the Dr. Sebi approved diet plan. Along with that, you should also think about taking black seeds, mulberry leaves, and fig leaves. Research on black seeds has found that taking as little as two teaspoons of the powder each day can reverse diabetes.

Figleaves are the top alternative medicine for diabetes on the market today. Mulberry leaves are a common treatment for diabetes in the Middle East. These can be made into a tea, and you can mix in some black seeds as well.

Some other foods that you should consider adding to your diet are ginseng, okra, ginger, fenugreek, red clover, Swiss chard, avocado, and bitter melon.

Chapter 8: Difference between Phlegm and Mucus

Mucus and phlegm are not identical, although most people consider them to be one. Let me explain, mucus is produced by our natural body as a defense mechanism. For example, mucus traps bacteria, so they do not enter the body. But if you eat too many unnatural foods that cause excessive mucus production by your body, it will be a problem because the cells and organs will be deprived of oxygen.

Phlegm Carries Disease

On the other hand, phlegm is very difficult to expel from the body. The presence of phlegm in the body is an indication that there is a disease lurking around somewhere in the body. When phlegm is excreted in the body, mucus accompanies it as well as bacteria. This is the more reason why phlegm is more problematic to the body.

Mucus Disease

It is ideal to know the concept of diseases, the environments where it thrives, and the causes. With this knowledge handy, it will be difficult for us to fall sick. This is the key to staying away from diseases and illnesses that your doctor will never tell you about. When we know these things, there won't be the need for a healer as getting sick will be a rare occurrence.

Mucus Is The Cause Of Every Disease

Diseases are found in the body when you have ingested an uncomplimentary substance into our body. This substance will conflict with our genetic structure, and this will eventually lead to us getting sick and weak. Almost everyone usually gets sick due to excess mucus in the body. The cause of most diseases is the presence of excessive mucus in the body.

When mucus accumulates excessively in the body, the mucus membrane breaks down, and cells get covered by the excess mucus. In essence, the mucus membrane is to protect the body from the invasion of aerobic bacteria.

Mucus and Phlegm Cause Disease

When our diet is made up of acidic food, the mucus membrane breaks down, and the already secreted mucus gets into the bloodstream. When this happens, the other groups of cells that belong to the organs get deprived of oxygen. If the mucus travels to your nostrils, it is referred to as sinusitis, when it flows to a bronchial tube, it is called bronchitis, and when it enters the lungs, and it is called pneumonia. If mucus manages to get into your eyes, there will be a problem with vision.

There you have it, three different diseases caused by mucus. There are more diseases; on the long list of other diseases caused by the invasion of mucus into various organs of the body are:

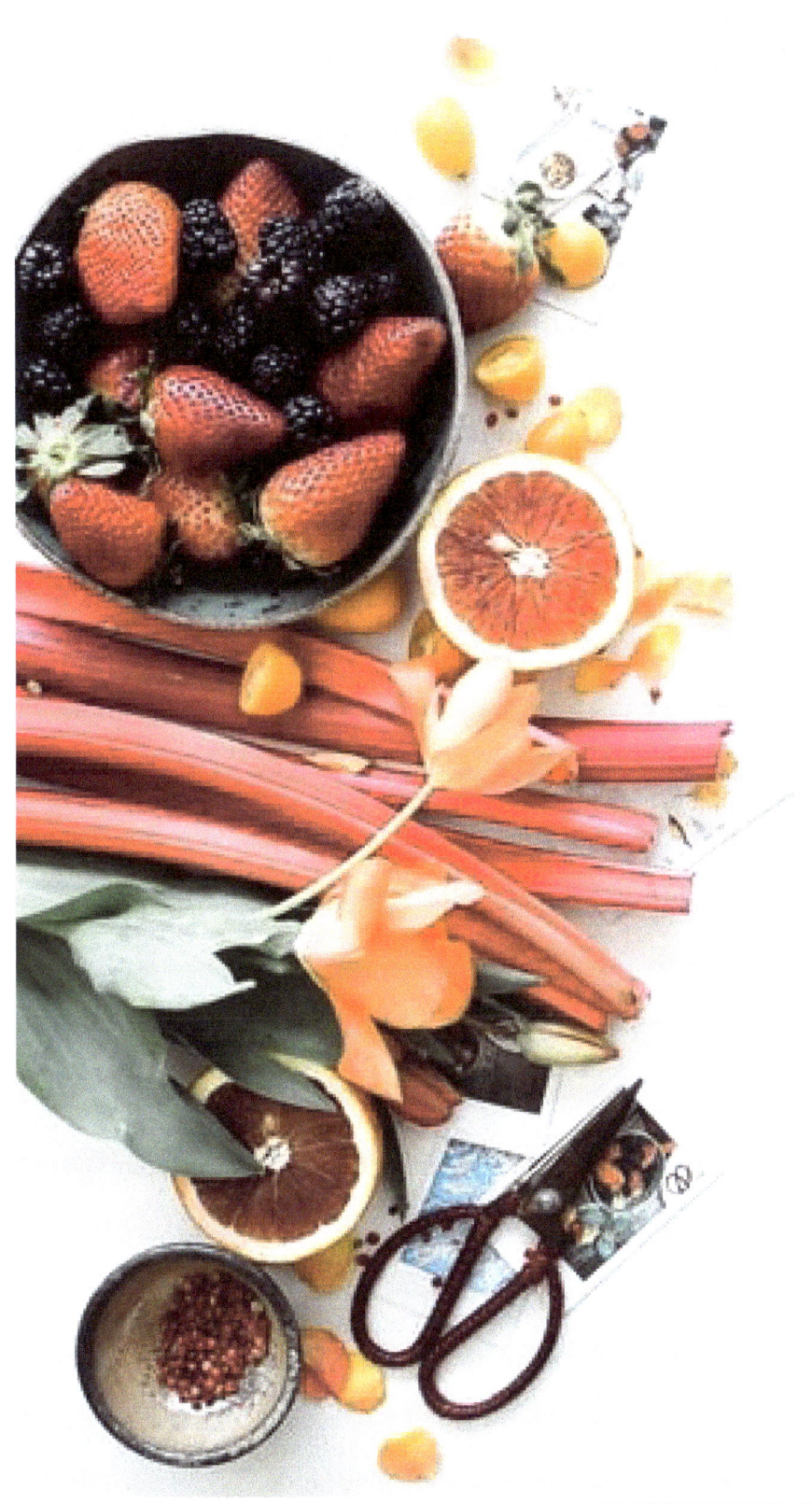

- Prostatitis – when mucus gets into your prostate gland
- Endometriosis – when mucus gets into the uterus of a woman (this can lead to yeast infection and vaginal discharge).

When you have the symptoms of any of these diseases, excessive mucus production caused by an inadequate diet is the underlying cause.

Phlegm After Eating

Humans experience phlegm every other time. When you cough out phlegm after eating, it is as a result of you consuming acidic food. Now you understand that the excessive acidic food that you consume is the cause of you coughing out phlegm. One of the significant factors that contribute to the excessive production of phlegm in the body is the consumption of processed foods. The body does not notice these foods, and it in turn results in a conflict. If after eating a particular type of food, you find yourself producing a lot of phlegm via cough, you need to stay away from such food. The production of excess phlegm due to the consumption of a particular type of food is an indication that such food is unhealthy. The secretion of excessive phlegm will deprive the body of oxygen as well as other parts of your internal organs.

Symptoms of Constant Mucus in the Throat

Acidic foods do not compliment the biological structure of the human body. The body's reaction to this is to produce more mucus every time you eat acidic foods. Excess mucus in the longs will extend to the throat. This situation will lead you to cough out phlegm after every meal you take.

A temporary solution to this condition is to gargle saltwater, but a diet change is what is needed to stop the body from producing excess mucus. If you refuse to change your diet to one that will eliminate the excessive production of phlegm, there will be more of it to cough out every time you consume acidic food. Every organ of the body that hosts this excessive mucus will experience one disease or the other.

Common remedies to clear mucus:

- Have a 2-7 days juice fast to enable your body to scrub and flush out the bodily fluid/mucus joined by a blended diet of foods grown from the ground suggested by Dr. Sebi.
- Boiled a quart of water, include half tsp. Of lobelia, and let it steep. At the point when it is tepid, strain it, and drink as much as could reasonably be expected. Stick your finger down your throat so you can regurgitation to free your stomach from mucus and bodily fluid.
- Take a hot shower, before this, quickly make the water cold and run it on your body. Hit the hay, at that point have somebody give you a hot fomentation to your chest and spine, and finishing it with a cold on - this is to diminish blockage.
- Remember, changing your eating regimen is the most significant thing you can do to help your body from delivering abundance mucus and bodily fluid.

Chapter 9: Detoxing the Liver

Different liver weight control plans are floating near. One can find an eating routine of this nature online adequately. A couple of nourishments simply last several days while others keep going up to three weeks. Most liver detox consumes fewer calories include eating commonly uncooked results of the dirt nearby whole-grain sustenance's. Water also expects a critical activity in any liver detox diet. A person that is going on such an eating regimen should savour any occasion eight cups of water each day for it to be powerful. Inferior quality sustenance's took care of sustenances, alcohol, coffee, and medications must be given up while going on a liver detox diet.

The Seven Day Liver Detox Diet Plan

- **Day 1-Day 3:** This period of this diet includes drinking just fluids. An individual, that sets out on this specific diet; should confine oneself to just drinking new lime squeeze and loads of water. This stage is one of the most troublesome, as an individual is fundamentally fasting and will feel feeble and tired. One can, on the off chance that the person wants, do some light exercise while on this period of the liver detox diet. It is important to enabling a lot of time to rest and not exaggerate.
- **Day 4 - Day 6:** This period of the liver detox diet is a lot simpler to deal with. An individual can eat every homemade food grown from the ground. Entire grain nourishments and bubbled vegetables are additionally permitted. Nonetheless, while an individual can eat certain nourishments at this phase of the detox diet, the person in question will likewise need to keep on drinking a lot of fluids. Fluids that are allowed at this phase of the menu are juices, home-grown teas, and handcrafted products of the soil juice.
- **Day 7:** One can eat similar nourishments that are taken into account days 4 - 6. One can likewise steam their vegetables as opposed to eating them either crude or bubbled. Herbs that are prescribed for this phase of the diet are Rosemary and Dandelion.

While going on a liver detox diet is an extraordinary method to enable the liver to wipe out poisons from the framework, it can likewise have negative symptoms. A separate ought to counsel their PCP before setting out on this kind of purging. A person that was encountering indications, for example, retching and agony should stop the diet promptly and look for medicinal assistance.

The Most Effective Method to Cleanse Your Liver

There are numerous ways on the most proficient method to detox your body, and in spite of the truth that it very well may be exceptionally testing, it isn't really inconceivable. Vital nourishment for the liver detox is; as of now referenced previously. Make sure to remember that nourishment for the day by day diet and drink loads of water each day. Liver detox is an incredible method to filter the liver from every one of the poisons present in the body. If the liver gets exhausted and an individual neglects to detox his/her liver, the liver may all of a

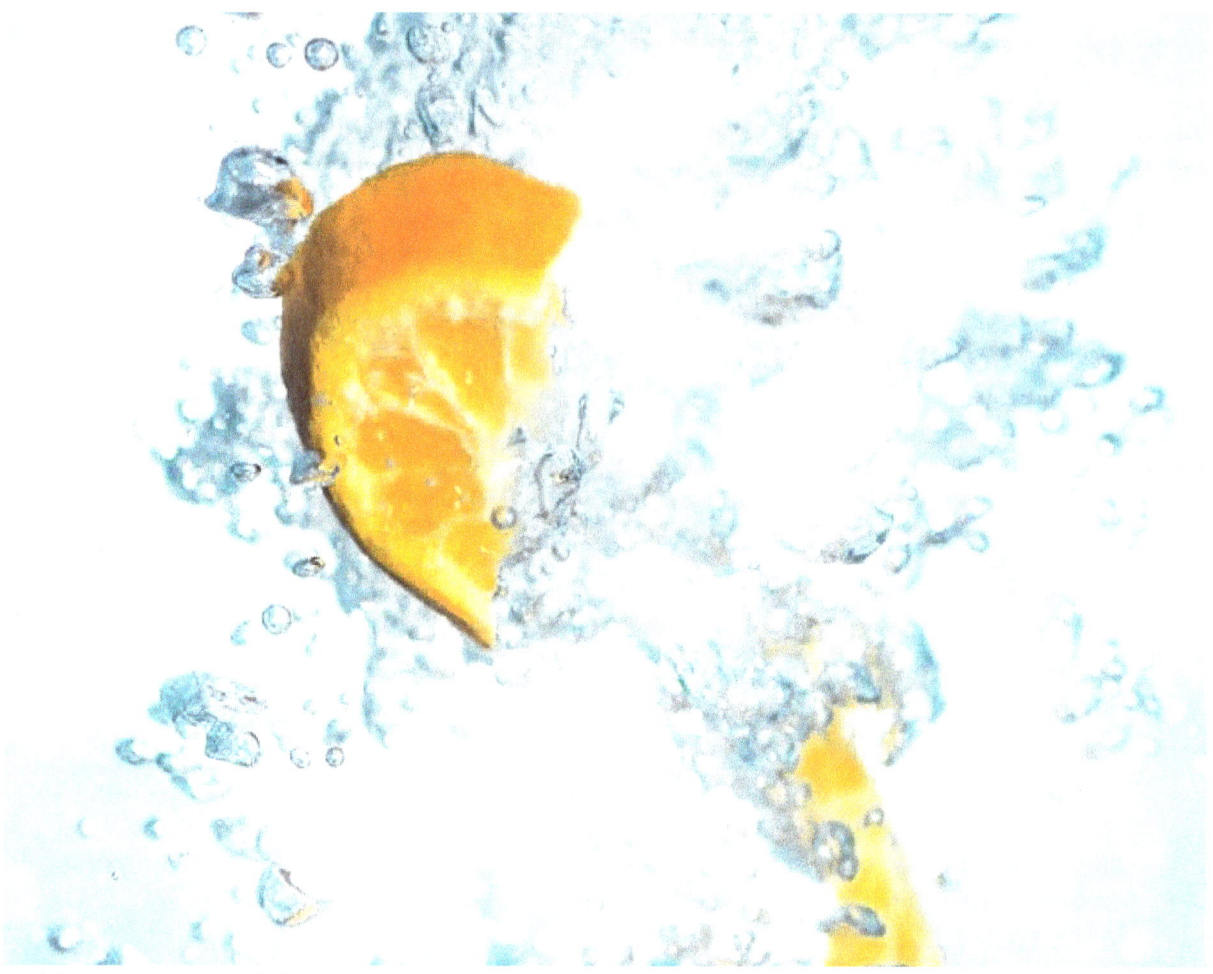

sudden separate and discharge a pool of smelling salts into the blood. This is hazardous and can prompt the severe harm of the sensory system, liver, mind, and kidneys. The body may likewise discharge lactic acid, which can cause constant weariness, hurting muscles, cerebral pain, tension, alarm assaults, and hypertension.

Step by Step Instructions to Start a Liver Detox Diet

A healthy liver can be acquired with the best possible measure of the correct sort of diet. The liver purging diet is presently a need in the general public because most nourishment that individuals eat nowadays contains additives and fake added substances that are significant for long stockpiling period yet destructive for our liver. To have a productive and successful liver purging diet, you should begin the correct way. So how are we going to start our liver purging food?

Before beginning a liver detoxification diet, make an agenda on the side effects (hypersensitivities, stench, nervousness, asthma, swelling, hypertension, low blood method, cold feet and hands, desires, stoppage, misery, looseness of the bowels, dry hair, dry skin, low energy, unpredictable glucose, weight addition, peevishness, and others) that you are presently encountering. Screen your body once per month to note if your body has come back to its best condition. It is additionally useful to make a rundown of nourishment that you expend to figure out what food should be dispensed with and what is to be kept up.

Seven days before the beginning of executing your liver purifying diet, you should quit smoking and drinking mixed drinks to avert over-burdening the liver that may cause trouble in wiping out harmful squanders that have gathered our body. Additionally, have a healthy diet by taking up crisp products of the soil and lessen the utilization of nourishments with a high measure of additives and other prepared food sources. Recollect that enormous numbers of the nourishments we expend every day contain unnatural poisons, for example, cancer-causing agents, anti-infection agents, pesticides, hormone medications, and fake sugars that may harm our liver.

Body condition is fundamental before a liver purging detox. Significantly, your body is decidedly ready to take a detox since you won't be permitted to devour healthy nourishments during a detox diet. It is additionally prudent to examine with your doctor the liver detox plan that you are going to take to evade different inconveniences to happen. Legitimate exercise will likewise have a molded body when a detox diet.

Light fasting seven days before your purging diet can be beneficial. The light diet contains heaps of water, crisp organic product juices, raw vegetables, and new natural products. New nourishments include more compounds that are fundamental in your liver purging diet. It additionally makes sure to eat at the correct time to abstain from overemphasizing your liver during the body melding. When your body is adapted, the danger of encountering undesirable reactions will be diminished.

Body detoxification can be begun with lessening your utilization of nourishments that has a high amount of poisons, for example, prepared food sources, liquor, artificial sugar, and espresso and increment your measure of admission of new leafy foods.

How important Is Your Liver's Health in Weight Management?

How significant is it to have a healthy liver when following a weight loss program?

- Non-alcoholic fatty liver disease is, at present, the most widely recognized liver disease around the world.
- All phases of non-alcoholic greasy liver disease are presently accepted to be because of insulin obstruction, a condition intently connected with heftiness.
- Tests show that in individuals with liver issues, the higher an individual's BMI (Body Mass Index), the more prominent the liver harm.

Perhaps the best worry in this nation is obesity in children. Furthermore, wouldn't you know it, so is youth NAFLD (Non-alcoholic Fatty Liver Disease)?

- Losing abundance weight is the foundation of the treatment of non-alcoholic greasy liver disease. There are meds that specialists can use to treat NAFLD; however, shedding pounds through diet and exercise is as yet the absolute best treatment. Nonetheless, this might be quite difficult. We live in a general public where high-fat, high carbohydrate, unhealthy nourishments are the standard, and exercise is an exertion. Diabetes is a scourge, and it is evaluated that 90% of individuals with Type 2 diabetes have greasy liver disease.

- Insulin Resistance is the most significant contributing component of stoutness. Stomach fat is the snitch story indication of Insulin Resistance. How would you look? You may require some assistance, yet diabetes and weight increase can be overseen. At last, advancing healthy dietary patterns and a functioning way of life, particularly in children, will most completely counteract NAFLD (greasy liver disease) and Type 2 diabetes.

- Greasy liver in itself is nothing to stress over and will vanish with loss of weight. The ideal approach to test is through a straightforward blood test to check whether liver chemicals come back to ordinary after weight loss. If they do, you can be quite well sure NAFLD (non-alcoholic greasy liver disease) was the issue. In any case, to be satisfied, solitary a liver biopsy can tell, which is costly and nosy, and for the most part, not worth the dangers.

Artichoke and Sarsaparilla are an incredible mix of liver health.

- Artichoke improves liver capacity, including bile generation for fat digestion; Increases the excellent HDL cholesterol; Lowers raised blood lipids, cholesterol and triglycerides; and Detoxes the liver and different organs of the body.

- Sarsaparilla cleanses the blood, helps in bladder health and hormone balance in the two people.

Look at it. It is anything but a regular thing. On more than one occasion per year should keep most everyone's liver running right, particularly on the off chance that they are eating right and practicing and not manhandling their liver with broad liquor utilization.

Control your weight and secure your liver simultaneously. Your health may rely upon it.

If you or somebody realize has over the top tummy fat, truly consider NAFLD. This impacts children, just as grown-ups and may require prompt consideration.

Outside Toxins and the Effect They Have on the Liver

We have seen the need to eat nourishments that will help detox the liver, and how infrequent liver detoxification to flush poisons out of the framework is useful. In any case, how would we maintain a strategic distance from these poisons in any case? You may be acquainted with a panic that has turned into a web sensation over the harmful impact of a vehicle's cooling framework; there is a considerable amount of disinformation out there also. I won't go into it here, yet teaching yourself on every one of these issues will assist you with expelling these bits of gossip.

In any case, it is evident that we all, and particularly those with persistent liver disease, ought to be wary against significant levels of natural poisons. We can have more noteworthy genuine feelings of serenity to lessen our introduction to toxins are:

1. Maintain a strategic distance from all tobacco smoke. By not smoking, yet evade all recycled smoke too. The vast majority comprehend the harm tobacco smoke can do to the heart and lungs. However, it likewise negatively affects the liver. The poisons in smoke lead to constant aggravation and scarring in the liver cells, which can prompt cancer and liver fibrosis.

2. Farthest point gas smolder presentation. Those vapors indeed are terrible for you. The liver will evacuate these poisons, yet on the off chance that severely strained, the liver may become overpowering. Much will rely upon the length and power of the presentation, yet the more that can be stayed away from, the better. There are filling stations now that have fume recuperation frameworks to catch the exhaust. This incorporates maintaining a strategic distance from gas contacting your skin.

3. Comprehend that benzene-containing synthetic compounds are unsafe. You can smell them with solvents, artistry supplies, and paints. This is frequently because of benzene, which is a lethal synthetic that can add to an over-burden of liver danger. It used to be utilized as an added substance to gas, yet has been diminished in on-going decades. Items that contain benzene be sure the region is all around ventilated.

4. Breathing in exhaust vapor can be dangerous. Is you are sitting in rush hour gridlock; there might be little you can do to abstain from breathing these exhausts. One choice is to hold the windows down and change your vehicle's ventilation framework to re-course. There will, at present, be some poisonous vapour in this air, yet positively not almost to the degree the outside fumes exhaust from sitting vehicles.

Chapter 10: Deconstructing the Plant-Based Diet

I was alright with my piscatorial diet. I didn't think there was substantially more that I could do, however, I was still keeping watch for new information. In a matter of seconds, before I embraced a plant-based eating routine, I felt an earnestness to discover something that would for the last time manage my clog and medical problems. I chose to give a soluble plant-put together eating regimen based with respect to Dr. Sebi's philosophy an attempt.

Hybridization and Genetic Manipulation

Dr. Sebi's approach not just stays away from the utilization of meat, dairy, and handled nourishments, it additionally evades profoundly hybridized, bland, and hereditarily altered plant nourishments. I follow the Dr. Sebi dietary guide which maintains a strategic distance from profoundly hybridized, bland, and GMO nourishments, related to utilizing spices in Dr. Sebi's African bio-mineral balance to re-establish the soundness of my body. Hybridization is where at least two plants join to frame another plant. Now and again this is a diagnostic procedure, and ordinarily, hybridization happens unnaturally and is maintained a strategic distance from.

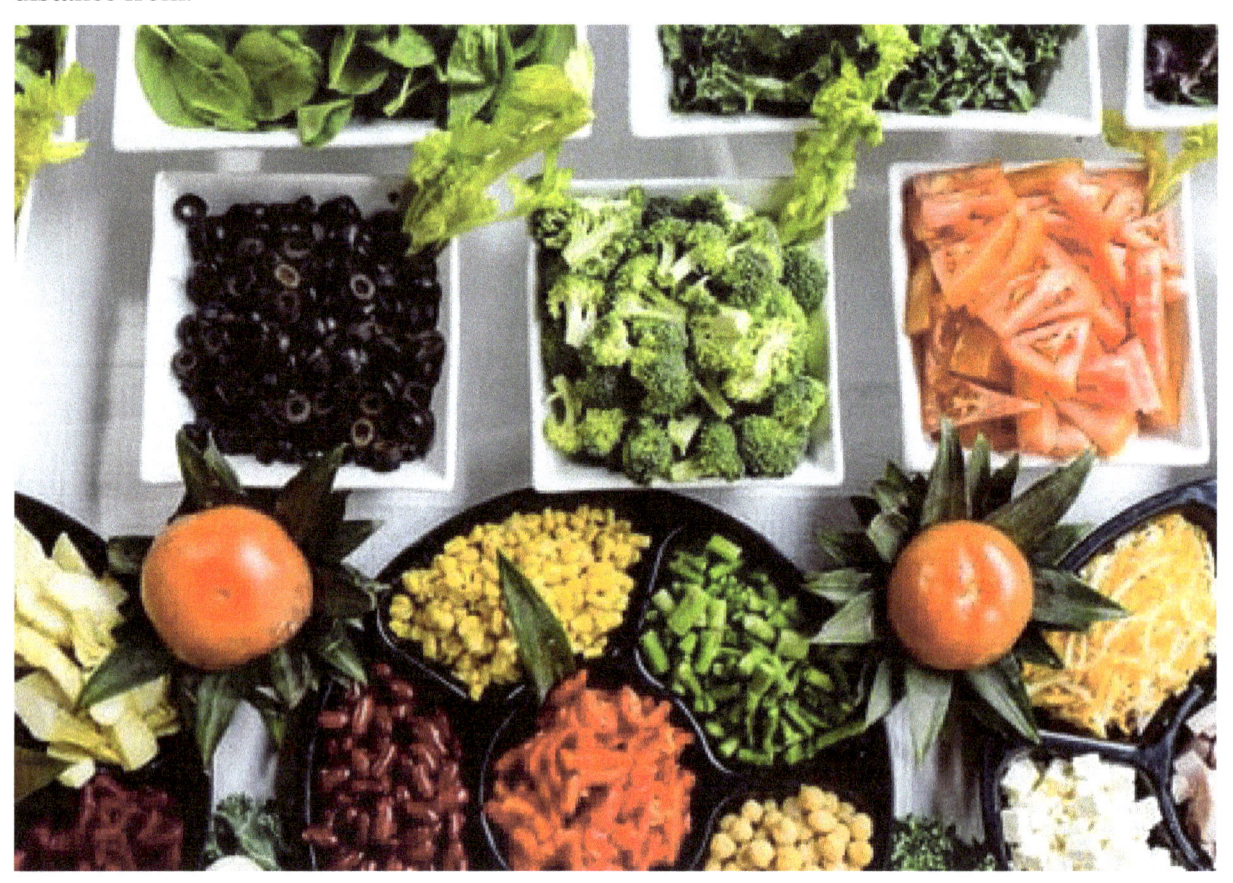

The procedure of constrained or unnatural hybridization adversely impacts the first piece and the proportion of plants' supplements. This outcome in food, that; was normally acclimatized by the body and appropriately bolstered homeostasis, to food to be less conspicuous by the body and results in destructive side-effects during processing. This procedure regularly brings about profoundly boring nourishments that are hard to process and remain in the stomach related tract excessively long. The starches overload certain microorganisms, toss the equalization of vegetation messed up, and bargain the uprightness of the digestive organs.

Basic half and a half and GMO plant nourishments, for example, "normal wheat," was left off the guide since they are destructive. Numerous individuals today have wheat-and gluten-related diseases, and the number continues developing. Individuals have expended wheat for a large number of years, yet it isn't until present occasions that wheat utilization has gotten dangerous. The liberal guilty party is the hybridization and genetic alteration of wheat that has created regular wheat. The hybridization and hereditary change of wheat have brought about the present normal wheat and transformed it into a corrosive shaping food.

Basic wheat was hybridized to adjust the arrangement of its gluten and to deliver more gluten. This is likely a purpose behind the ascent of wheat and gluten diseases. Most regular wheat has short stems, which is the consequence of RHT-overshadowing qualities brought into wheat. Norman Borlaug embedded RHT qualities into current wheat assortments during the 1960s. These adjustments to wheat's genetic structure make it not quite the same as the wheat individuals stayed alive on for a huge number of years, and are the presumable purpose behind its adverse effect on individuals' wellbeing. Shirking of half breed nourishments and adhering to the utilization of nourishments on the Dr. Sebi healthful guide is a significant differentiator in the manner I approach a plant-based eating routine contrasted with numerous others' methodology.

Hereditarily Modified Organisms

GMOs are hereditarily altered life forms and are the immediate control of qualities in nourishments. 80% of hereditary change to crops is done to make them impervious to pesticides. A little level of hereditary control is done to make the look and smell of items all the more speaking to buyers. GMOs exist outside the common law of God/the source of life/nature. They didn't create because of the savvy request of life. Their organization isn't regular and the body doesn't acclimatize them appropriately.

Bioengineer's contention is the hereditary control just influences the focused on the characteristic of the food and that's it. Actually bioengineers don't realize that is valid; in light of the fact that they don't have a clue how the change influences each other quality and part of the controlled food. Parts in the food we eat create corresponding to one another, and bioengineers have no clue about how controlling one quality influences others and how the utilization of the altered food influences the body. GMO nourishments frequently advance toward the food flexibly without appropriate outsider long haul considers being performed to decide the wellbeing results of hereditary adjustment.

Gilles-eric Seralini played out an investigation of the drawn-out impacts of Monsanto's GMO corn, which was at that point endorsed and available. He took care of rodents' Monsanto's roundup ready corn, and they grew enormous tumors, and some kicked the bucket. The examination was distributed in the diary food and chemical toxicology. Seralini confronted an invasion of analysis since he apparently utilized rodents that would in general create tumors (the Sprague-Dawley strain), and he utilized too hardly any rodents. The diary withdrew the investigation, and established researchers endorsed the business-driven censorship.

Seralini played out a similar report Monsanto used to get the GMO corn endorsed. Seralini utilized a similar strain of rodents and the same number of rodents from the Monsanto study did. The Seralini study was additionally distributed in a similar diary as the Monsanto study. The distinction being Seralini ran his investigation for a more drawn out time. Monsanto's momentary investigation indicated no proof of strange tumor advancement, while Seralini's drawn-out examination demonstrated the Monsanto study was halted rashly and didn't give enough an ideal opportunity for the tumors to creating.

Through control, such as getting the Seralini study withdrew, the discussion regarding whether GMOs are hurtful proceeds. Yields like soy are GMO designed to be impervious to poisonous pesticides, which permits them to be showered straightforwardly with the harmful pesticides. These yields end up in the commercial center, debased with a lot of destructive pesticide residue.

Clinical tests have demonstrated that Monsanto's ready roundup pesticide has dangerous harmful and hormonal effects. Past tests done on creatures have indicated that glyphosate, the principle fixing in the roundup, contrarily influenced early-stage advancement, upset hormones, and meddled with male fruitfulness. Later tests were finished utilizing the secluded glyphosate, and those tests demonstrated that glyphosate without anyone else didn't have a very remarkable poisonous impact on human cells. In spite of the fact, that glyphosate is the fundamental fixing in roundup, it isn't the main fixing. Different fixings in roundup permit the glyphosate to infiltrate human cells and cause damage. Roundup was seen as multiple times more harmful than its dynamic fixing glyphosate and was among the most poisonous pesticide items tried, however, it is usually accepted that roundup is among the most secure herbicides used.

The legitimate level for build-up levels of glyphosate in nourishments had been at 0.1 to 0.2 milligrams per kilogram. The build-up levels of glyphosate found in GMO soy crops surpass as far as possible by a normal of 2,000 percent. Though the contention proceeds with respect to in the case of altering the genetic structure of food is hazardous to the body, it is obvious that pesticide-safe GMO crops are unsafe.

Prepared Foods

The kind of plant-based eating routine individual practices will create various outcomes. Handled plant nourishments can be as unsafe as prepared creature food sources. Prepared plant-based nourishments contain harmful added substances and additives and can incorporate mostly hydrogenated oils, handled starches, high-fructose corn syrup, manufactured sugars, and unnatural concoction additives. Sorts of prepared plant nourishments can incorporate baked goods, bread, oats, and vitality drinks. Types of handled creature food sources incorporate cheeseburgers, franks, and inexpensive food meat.

In Part Hydrogenated Oils

Essential vegetable oils are handled and controlled to create counterfeit Trans fats called somewhat hydrogenated oils. Increasingly strong, give them a progressively alluring taste and surface, make them increasingly decent to profound fricasseeing, and add time span of usability to nourishments. Somewhat hydrogenated oils are the essential wellspring of trans fats in the standard American diet (sad), yet they are as yet utilized even with the FDA requiring trans-fat food naming in late 2006. The FDA's drive has diminished the utilization of Tran's fat; however, numerous individuals do, in any case, intensely devour this wellbeing hurting substance.

The utilization of incompletely hydrogenated oils raises low-thickness lipoprotein (LDL) cholesterol and brings down high-thickness lipoprotein (HDL) cholesterol. Consuming mostly hydrogenated oils increment the danger of creating coronary illness and stroke. Heart sickness is the main executioner in the United States, representing 25 percent of all deaths. Though unnecessary LDL cholesterol in the circulatory system advances coronary illness, some LDL is expected to help legitimate cell work. LDL cholesterol was given the expression "terrible cholesterol" since it contains progressively fat and less protein, contrasted with HDL cholesterol. The body needs some LDL cholesterol and will conveyance to any place it is required. The blood it gets stored in the dividers of supply routes. Since HDL cholesterol contains not so much fat but rather more protein than LDL cholesterol it goes about like a vacuum, and gets abundance LDL cholesterol as it goes through the circulation system.

The utilization of cholesterol isn't important and has inconvenient outcomes. The sad eating routine is high in cholesterol and fat, and a portion of the devoured LDL cholesterol stalls out on supply route dividers and compromises their trustworthiness and homeostasis. This triggers the body's safe framework to convey white platelets to evacuate the LDL cholesterol adhering to conduit dividers. White platelets encompass the LDL cholesterol so as to kill and expel it from supply route dividers and simultaneously, convert it into a poisonous, oxidized type of cholesterol.

After some time, more LDL cholesterol, white platelets, and different cells adhere to the undermined zone of the corridor dividers and start a procedure of constant irritation that further damages the supply route divider.

Chapter 11: Classification of Foods

Foods are classified into different forms depending on whether they contain acids, and alkaline. Examples of foods are hybridized food, raw foods, live food, genetically modified foods (GMO), drugs, and dead foods.

Hybridized Foods

They are foods that are not natural. They are created and formed by cross-pollination. The vitamins and mineral levels cannot be quantified and they cannot be grown naturally.

Foods that are cross-pollinated (hybridized) lack proper mineral balance that is present in wild foods. Consumption of hybridized foods results in a lack (deficiency) of minerals in the body.

Fruits and vegetables that are hybridized result in excessive stimulation of the body which subsequently results in loss of minerals in the body.

It is reported that hybridized foods lack electrically charged components. This is because of most soils in the world especially the United States, lack minerals thereby affecting the foods that are planted on them. In as much as the soil lack minerals, the crops planted on them will automatically lack minerals.

This implies that most foods we eat daily are junk. Junks foods are reported to be void of nutrition and this result in several health problems.

Hybrid foods are mostly sugars that cannot be identified by the body's digestive system. Examples are cows, pigs, watermelon, chicken, sausage roll…and many others.

The engineers that are involved in producing hybridized foods always conclude that they are doing it for individual to get enough food for consumption but unknowingly, they are causing us more harm than good.

Raw Foods

Raw foods are living foods that have not undergone processing and they are undercooked. They are foods that are dried with the use of direct sunlight and are majorly organic foods.

When raw foods are eaten, there is a high tendency that the individual loses weight because it helps the digestive system to digest the foods quickly. This implies that raw foods are beneficial for those who have the intension of losing weight and are ready to keep lean and clean.

These foods also contain many components needed for the digestion process and are destroyed within a short time if not properly dried.

Raw foods help in the improvement of overall health and can help in fighting against disease-causing organisms. Many individuals that inculcate the habit of eating raw food spend little or zero monies in the hospital because their immune system is competent.

However, other dieters believe that raw foods could contain poison that might cause harm to the body. They, therefore, advise that raw foods should be cooked to remove some toxic substances in it. Such foods include undercooked meat, chicken, fish...and more. They concluded that cooking food helps in killing every viable bacterial and other disease-causing organism that may be present in them.

Live Foods

Live foods are nourishments that are not dead without consuming them. All live foods do not contain toxic components when they are left to undergo fermentation.

They are foods that are not processed, cooked, microwaved, irradiated, genetically modified, drenched with chemicals (pesticides, insecticides, and preservatives).

More so, living foods do not undergo destruction when they are not in their environment. The materials required for the process of digestion are embedded in the living food which contains almost the same pH with water.

Live foods are the only type of nourishment that could restore the micro-electrical potential of the cells in the body. The electrical potential of the body's materials and cells is a direct result of the aliveness of our cells.

Live foods develop the electrical potential in cells, between cells, at the interface of the cells, and with the micro-capillary.

Therefore, live foods help the body to become re-energized and cause it to be in the state that is fit to fight any disease. It is also important in detoxifying the body in the intercellular and intracellular level.

Genetically Modified Foods (GMO)

These are food improved by a man with the use of genetics. They mostly damage the immunity in the body. These foods form an unusual approach in humans and also cause genetic consequence in the body.

Genetically modified foods contain genes of allergen which facilitates allergic reactions in the body. Excess consumption of genetically modified foods is reported to be associated with the inability to resist bacteria in the body.

Examples are foods that are grown hastily, weather-resistant foods such as corn, yeast, brown rice...and many others.

Drugs

Many drugs are dangerous and harmful to the body. They are extremely toxic and acidic. Most of them are extracted and are synthetic.

Drugs can influence and affect several body organs thereby reducing the immune system, increasing the susceptibility of infections and diseases, as well as causing cardiovascular problems.

Examples are cocaine, sugar, all prescription drugs, heroin...and many others.

Dead Foods

These are foods that when fermented become toxic and they have a prolonged life span. They are overdone and over-processed foods.

Dead foods are associated with the risk of having depression, cancer, untimely death, cardiovascular diseases and problems, poor digestion as well as diabetes.

Dead foods facilitate the accumulation of fatty tissues in the body which could result in the above-listed health problems.

Dead food is void of nutrients because the refining process has taken almost all the nutrients (fibers, vitamins, minerals) available in it.

Most of the dead foods are very tasty and inviting in that you continue eating them without stopping. As a result, you become fat and feel sick.

Examples are deep-fried foods, synthetic foods, white rice, sugar, soft drinks, snacks, desserts, alcohols, sugars...and many more.

The Importance of Dr. Sebi's nutritional Diets

All Dr. Sebi's recommended diets are majorly live foods that add benefits to the body and also improve the overall health.

Hence, the benefits are:

It helps in the inhibition and treatment of cancer.

It helps in the prevention and cure of stroke.

It aids in the prevention and treatment of high blood pressure.

Cholesterol is absent in his diets.

Alcohol is absent in his diets.

It contains very low saturated fats which also prevent major heart-related diseases.

It helps in the prevention and treatment of diabetes.

It helps in weight loss.

It contains very low fat which prevents heart diseases and other heart malfunctions.

It contains no processed sugar.

It helps in controlling your appetite.

It helps in the reduction of susceptibility to diseases.

How to Embrace Dr. Sebi's Diet

Drink one gallon of alkaline water in a day.

Do away with foods that are canned and processed.

Eat foods that are listed in the recommended food list.

Do not prepare your food with the use of microwaves as it could cause damage to your health and reduce the nutrients present in it.

You must not engage in the intake of alcohol.

Gradually switch to the alkaline diet if you are so accustomed to junks.

Foods that are hybridized should be shunned.

Chapter 12: Herbs

Irish Sea Moss

Also known as – carrageen moss, sea moss

Latin name – Chondruscrispus

Origin – Atlantic coast of North America and Europe

Parts used – whole part of the plant

Irish Moss Benefits

One of the most undervalued and important benefits of the Irish Sea moss are its ability to help balance the thyroid hormones of the body. It contains the important thyroid precursor di-iodothyronine (dit), and the tri-iodothyronine (t3), and the thyroid hormones thyroxin (t4). The failure of the thyroid to produce these hormones would harm the body's metabolism and other bodily systems. These iodine compounds are organically present in the brown sea moss (Irish moss)

Respiratory Health

Irish moss is a great source of potassium chloride. This means that it can dissolve phlegm, catarrh, helping to clear the lungs of any phlegm that is present and causes the common cold, while it also soothes inflammation of the mucus membrane to prevent congestion.

Because it possesses expectorant qualities, it helps prevents the common cold from turning into pneumonia and can handle all other respiratory problems like bronchitis. Irish moss also possesses antiviral properties, which helps to prevent or treat a myriad of disorders like sore throats, flu, coughs, and many more.

Weight Loss

Irish moss can reduce appetite due to its ability to take in moisture, filling its volume and increasing the intestinal tract with a huge type of material, thereby increasing the urge of fullness. Its calm laxative feeling can increase the removal process of waste via the gastrointestinal tract. This content will boost metabolism, which will increase energy and help improve weight loss.

Digestive Support

Irish moss possesses a mild laxative effect with a soothing effect on inflamed tissues within the intestinal tract, which provides relief from a wide range of intestinal disorders.

Side Effects

There is currently no side effect while using Irish moss at this time of writing.

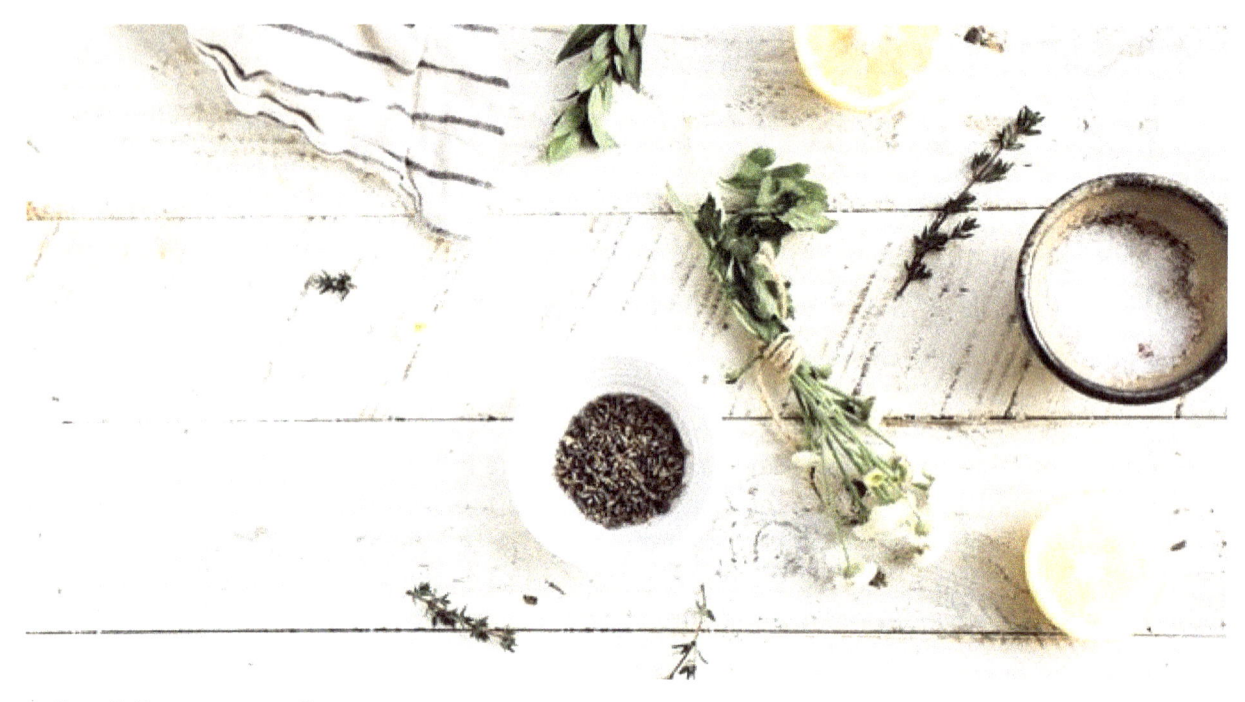

Bladderwrack

Overview Information

Bladderwrack is a form of seaweed. The whole plant of these herbs is used to make medicine by people.

It is used for many conditions, but as far as medical research has gone, there isn't enough evidence to show that it is effective for them. Bladderwrack is also used to treat iodine deficiency, over-sized thyroid gland (goiter), underactive thyroid (myxedema), obesity, joint pain, digestive disorder, arteries, and heartburn.

It also functions effectively when used in the treatment of urinary tract disorder, anxiety, bronchitis, constipation, and emphysema. Several people testified it helps in immune system boosting and also increases energy.

A lot of people also used bladderwrack in the application of skin diseases on the skin, burns, insect bites, and aging skin. Bladderwrack mustn't be confused with bladderwort.

How Does It Work?

Bladderwrack, like other sea plants, possesses a different amount of iodine, which is used in the application of thyroid disorders. Products containing bladderwrack may contain a varying quantity of iodine, which makes it quite an inconsistent source of iodine. Bladderwrack contains algin, which is utilized as a laxative in helping stool pass via the bowels with ease.

Uses and Effectiveness
- Iodine deficiency
- Blood cleansing
- Arteriosclerosis (hardening of the arteries)
- Rheumatism (achy joints)
- Obesity
- Constipation
- Arthritis
- Digestive problems
- Thyroid problems which include goiter (an oversized thyroid gland)
- Other conditions

Side Effects

Bladderwrack is safe when it is applied directly to the skin. Bladderwrack might be quite unsafe if taken via the mouth. Due to its high concentration of iodine, it could cause or worsen some thyroid problems.

The prolonged intake of dietary iodine is related to goiter and increases the risk of thyroid cancer. Like other sea plants which serve as herbs, bladderwrack is filled with toxic heavy metals like arsenic from the water it lives in.

- Pregnancy and Breastfeeding

    Intake of bladderwrack might seem unsafe during pregnancy and breastfeeding, don't use it.

- Bleeding Disorder

    This herb slows down blood clotting. Which means that if you have a bleeding disorder, bladderwrack might increase your risk of bleeding?

- Infertility

    Frankly speaking, too much intake of bladderwrack might make it harder for women to get pregnant and conceive.

Cascara Sagrada

Cascara sagrada is known as a shrub. The back of the cascara sagrada is dried, and it is used to produce medicine. It has compounds referred to as anthraquinones that possess powerful laxative effects.

It has been listed on the USA pharmacopeia ever since the 1890s and got first approval from the USA food and drug administration (FDA) for use. Other names of cascara sagrada include California buckthorn, yellow bark, sacred bark, and bearberry.

Uses of Cascara Sagrada

Cascara sagrada is used mainly for medicinal use as the dried back is used to produce medicine. The medicine, in return, serves as an avenue for the treatment of various illnesses.

Benefits of Cascara Sagrada

Cascara sagrada is used to treat constipation. It is perceived that the anthraquinones found in the bark hold back the absorption of electrolytes and water in the intestines. Due to this, the volume of stool increases because it sucks up the excess water, which in turn increases the pressure around the intestine. This results in the stimulation of muscle contractions in the colon, quickening the clearance of the bowel.

Cascara sagrada is also perceived to be able to cure or prevent liver problems, fissures, cancer, hemorrhoids, and gallstones.

Cascara sagrada aids to cleanse the colon of damaging toxins and waste products in the body, and by so doing, it acts as an element in several detoxes and cleanses herbal formulas.

Since the dried bark of the cascara sagrada is rich in emodin, an anti-fungal and anti-microbial factor, it is then capable of eliminating parasites from the body.

Side Effects of Cascara Sagrada

Since it is meant for short term use only, if cascara sagrada is used frequently to cure constipation, it may likely cause abdominal pain and cramp.

Cascara sagrada is also likely to result in a condition referred to as melanosis coli, which is known to be a discoloration of the lining of the colon.

Cascara sagrada can also result in severe dehydration and quick loss of electrolytes which include potassium, chloride, and sodium. This way, you are likely to experience the below:

- Energy loss
- Headaches
- Cramps or spasms
- Depression
- Severe nausea

Blue Vervain

Blue vervain is a flowering plant found in the family of vervain, referred to as verbenaceae. The blue vervain is also an herb that possesses opposite, easy leaves which contain double serrate margins, borne on awkwardly erect, branching square stems. It is a purple flower that springs up during the summer, and it is a popular plant found across North America.

Its scientific name is known as verbena hastata, and also by the name swamp verbena. The blue vervain is robust and it can resist drought. Herbalists and traditional medicine men mainly use blue vervain.

People can take the blue vervain as a warm infusion of leaves, flowers, roots, and also as tea.

Uses of Blue Vervain

Blue vervain is used for a lot of purposes like detoxifying the body because it helps in the release of urine from the body system. It can also be used to remove toxins from the body together with excess fat, salt, and water.

Benefits of Blue Vervain

The blue vervain aids in protecting the liver and kidney by lowering the existence of toxic substances that builds up in the body. For instance, your bladder has been infected, and blue vervain can be of help to cleanse your bladder.

Blue vervain eases symptoms of respiratory disorders. In certain people that often experience chest congestion, chronic bronchitis, respiratory inflammation, and sore throats, blue vervain tea can help remove irritation and tracts.

Blue vervain stables your nervous system and keeps them healthy. The contents of the blue vervain can cure numerous illnesses, which include chronic anxiety, stress, nervous disorders, and sleeplessness. Drinking a cup of blue vervain tea can aid in cooling our nerves and making sure our body does not experience any disorder.

Blue vervain is also beneficial for people suffering from depression. The herb is capable of instigating positive thoughts and improving your mood positively.

Blue vervain also helps women suffering from severe periods. It is capable of lessening general discomfort and cramps, especially in women.

Other benefits of blue vervain include helping in oral health, reduction in inflammation and pain, and anti-parasitic activities.

Side Effects of Blue Vervain

- Gas and indigestion
- Redness and rash
- Severe anaphylactic reactions

Burdock Root

Scientific name: Arctium

Family name: Asteraceae

Order: Asterales

Subfamily: Carduoideae

Burdock root is a biennial plant found mostly in Asia and Europe, but it recently grows in the USA. Burdock deep roots coming from the burdock plants are so long and can be brown or black on the exterior layer.

Burdock root has been in use for 100s of years for medicine to cure different aliment. In traditional mode, burdock root was majorly used as a diuretic as well as digestive assistance.

It has oils and compounds referred to as plant sterols and tannins. Burdock root can be used as a tea, herbal tincture, and in a powdered form that individuals can consume in pill form, as a decoction, which is known to be a watery form produced from boiling the herb.

Benefits and Uses of Burdock Root

Burdock root eliminates toxins from the blood: in recent years, burdock root is always known to purify the blood and it can eliminate toxins found in the blood.

Burdock Root Can Inhibit Some Kinds of Cancer

It can assist in curing skin diseases: skin problems such as acne, eczema, and psoriasis can be cured by burdock root. Since it has antibacterial and anti-inflammatory properties, the treatment of the skin is very much possible.

It houses antioxidants such as luteolin, phenolic acids, and quercetin, which guides the cells in the body from harm and can prevent various health problems.

Side Effects of Burdock Root

It may lead to rash when applied to the skin.

May lower blood sugar levels too much

Chapter 13: Dr. Sebi's Mucus Diets

Dr. Sebi's bodily fluid weight control plans are eating less that help in expelling overabundance abstains from food in the body that could frustrate the assurance of the surface linings encompassing and greasing up organs that forestall and fix infections in the body.

Dr. Sebi utilized the utilization of certain antacid spices and diets that are fit for evacuating overabundance bodily fluid in the body to improve solid living. Dr. Sebi's weight control plans additionally help in the evacuation of irritations in the body.

Dr. Sebi suggested that detoxification and purifying are significant in battling abundance bodily fluid in the body. He additionally said antacid spices and diets are viable against the over-creation of bodily fluid in the body.

Along these, let us take a gander at the detoxification technique fundamental for the evacuation of overabundance bodily fluid to stop the over-creation of bodily fluid in the body.

Dr. Sebi's 14 Days Fast Detoxification Herbs to Remove Excess Mucus, and Remove Acid

Dr. Sebi in one of his talk said "detoxification is at the core of disposing of bodily fluid out of the body; there are no different ways that will bring the necessary outcome. Bodily fluid is a significant motivation behind why individual contact infections in the body. It resembles the entryway that opens foreign bodies into the body when it is in overabundance."

In this manner, fasting is a fundamental factor that can help detoxify the body. At the point when you quick, the body experience purifying and detoxification process. For you to accomplish the fix of a few ailments and get more fit, you have to give in enough penance like the one you are going to experience. Decreasing bodily fluid from your body is a groundbreaking approach to recuperate your body from all maladies that you may look in the body.

Sickness brought about by surrendered bodily fluid can be expelled by detox from your body contingent upon how genuine you participate in the techniques since they are difficult to discharge out of the body. In this way, your body needs to remove it out by awakening them by means of fasting and detoxification and free them out.

The Spices Utilized for the 14 Days Detoxification of the Body Are

- Burdock root.
- Stinging bramble root.
- Cascara sagrada.
- Hydrangea root.
- Sea greenery plant.
- Nopal plant.
- Elderberry.
- Red clover spice.

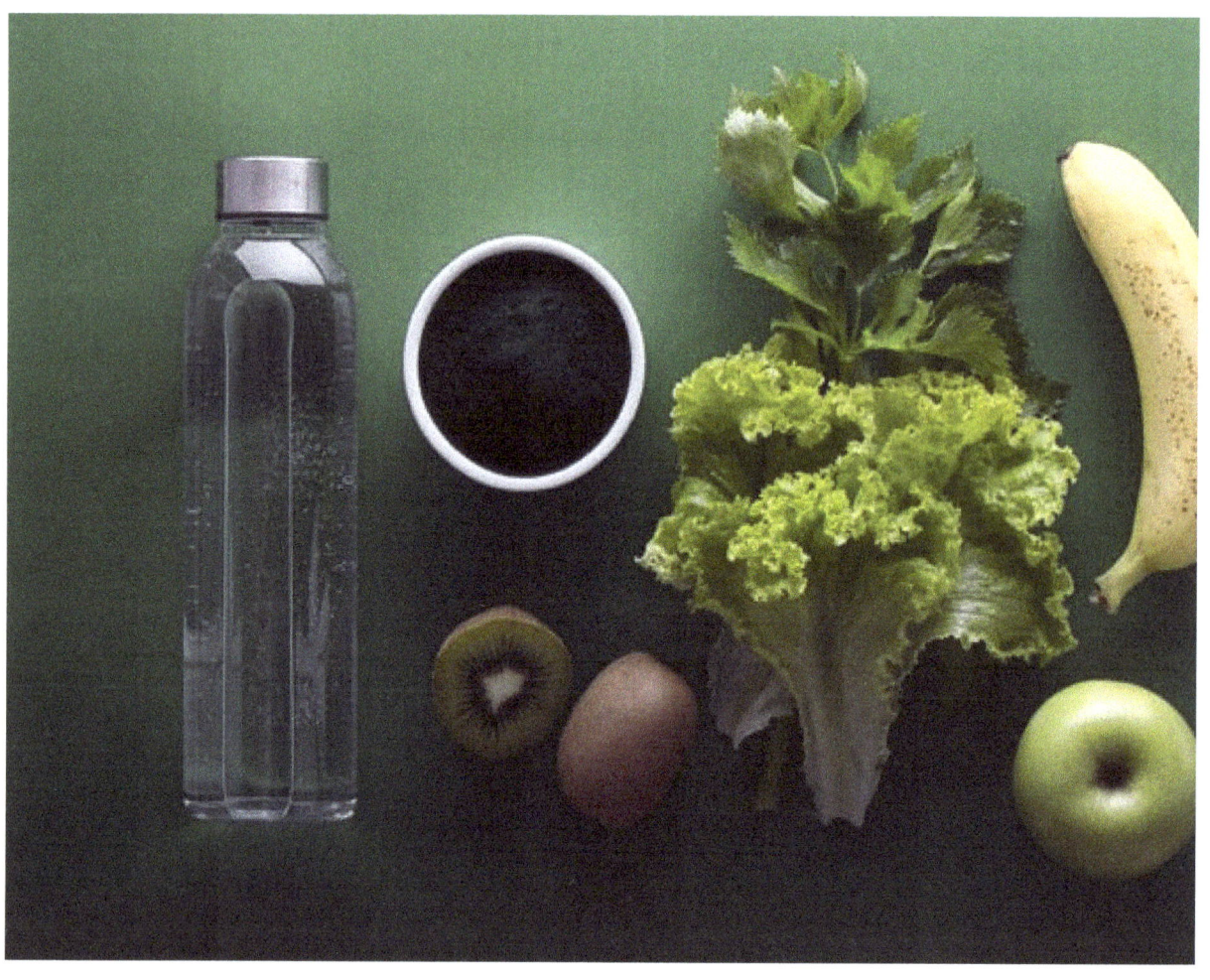

Directions to Prepare the Herbs and Doses

- Ensure the plants are very much dried and safeguard in a dry and clean holder.
- Grind them into powder structure.
- Collect one tsp. of every one of the above plants and include two cups of antacid or spring water.
- Place it in a wellspring of warmth and permit bubbling.
- The bubbling ought to be done inside 3 minutes or until you see that the concentrates of the plants are as of now coming out and the shade of the water is changed.
- Bring it out of the warmth source and leave it for a couple of moments to get cool.
- Drain it before drinking.
- This ought to be taken in the first part of the day and before hitting the sack for

- 14 days.
- Some different foods grown from the ground are affirmed by dr. Sebi you can take during this procedure this incorporates watermelon, berries, mushroom, zucchini, desert flora plants, and verdant green. You can likewise take tamarind squeeze and water.
- You are not required to take any strong nourishment regardless of whether recorded in the food records inside these 14 days of detoxification.
- Some of Dr. Sebi's items utilized for purging and detoxification are bio-ferro, viento and chelation.

The Benefits of Dr. Sebi's Detoxifying Herbs

- Remove abundance bodily fluid and irritation.
- It gives vitality to the body.
- Revitalize the body.
- Remove harmful waste from the body.
- Multiply cells in the body.
- Provide the body with irons.
- Cleanses and advances blood.

Dr. Sebi's Detoxifying and Cleansing Diets to Remove Infected Mucus

Dr. Sebi's detoxifying and purifying eating regimens are principally made out of all the affirmed basic restorative spices for sustenance to at first slaughtering all the reasonable germs contaminated covered mucosa layer of guts, lung tracts or nose channel: expel all the infected bodily fluid out of the energetic body to improving assimilation and discharge; and in a flash supplant the tainted bodily fluid with a sound bodily fluid to forestall aggravation of the epithelial layer, ulceration, indigestion, chest torment, excruciating ingestion of food, loose bowels, drain (stooling of blood) or hemorrhoid (bulge of butt with bodily fluid release and challenges in poop) ... and numerous others.

In this manner, it will do you an incredible kindness, on the off chance that you carefully hold fast to the arrangement and the suggested amount of every specific formula for each diet.

They have been utilized a few by numerous victims with different signs and side effects of infections related with a wholesome waterway from mouth to butt, pancreas, lungs, liver, kidneys, heart, uterus, scrotum, blood tubules... and numerous others returned to affirm the great quick recuperation they encountered during the utilization of the eating regimens.

Chapter 14: Dr. Sebi's Alkaline Diet Tips and Tricks

The Alkaline Diet: A Little-Known and powerful Weight-Loss Plan

What if you heard of a reduction of weight plan to help you reduce weight and look younger? Will you try? Should you try? Alkaline diets and behaviors have been around for more than 60 years, and many people don't know about their normal, healthy, and tested weight-loss properties!

The alkaline diet is not a fad or a gimmick. It is a safe and quick way to experience higher fitness rates. This will inform you what this diet program is, what makes it special, and how it will result in life-changing outcomes for you, your tail, and your wellbeing.

Will you love today a lean and beautiful body? You are in the minority, if so. Unfortunately, more than 65% of Americans are overweight or obese. If you are weighty, it is possible that you suffer poor health conditions such as weakness, stiffness, swollen muscles, and a variety of other illnesses.

Worse still, you still have the impression that you still love the body you like and deserve. Maybe you were told you are growing older, but that's just not the truth. Don't give into that myth. Don't fall into that myth. Many communities have strong, lean older adults who go to great health in their 1990s!

The reality is that the body is a computer of a genius architecture, and if you experience some adverse health effects, that is proof that the blood composition is too acidic. The signs are a call for assistance. That is for one day; the body will not break down. Rather, your wellbeing is gradually eroding over time, finally slipping into 'disappointment.'

What's wrong with the Way You're Eating Now?

S.A.D relies on processed foods, fats, caffeine, meats, and animal goods. All of these products are extremely acidic.

In brief, our S.A.D lifestyle upsets our species' normal acid-alkaline equilibrium. This illness induces malnutrition, higher rates of aches and pains, colds and flu, and disease inevitably develops.

We missed our path. We lost our way. It is where an alkaline diet will lead to improving our wellbeing.

I'm confident that you recognize the word PH relating to the acidity or alkalinity of something. Alkalinity on a scale is calculated. You should take a quick and economical home check to see where your alkalinity is and to track your alkalinity periodically.

Scientific doctors and scientists have understood this lesser-established reality for at least 70 years... your body requires a certain PH degree or delicate equilibrium of the acid-alkaline levels in the blood to ensure the wellbeing and longevity is optimum.

Perhaps You Wonder, "Why Do the PH balance and Alkalinity Mean to Me?"

Two definitions would be used to demonstrate how acid and alkalinity are essential to the body.

1. We also realize that there is an acid in our throats. This acid is necessary for conjunction with enzymes to divide food into simple elements that can be ingested by the digestive tract. What if we have no fat in our belly? We can die of starvation in no time since the body can't use a whole slice of meat or whatever! Can you make sense?

2. Various body parts need varying acidity or alkalinity amounts. The plasma, for example, needs a bit more alkaline than the stomach acids. What if you have so much acidic blood? This can nearly chew into the nerves and lungs, triggering major internal bleeding!

Although these explanations demonstrate that the various components or structures of the body need specific pH values, we should not think about this.

Our question is simple because it's that we're all mostly acidic. If you want to know more about pH, just check the word for lots of knowledge on the internet.

It is the most critical thing to remember. If the body becomes too acidic after a long period of time, it contributes to other diseases such as obesity, diabetes, lack of bone mass, high blood pressure, lung failure, and stroke. The list is infinite, as the organism eventually gives up the battle for life and falls into the state of survival as long as possible.

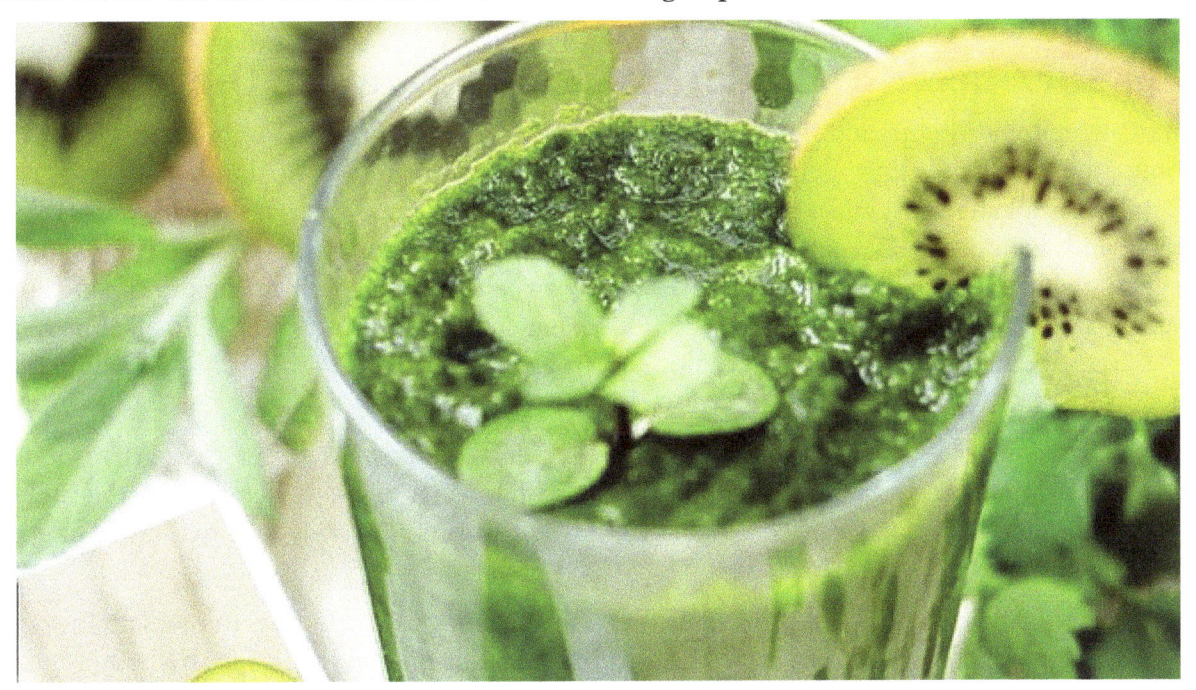

What's the Alkaline Diet Like, and What Would You Expect?

Like other adjustments in diet or lifestyle, a phase of transition may take place. Yet if you're eating the cleanest food your body needs, you won't really have to feel thirsty, unlike other diet strategies. Plus, once you're full, you can consume all you want. You won't have to count calories, either. And you can appreciate a lot of variety, so you're never going to be bored with cooking.

Find an alkaline diet as a kind of "juice fast" for the body. It's just not that serious. You consume rich and readily digestible foods that your body longs for. Once you supply all the cells in your body that it wants so badly, the appetite goes out. Yet dull vegetables don't have to fret, as there are plenty of tasty recipes on the internet and in books.

What Would You Find an Alternate Strategy, Including an Alkaline Diet for Other Eating Plans?

If correctly practiced, you should assume that the fat can dissolve more quickly than for traditional plans. There are also accounts where individuals claim they drop more than two pounds a week. (And with most food plans, the weight will not be wise). When your skin becomes lighter, your vitality improves, and you would look younger.

Furthermore, the alkaline diet does two items that are essential to conventional diets.

1. It provides superior nourishment to your body's cells.
2. It naturally helps to detoxify and cleanse the cells, too.

All of these factors illustrate why an alkaline diet operates both quickly and comfortably.

Tips for Successfully Following the Alkaline Diet

Often, stretching for the additional mile, you get to the areas you had only dreamed about. Going well on an alkaline diet will be the battle that ultimately contributes to a balanced lifestyle. An alkaline diet is an assumption that certain products, such as berries, vegetables, roots, and legumes, leave an alkaline residue or ash behind in the body. The body is strengthened by the key ingredients of rock, such as calcium, magnesium, titanium, zinc, and copper. The avoidance of asthma, malnutrition, exhaustion, and even cancer is an alkaline diet. Conscious about doing something like that? Here are ten strategies to adopt the alkaline diet effectively.

1. Drink water - water is probably our body's most important (after oxygen) resource. Hydration in the body is very important as the water content determines the body's chemistry. Drink between 8-10 glasses of water to keep the body well hydrated (filtered to cleaned).
2. Avoid acidic drinks like tea, coffee, or soda - our body also attempts to regulate the acid and alkali content. There is no need to blink in carbonated drinks as the body refuses

carbon dioxide as waste!

3. Breathe - oxygen is the explanation that our body works, and if you provide the body with adequate oxygen, it should perform better. Sit back and enjoy two to five minutes of slow breaths. Nothing is easier than you can perform yoga.

4. Avoid food with preservatives and food colors - our body has not been programmed to absorb such substances, and the body then absorbs them or retains them as fat, and they do not damage the liver. Chemicals create acids, such that the body neutralizes them either by generating cholesterols or blanching iron from the RBCs (leading to anemia) or by extracting calcium from bones (osteoporosis).

Chapter 15:   Risks and Concerns

The ideal pH level throughout your body should be between 7.2 and 7.4, which is actually a slightly alkaline state for your organism. While it's not good to have an overly acidic body, it's equally wrong to reach a high level of alkalinity. That state is also known as alkalosis, and it occurs when you have excess alkali or base in your body.

You can get too alkaline if you have higher bicarbonate or lower carbon dioxide levels. The first one is also called metabolic alkalosis, while the other is known as respiratory alkalosis. You can also suffer from hypokalemic alkalosis (extreme lack of potassium) and hypochloremic alkalosis (severe lack of chloride).

Symptoms of Alkalosis

There are certain symptoms you can notice that might be related to alkalosis. The first one is confusion, which is dangerous because it can lead to fainting or even coma. You might also feel hand tremors, prolonged muscle spasms or muscle twitching. Numbness in your arms, legs, and face, as well as tingling, are also symptoms that can occur during alkalosis. You can also feel nausea and even start vomiting, or you can be unable to catch your breath. You can try to help your breathing by using a paper bag to breathe into it. Aside from that, the best way to correct the imbalance caused by alkalosis is to take medications, so make sure to call your health provider if you experience any of the symptoms.

Hypokalemia

Alkalosis can cause hypokalemia, which is nothing else than an extreme lack of potassium in your body. Potassium is crucial for our organism to properly conduct various processes, such as proper cell function, including muscle and nerve cells. Aside from eating and metabolic disorders, medications can cause hypokalemia. You should avoid chewing tobacco that contains glycyrrhetinic acid, as well as drinking a lot of herbal teas and eating a lot of liquorice. Symptoms of hypokalemia include fatigue, constipation, and paralysis of vital body organs.

Arrhythmias

Heart arrhythmias can occur if you reach alkalosis. In case you don't know, the arrhythmia is irregular heart beat (it can be both too slow and too fast). Symptoms of arrhythmia include chest pain, heart palpitations, fainting, and shortness of breath. You may notice that you are sweating more than usual and that your skin became pale. If not taken care of, arrhythmias may lead to heart failure, heart attack, or a stroke that can even be fatal.

Coma

If your blood has excessive alkaline levels, you may go into a coma, which is a deep and profound state of unconsciousness. Comas can last up to three or four weeks (rarely longer), and you can completely recover when it comes to awareness. However, more often than not, people that wake up from a coma suffer intellectual, physical or psychological problems. In some cases, people don't recover their awareness completely, and they stay in a partially vegetative state. That is why you should be especially careful not to have excessive alkalosis levels in your body.

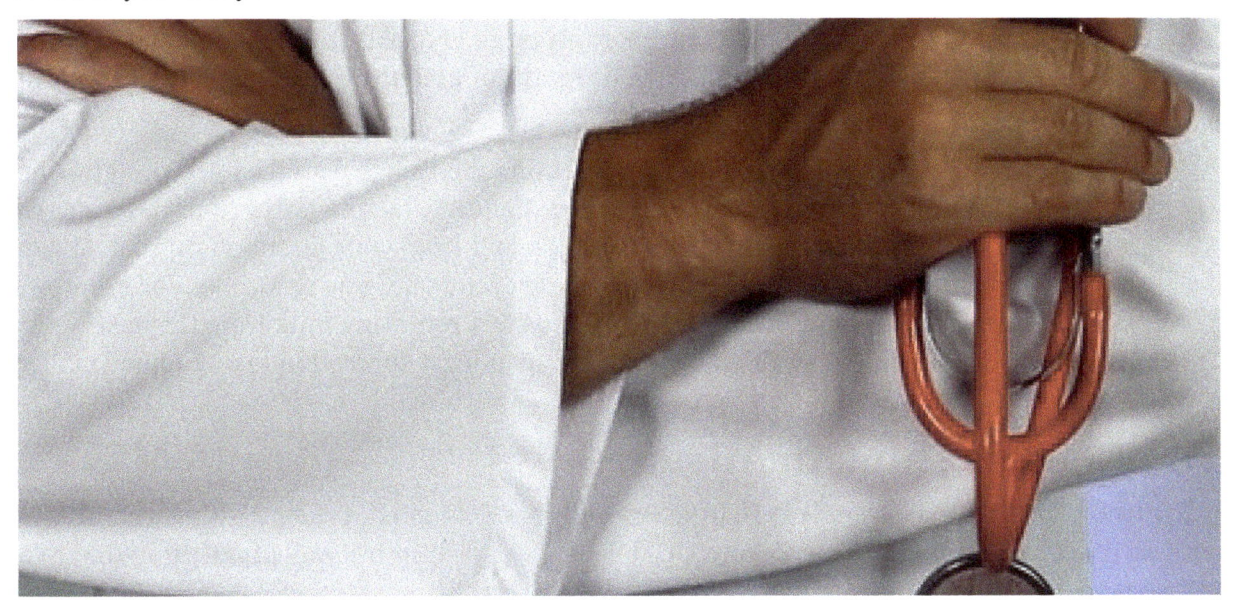

Mistakes Beginners Starting Alkaline Diet Often Make

Now that we've covered health risks let's focus on some mistakes beginners usually make when they start with the alkaline way of nutrition. That way, we can secure that you won't repeat these mistakes and that you will be on your way to achieving an alkaline lifestyle:

- You can't reach perfection immediately

- Whenever people start a diet, they have in mind that they need to strive for perfection. Whether a person is a young artist or an experienced engineer, they want to reach the alkaline goal immediately and be perfect from day one.

- The truth is – it's extremely hard to conduct any diet from the beginning entirely. Expecting too much is a sure way to failure. Starting the basic nutrition means that you should change your way of life and that is not something you can easily do. Furthermore, it just takes extreme effort and brings almost no fun and enjoyment.

- Believe it or not, the fastest way to make a change in your life is to take it one step at a time. Remember, you are not only trying to implement new eating habits and foods, but you are also trying to give up the old ones. That requires a lot of work and persistence. That is why it is important to appreciate all the small steps you've made.

- It's only natural that you will have an occasional setback. People often throw out the window everything that they have done up until that point once they make their first mistake. That's wrong!

- The pressure is enormous – you need to fight the cravings, change your habits, fight

- your brain not to desire particular foods, and go through the everyday stress and work and in your private life. That is just too much to handle at once, so make sure to appreciate on everything you managed to do.

- When it comes to alkaline diet, the important thing is to take care of some basics, such as staying hydrated and securing that your intake of green vegetables and minerals is at an adequate level.

- It might be good advice to focus on implementing the things you like into your alkaline diet. Of course, these need to be the things that are in line with your new way of nutrition, but make sure to know what you like and keep your attention on that. If you need to eliminate a lot of highly acidic foods, try removing one at a time. For example, don't drink coffee anymore from this week, and start removing milk from the next week. When you are keeping it gradually, make sure to at least succeed in taking these smaller steps.

You Need to Think in Advance

If I learned something from people that successfully implemented a diet, it's that you always need to think in advance. I've personally faced a sudden crash in my way of nutrition due to a simple reason – I wasn't prepared.

A particular way of nutrition requires you to have certain meals. But when you've just come home from a stressful day at work, and you notice that there is nothing to eat, everything goes down the drain. If you add that it's rainy and cold outside and you don't feel like going to the store, ordering a pizza seems like a very good idea. And while you are waiting for it to arrive, you grab than convenience food that has been in your cupboard for weeks.

Thinking in advance first means that you need to have enough of raw ingredients in your refrigerator to be able to whip up a meal whenever you need it. The other important thing in preparation is to know what you are going to cook. It's virtually impossible to invent a meal in a short amount of time, especially if you are looking for an alkaline-friendly dish that should also be tasteful.

My advice is to prepare a bunch or recipes that are easy, tasteful and alkaline-friendly. These meals should be dishes that you can always rely on. You should make sure to perform shopping regularly to secure that you have enough ingredients in your fridge.

A good idea is also to make a nutrition plan in advance. You don't just need to know what you are going to eat for lunch, but you also want to plan what you will eat for dinner tomorrow or two days for now. That's why it's important to make a menu of things you like and plan ahead.

Whether you are on the alkaline or any other type of diet, it's crucial not to leave things to fate. Shopping and eating day-to-day is a big mistake – hunger, tiredness or any other reason will eventually cause you to disrupt your diet just because you weren't prepared. Instead, make sure that your refrigerator always has about a dozens of ingredients you can use to make different alkaline meals or snacks in a matter of minutes.

Chapter 16:   Before You Begin

There are many different types of cleanses, from fasting to whole foods, but they all aim to accomplish the same thing, and that is to get rid of inflammatory substances and toxicity. Then they provide your body with pure forms of nutrients. The goal of a cleanse is to heal and restore your body to its optimal health and give its powerful detoxification systems to work without the blockages that are normally there.

The occasional detox is great for the body, but you should never just jump straight into a detox. Getting your body ready for the detox is just as important as the actual detox. If you already follow a very healthy and clean diet, then you won't have as much to do to get ready. But if you are like most people and follow a standard American diet, then you will have some work to do.

Cleanse and detox are words that tend to be used interchangeably, but they aren't quite the same thing. A cleanse is something that you do that will cause detoxification. Your body detoxes naturally as soon as your food has been digesting. This is where it will remove toxic and foreign materials.

Unfortunately, the regular lifestyle and diets of most people cause them to accumulate more toxins than the body is able to purge. Because of this, we need to, on occasion, do a cleanse or fast where we consciously reduce the number of toxins that we are consuming so that the body is forced into a natural detoxifying state.

A cleanse could be a complete abstinence from food or toxic activities, and you only consume water. This type of fast might be helpful, but it's pretty hard to keep up. The Dr. Sebi detox won't require you to stop eating altogether, but if you want to try that type of cleanse, feel free to because it can do amazing things to your body.

Starting just a few days before you plan on beginning your detox, you will want to start changing how you eat. You will need to eat simple, light foods like salads, soups, or veggies. You will want to focus on raw veggies and leafy greens. This is especially true if you haven't been much of a clean eater. You need to give your body a chance to get ready for the cleanse. Take little steps by slowly cutting out processed and sugar foods, and star to increase your intake of fresh foods and grains.

Taking these small steps will increase your body's alkalinity to help it get ready for the deeper cleanse of your detox. During the detox, your body is going to end up releasing toxins that are stored in your tissues. These toxins may enter your bloodstream and can end up causing trouble sleeping, mood swings, body odour, bad breath, aches and pains, or rashes. By preparing for your detox, you can minimize your chances of developing these side effects.

To help you out, we will go over some tips on getting your body ready for your detox.

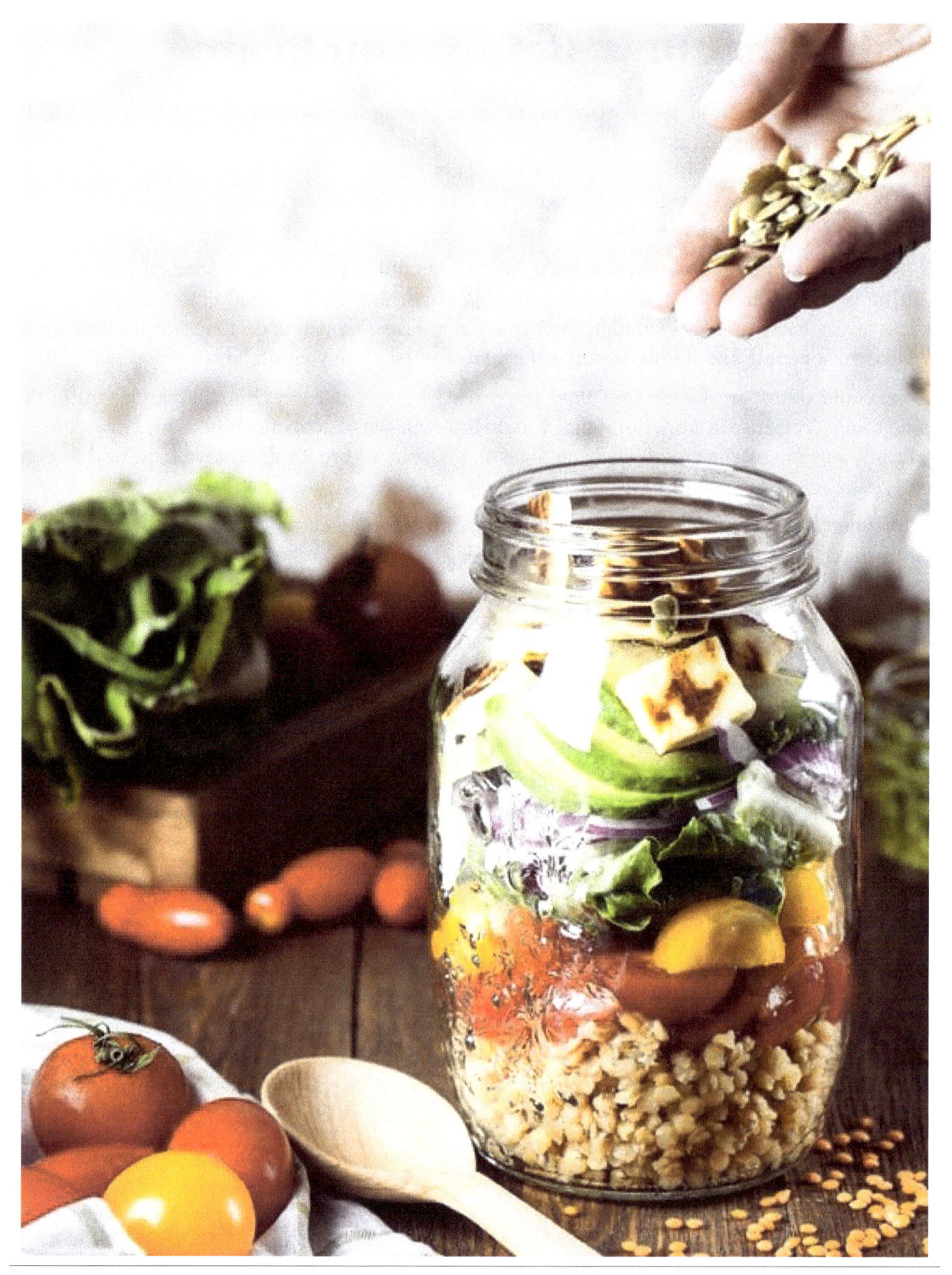

Dietary Changes

- Begin Your Day Right

You should start adding in a glass of warm lime water to your daily routine. This helps to jump-start your digestion and boost your metabolism. Lime juice is very alkalizing to your body, rich in vitamin C, and helps to cleanse your liver, which are all very important parts of detoxification.

- Switch Up Your Drinks

You will want to start drinking more spring water during the day, and start adding in some cleansing herbal teas, such as burdock, dandelion root, or nettle tea. This is also the best time to switch from regular tap water to spring water. You have to drink spring water while on Dr. Sebi's detox.

If you drink alcohol or coffee, you need to start cutting back on your consumption of them. You won't be able to have them on the detox. To let go of coffee, a good alternative is an herbal or green tea. While green tea does contain caffeine, it is full of antioxidants, which will help your detoxification. Sodas and energy drinks should also be eliminated.

Water will play a very big part of your life, so beginning your day with two glasses of water is helpful in getting ready for your detox. If you choose to do the hot lime water that counts towards a glass.

- Keep Things Simple

Start to change your meals to something that is very simple and easy to make. You should opt for dishes that are heavy in natural fruits and vegetables and start weaning yourself off of meats, if you are a meat eater. Include a lot of foods that are rich in chlorophyll because these aid in detoxification.

This can also include drinking veggie soups and broths. If you find it hard to eat enough vegetables, you can get your veggie intake through smoothies or juice. An easy way to add more fruits and veggies into your current diet is by adding a piece of organic fresh fruit to your breakfast each morning. You can also turn to fresh fruits as your mid-afternoon snack instead of heading to the vending machine. When picking out your fruits and veggies, go with organic, seasonal, and local produce when you can so that you avoid pesticides.

- Reduce Your Animal Product Intake

You are going to have to cut out animal products completely on Dr. Sebi's fast, so leading up to it, you should start weaning yourself off of them. The first place to start is to stop eating processed and red meats. This includes things like cured meats and sausages. Choosing leaner meats and fish is a better choice during this time. When picking fish, stay away from fish that are high in mercury, like mackerel and tuna. Fish like salmon, scallops, anchovies, and shrimp are better options.

- Check Your Oils

    A lot of people will cook with vegetable or canola oil because the health industry tells you they are better because they are lower in fat, but they aren't. You need to start using olive oil, avocado oil, coconut oil, and grapes seed oil. Coconut and olive oils should not be cooked and should only be used raw. You can also use these oils along with some lime juice and herbs to create your own salad dressings.

- Up Your Grain Intake

    Right now, you don't have to worry about eating Dr. Sebi approved grains. All you need to worry about is increasing how much whole grains you eat. Start eating more brown rice or spelt, and also start eating more pseudo-grains like quinoa. You need to start reducing how much refined foods like pasta and bread you consume, and that includes whole-grain bread or pasta. Do your best to avoid wheat wherever you are able to.

- Get Rid of Refined Sugar

    You have to start reading nutrition levels to make sure that foods aren't hiding sugars. Before the detox, you can pick healthier sugar alternatives in moderation. Maple syrup, raw honey, rapider sugar, coconut blossom syrup, coconut sugar, or agave nectar are great alternatives. Once the detox starts, you will only be able to have agave nectar.

- Get Rid of Table Salt

    Table salt does not provide you with any nutrients. Your body also has a very hard time metabolizing table salt. While you are checking nutrition labels for sugars, check and make sure they aren't hiding any table salts. The majority of processed foods will have large amounts of chemically processed salts. You should use sea salt as your salt source. It is full of minerals and they are able to help get rid of heavy metals within your body.

- Cut Out Unhealthy Foods

    Leading up to the detox, you should slowly start cutting out unhealthy foods that you like to eat. This includes things like store-bought cookies or muffins, chips, and fried foods. Choose, instead, to snack on homemade dried fruit, seeds, and unsalted nuts. Before the detox, feel free to try some raw chocolate to help you with your chocolate fix.

Get Your Mind Ready

But what should we do about the mind? There is a lot of evidence that has found that our mental state, from stressed to relaxed and all that is in between, has a large impact on our wellbeing and health. While you can do a cleanse for a week without changing anything else about your day, and you may feel pretty good after but, when you add mindfulness into your cleanse, you will uncover some amazing opportunities to move your focus inwards to create as much space in your emotional body and mind as you can in the physical body.

You could possibly be at a time of transition and you're looking for a fresh start to push yourself into the succeeding phase. You could be holding onto something, such as a loss, fear, resentment, or unhealthy relationship that you want to get rid of. Maybe most of your day is spent focusing on and caring for other people and feel like you need to do something for yourself. A lot of use resist turning in and may even fear it. You could have an inner voice asking you to stop distracting yourself in order to listen to your intuition.

In order to get the most from your cleanse, it is a good idea to like what you want to get rid of other than the junk in your diet and why you are drawn to this cleanse.

- Relax and Meditate

    Getting ready for the cleanse doesn't just mean getting your belly ready for the change in foods, but it also means making sure your mind is ready for the change. Relaxation and mediation are a big part of detoxing because they can help you to reduce or eliminate your stress. Stress is the number one cause of so many unhealthy habits, such snacking on junk food or overeating. If you simply set aside some time each day to simple sit and be still, it will help to quiet your mind. This will help you to remain focused on what your goals are.

- Start Journaling

    It's also a good idea to start keeping a detox journal. While you are getting ready for your detox, you can take the time to write out the guidelines for it, or simply write out what you hope it will do for you. In it, you should also make sure you schedule rest time. Your body will be doing a lot of work, and it's common to start feeling tired. Making sure you have rest time set aside will help to combat any fatigue you may experience. While detoxing, you can expel mental toxins by writing in the journal. You can write anything you want so that you mentally cleanse yourself. Let the words flow and don't worry if it makes sense, is grammatically correct, or what have you. Simply writing things out on paper is very therapeutic.

- Clear Your Space

    While this might not seem important, but before you start cleaning your insides, you should also clean your outside. It has been proven that the health of the mind is greatly impacted by your surroundings and all of the environmental toxins lurking in your space. Take the time to vacuum the floor, give your sheets a change, and use an air filter. You should also create your own sanctuary that you can use during your cleanse. This could be an entire room in your house if you have a spare one, or it could simply be a comfy chair placed to a window. Wherever you place your sanctuary, remove all of the clutter and place a vase of some of your favorite flowers or simply a photo that makes you happy. You can also choose something that calms or inspires you.

Chapter 17: Alkaline-Plant-Based Diet

The Health Benefits of Alkaline Plant-Based Diet

If you are a vegetarian, vegan, or aiming to move in this direction, the alkaline diet is ideal. While all dietary plans can be built on a strong foundation of vegetables and fruits, a plant-based diet is one of the best options for adhering to this way of eating. Not all vegan or plant-based diets are alkaline; a lot of foods that are free of animal products can be processed and contain acidic ingredients, though once digested, many "acidic" fruits and vegetables become alkaline. One of the most beneficial, nutrient-rich foods for an alkaline diet is soy. Soybeans (edamame beans) are a great snack on their own, as is tofu, tempeh, miso, and other soy-based foods. When choosing soy products, look for organic, natural options, and avoid preservatives as much as possible.

Why Choose a Plant-Based Diet?

There are many reasons for moving to a plant-based diet, from reducing meat in your diet overall, to implementing one or two "meat-free days" each week. If your current diet is very meat-heavy, this will take some major adjustment, so it is best to not make the switch from red meats to full veganism overnight. Veganism or vegetarianism works best when whole, natural foods are chosen instead of packaged or processed options. A lot of marketing is involved in promoting meat-free packaged snacks and condiments, though many of these may contain sugars, high amounts of sodium, artificial color, additives, and other ingredients that are unhealthy.

There is a lot of research to support a plant-based diet, and the high amount of alkaline in many fruits and vegetables means a good fit with the alkaline-based diet:

- The emphasis is on the whole, natural foods, which simplifies the process of shopping and selecting foods for your diet. This also makes meal preparation and planning much easier, as your focus will be on vegetarian-based eating, without meat as an option, and little or no dairy.

- A plant-based diet can help with weight loss, as vegetables and fruits are digested and used much more quickly than meat and dairy products. There are also fewer calories contained in vegetarian meals, even where the actual portion size is the same or similar to a meal, including meat.

- Meeting your goal weight is a great achievement, and maintaining weight is another task. This can be done much more effectively with plant-based eating, as there are not only restrictions on meat and dairy consumption, but on processed foods, which sometimes contain meat by-products (gelatine) and a high amount of preservatives and artificial flavors.

- Soy is a major staple of a plant-based diet. The amount of calcium, protein, iron, and nutrients in soy products is comparable to meat, and with a fraction of the calories and fat. Soy is also relatively inexpensive and easy to find in most grocery stores. Tofu, tempeh, and edamame beans are popular ways to enjoy soy in almost any type of meal.

- Enjoying a plant-based diet can reduce or eliminate food sensitivities to dairy and meat products, as these are no longer a part of the diet. Other food allergies or sensitivities may be less of a factor, once a more pH balance is established in your body, digestion becomes easier and health improves overall.

- The health benefits of a plant-based diet, especially vegan, where all meat by-products and dairy foods are eliminated entirely, are numerous, from improving heart health and cardiovascular function to preventing cancer, type 2 diabetes, and many other conditions. Prevention is a big factor in why choosing a plant-based diet, as many conditions and diseases can be avoided in the first place.

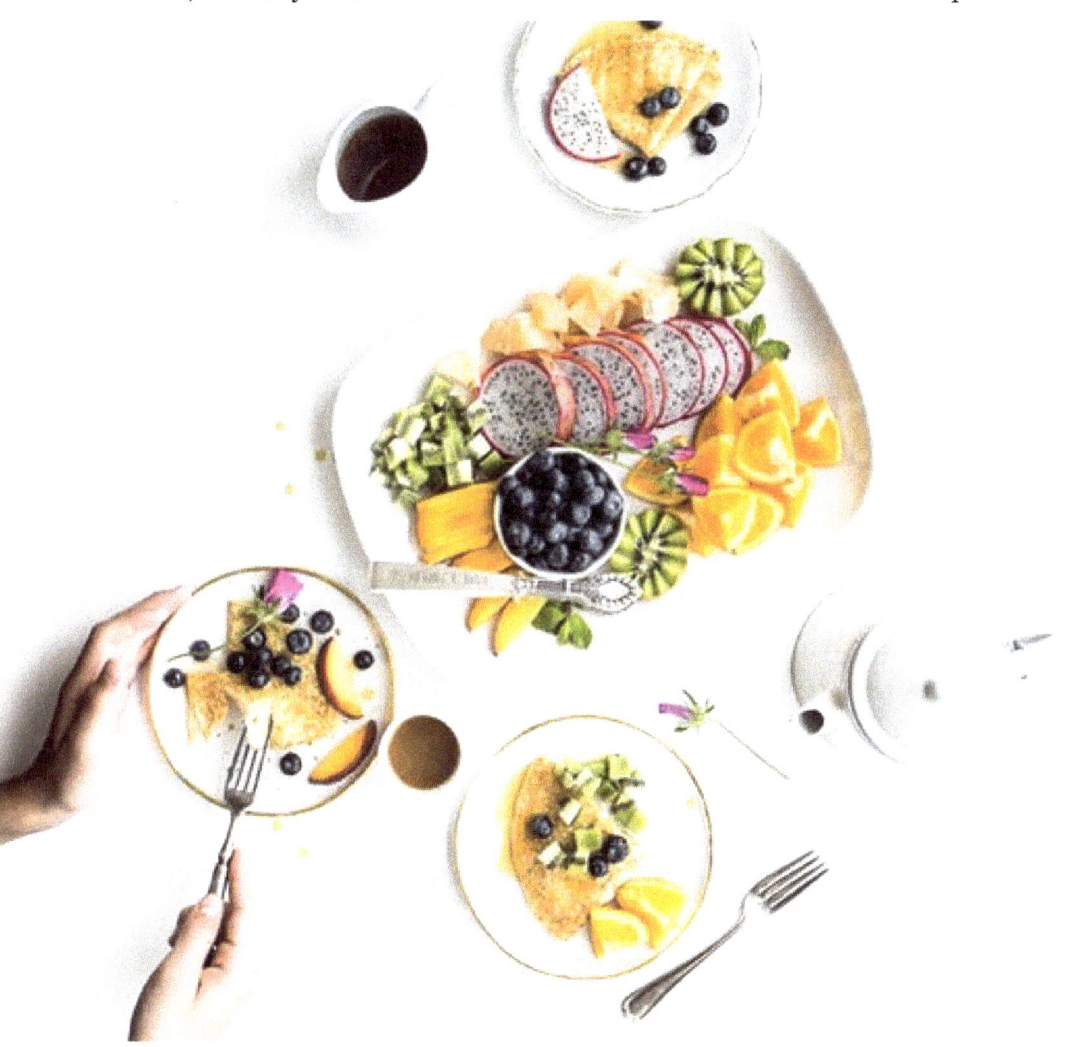

The Benefit of Soy in an Alkaline Diet

When it comes to soy, there are a lot of studies and findings that result in positive outcomes and benefits of eating soy on the dangers of increasing estrogenic and the impact of this on your health. Overall, soy is a healthy option for any diet, especially for plant-based vegan diets that avoid all meat products. For people with allergies to soy and soy-based products, some alternatives can be used to adhere to a vegan meal plan successfully. For most people, soy is a good option with the following advantages:

1. High in protein. Soy can provide just as much, if not more, protein in your diet than meat. In combination with a balanced diet that includes fresh vegetables and fruits, your body will receive more than the required daily protein.

2. Low in cholesterol. Plant-based foods are low in cholesterol, saturated, and Tran's fats, which makes them a good choice for good cardiovascular function and a way to prevent heart disease.

3. High in fiber. Soy, like all vegetables and fruits, is very high in fiber. Not only will you meet your daily protein, calcium, and iron requirements by switching to soy from meat, you'll also receive a good dose of fiber with each serving, which increases metabolism and keeps weight at a healthy, manageable level.

4. Vitamin B12 and other nutrients considered only available in meat and meat-related products are also found in some soy products. Fermented soy, such as miso and tempeh, contains a sufficient amount of B12 to meet dietary requirements.

5. Vitamin D is often an ingredient in dairy milk, due to being fortified, though this can also be found in various soy products as well. While only a small amount of this vitamin is required, it's important that it's a part of your diet.

6. Soy products come in many forms, textures, and flavors. Soft tofu varieties, for example, can be used to create puddings, cakes, and smoothies. Firm tofu and tempeh can be marinated and fried, baked, or sautéed with any combination of vegetables and ingredients. Soymilk is a great alternative to dairy and can be used with cereals, in smoothies, milkshakes, and as a refreshing beverage.

7. Easy to digest. While some people have reported bloating and mild issues with digesting soy, in general, it's easy food for the body to digest and break down for nutrients.

Alternatives to Soy for a Plant-Based Diet

If soy-based foods are not an option for your plant-based diet, there are many alternatives to choose from. These foods contain high amounts of protein, calcium, and iron, which are found in meats and dairy products:

- Coconut-cultured yogurt:

    Similar to dairy yogurt, vegan, coconut-based yogurt is made by cultivating bacterial culture from coconut to make a product with the same texture, nutrients, and a similar flavor to dairy yogurt.

- Vegan cheese:

  Most varieties of vegan cheese are soy-based, though a growing number of plant-based cheeses are made from vegetables and vegetable oils. The benefits of vegan cheese include a similar taste and texture to regular, dairy cheese. Vegetable-based cheese, as opposed to soy-based products, tends to melt easier, which makes this variety a preferred option for vegan grilled cheese and Mac-and-cheese dishes.

- Almond, cashew, and coconut milk:

  There are many non-dairy milk alternatives available at nearly every grocery store and local restaurant. Almond milk is becoming nearly as popular as soymilk, as well as other nut-based kinds of milk, including cashew milk. Some varieties include a combination of almond and coconut milk, or cashew and almond, for a pleasant, nut-like taste that works well in recipes, smoothies, and cereal. More people are ditching dairy milk and cream for non-dairy options for their coffee and tea as well. Other alternatives include hemp and rice milk.

- Nut Butters:

Peanut, almond, and other nut kinds of butter are an excellent source of protein and energy. Just one or two spoons of these kinds of butter will provide a good boost of nutrients before a workout or an active day.

- Other Soy Alternatives:

Nuts and seeds can be added to stir fry dishes and salads, instead of tofu and other soy foods to boost the protein and calcium content. Olive oil or coconut oil is both good alternatives for baking and cooking vegetarian dishes. Both oils have a neutral flavor that works well with any combination of ingredients.

Alkaline Fruits

Fruits are an excellent source of vitamins, fiber, and energy, with natural sugars that can easily replace the need for sweet snacks and processed foods. When we shop for fruits, we tend to choose from a small circle or group of fruits that we are familiar with and comfortable. The variety or limitations on what fruit we buy can depend on what's in season, how much of a budget we have to work with, and our cravings. Bananas, apples, oranges, and berries tend to be most popular, and for a good reason: they are delicious and easy to eat. Apples are best during autumn when they are in peak season and are available in many varieties that vary in texture, taste, and appearance. During summer months, it's the perfect time to enjoy fresh fruits, such as berries, bananas, and melons.

If you buy local, fresh fruits become less available during winter or colder seasons. Frozen fruits are another option to consider. They are just as healthy and more convenient, as they last longer and can be used at any time. Canned foods, even vegetables or fruits should be avoided, as they contain extra sodium and sugar, along with other additives.

Which Fruits are high in Alkaline?

All fruits have a significant amount of alkaline, which makes them all good choices for an alkaline diet. The amounts vary depending on which fruit, where alkaline is low, moderate, or high. Some fruits that contain acidic properties will convert to alkaline once digested, like tomatoes and citrus fruits, while others contain a high amount of alkaline before consumption:

1. Blackberries, strawberries, and raspberries. Berries are a great choice in an alkaline diet due to their high amount of vitamin C and antioxidants.
2. Nectarines, like peaches, are high in alkaline and make a great snack on their own or in a fruit salad.
3. Watermelons are not only high in alkaline but also contain a good amount of potassium and fiber. They are an excellent choice for a snack and especially refreshing during the summer season when they are more readily available.
4. Apples have more of an amount of alkaline that's more moderate to high, though they contribute a lot of nutrients that make them a preferred snack any time of the year. They can be enjoyed raw, stewed, or baked for a variety of dishes. Apples are also naturally sweet, which makes them ideal for desserts.
5. Bananas are high in potassium, fiber, and pack a lot of energy into just one serving. In fact, one banana can provide up to 90 minutes of energy, an easy and quick snack before a workout, hike, or going cycling.
6. Cherries, similar to berries, are high in alkaline and fiber. They also promote regularity and a healthy metabolism.

Are there any fruits to avoid? With an alkaline diet, virtually all fruits are good options, which makes the diet an easy process to follow.

Chapter 18: Eating Naturally with Dr. Sebi's Teachings

The Dr. Sebi diet is often referred to as the African bio-mineral balance. This was how he would cure people of a variety of diseases. It is basically a vegan diet that is made up of foods that he called "electric" or alkaline foods. It is suggested that, while following this diet, you also take his healing supplements.

You cannot eat any meat or animal products while on this diet, as well as foods that contain a lot of starch. The reason for this is that you are only supposed to eat alkaline-forming foods, and those foods form acids.

Meat products cause uric acid production, dairy products cause lactic acid, and starch causes carbonic acid. All of these acids will build-up, which causes a build-up of mucus. The mucus robs our cells of oxygen. However, if you eat electric foods, they feed the body. The human body is electrical, so it needs electric food to function.

This diet is made up of grains, teas, nuts, veggies, and fruits. Among the foods, you can eat wild rice, amaranth, quinoa, mushrooms, watercress, kale, dates, figs, mangos, avocados, and much more. These foods will help to nourish your body and won't end up causing an accumulation of mucus.

If you plan on really starting this diet, you must make sure that you really want it. The first thing you will need to do is to make some changes to how you eat. You will probably find that this is going to require you to be your best emotional state and the right state of mind.

Eating is a big part of our life and the types of things we consume form strong habits that can end up lasting our entire life. It can be very hard to break these habits and deal with the influence of family and friends. That means, before you jump right into this diet, you should take some time thinking about changing how you eat. You don't want to promise yourself this and then end up not being able to follow through just because you weren't prepared.

Instead, you should begin slowly. You can even talk to your family and friends. The reaction you can get from people when you talk to them about Dr. Sebi's diet will vary. Some will want to learn more, while others will write it off as bunk.

That being said, you shouldn't tire yourself by trying to convince everybody else before you make sure that it is right for you. Your vitality, health improvements, and cleaner outlook will show your family way more than just your words.

Once you do start making the transition, the first thing you need to do is to start reading food ingredient labels on everything. This will help you to stay conscious about what you are drinking and eating. When you are first starting out, before you live completely by the nutritional guide, this awareness is going to provide you with the incentive to change things as you continue on. Later on, if you do end up straying from the diet, you will still be able to remain conscious about what you are eating.

If you have long been a meat-eater, that may be the hardest thing to transition from. The best thing you can do is to start making the transition from meats by switching to eating only fish. Then you can slowly start eating less and less fish each week.

It is also important that you start making your own snacks. This will ensure if you do get the urge to snack, that you will have good snacks to eat. Approved nuts and raisins are a good choice.

Then you need to make sure that you are eating all of the right foods. That means you need to learn what foods are and aren't on the nutritional guide. You must stick to only those foods. At first, this will feel tough, and that is expected. In fact, it is very hard to do in our society when only the bad foods are pushed at us. This is the reason why I stressed that you must be emotionally ready.

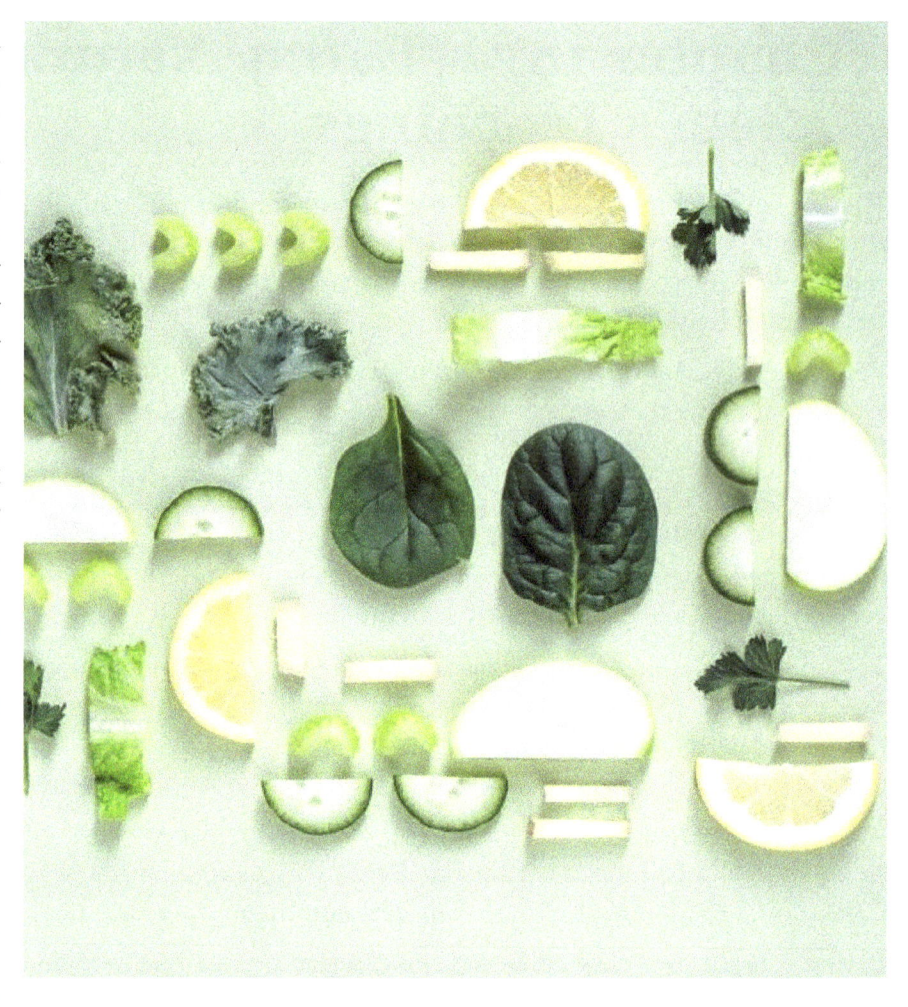

You also need to make sure you are drinking plenty of water. While we have all known for a while now that water is a very important part of our health, most of us are still not drink enough. Plus, there are a lot of Dr. Sebi products that you will be taking, like the Bromide Plus Powder, contain herbs that act as diuretics. That means you have to take extra care to make sure you don't allow yourself to get dehydrated.

Dr. Sebi suggests that you drink a gallon of spring water every day. Spring water has a naturally alkaline pH, whereas tap water can be high in chloride and many other contaminants.

You will also need to learn how to cook your own meals if you don't cook already. You aren't going to find too many pre-packaged foods that fit into the Dr. Sebi's diet. Once you do get the hang of cooking, you will find that you can change your favorite dishes into Dr. Sebi-approved dishes.

Chapter 19: How the Alkaline Diet Can Help You

When it comes to diets, you are probably all fed up with hearing about and then trying so many of them, with their promises of incredible results. These "potential" results are usually related to weight loss, and this is something this kind of diet doesn't focus on. The main purpose of the alkaline diet is to improve your health. Of course, if you associate the diet with intense workouts, you will also notice weight loss. And any time the body is functioning at its peak efficiency and health, there will be noticeable effects. Also, unlike other diets, the alkaline diet is best followed permanently, so it's not something to use for a limited period of time. Using the alkaline diet as a life plan may sound a bit discouraging, especially if you have to give up some of your favorite treats. Still, you are gaining a lot of health benefits by following this life plan. It's the smart way to live the rest of your life.

Anti-Aging Effect

There is no known substance that can completely reverse the aging process, but there are several tricks you can use to slow down this process. The alkaline diet is one of these tricks, but it is not a "Fountain of Youth," so you shouldn't expect miracles, as it doesn't add years to your life. It simply helps you feel and look younger and healthier because its effects can be noticed on the skin, nails, and hair. Your skin will regain its radiance and elasticity, your hair will be shinier, and your nails will become stronger.

Increased Vitality and Energy

There is no doubt that the alkaline diet improves your metabolism, and this enhances your vitality. Your digestive system needs the energy to process food and even more to handle acid-forming types of food. Drawing that energy from other body systems puts the whole body into a lethargic state. Balancing the acid/alkaline ratio in your body also increases energy levels because it frees up oxygen for different cells and thereby enhances their functioning. The alkaline diet stabilizes energy levels throughout the day, avoiding any kind of sugar rush resulting from the consumption of sweeteners, sweets, and sodas. Trying this life plan helps you impose self-discipline because you establish when to eat and what to eat, which will definitely lead to more restful sleeps. All of these factors produce a cumulative effect of increased energy and vitality.

Prepares Your Body for Weight Loss

This diet doesn't promise you phenomenal weight loss, but it can set the right conditions for your body to lose weight. The Alkaline Diet can help you reach the natural body weight or Body Mass Index (BMI). It's not designed as a slimming diet, but if you are overweight and have a sluggish metabolism, this diet can speed up your metabolism which can lead to weight loss. You will also eliminate toxins and therefore relieve the fat tissue of the load it's carrying, making it more available to be burned. The alkaline diet also boosts your energy level, which can give you extra motivation to work out and lose weight.

Decreased Bloating and Constipation

Another benefit of this diet, or cure, as some nutritionists like to describe it, is related to your urine and feces. After a short time of living according to the alkaline diet, you will notice soft feces and clear urine, as your body will function properly and you will become more regular in your bowel movements. Constipation is something anyone wants to avoid, so if you are experiencing this condition, you should know that the alkaline diet is better than any laxative. It will regulate your bowel movements and, with proper hydration, guarantee a soft stool. The way you eat can also have a serious impact on the work your digestive system does. If you chew your food enough, you make things easy for your digestive system which will be able to properly digest the food, relieving pressure on your stomach and avoiding constipation.

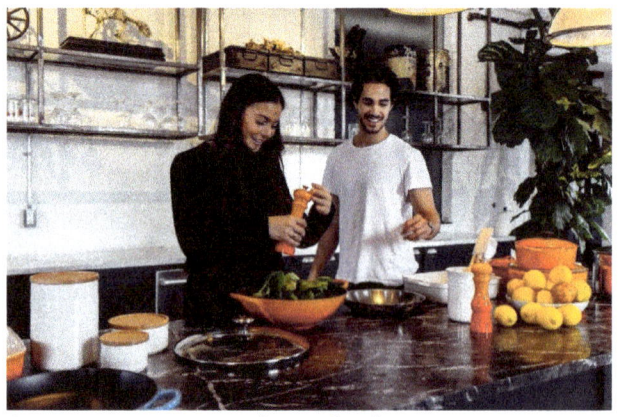

Better Brain Function and Mood

When you feel more energetic and healthier, you also feel better and have a positive attitude. A study conducted by Rudolph Wiley in 1987proved that acid imbalance can cause all sorts of disorders of psychogenic, psychological, psychosomatic, and stress-related natures. This study demonstrated that an alkaline diet decreased or completely eliminated a symptom's severity for more than 85 of participants. Also, this kind of diet consists of plenty of fruits and vegetables, which are rich in vitamins like B6, a very helpful vitamin for your brain function and mood. All the vitamins and minerals which come from the fruits and vegetables of this diet are very helpful for the proper function of your brain and body. Associating this diet with exercise (even if it's not intense) and avoiding as much as possible caffeine, alcohol, and processed food also help.

A Shield against Diseases and Allergies

There are plenty of allergies known today which are in fact just inflammation in the stomach. Probably the most common allergies are towards peanuts or milk proteins. In such scenarios, the problem-causing food has to be identified, and the system has to be cleansed from it. Then some alkalizing treatments have to be tried on the system. If somebody is experiencing allergies, comprehensive research can discover if the subject is vulnerable to diseases like diabetes, heart disease or even cancer. There are enough theories which claim that these diseases are favored by an acidic environment, and increased alkalinity can suppress these diseases in an early stage. Also, it is known that veggies and ripe fruits are great sources for antioxidants, which represents the best way to protect you from these kinds of diseases. Bottom line, your immune system is as healthy as your stomach is.

Stronger Bones

If you are experiencing any muscle or bone pain, then the alkaline diet is what you need. It will help you ease your pains and can even prevent or cure osteoporosis, as the diet decreases the bones' acidity with alkalizing minerals. Healthy bones are favored by an alkaline environment, calcium, vitamin D, and weight-bearing exercises.

Enhanced Fertility

Fruits and vegetables with high alkaline levels can seriously improve fertility, for both men and women. The consumption of these foods has amazing effects on the way the reproductive system performs. The body's hormonal system works better in an alkaline environment, leading to better cell function and better fertility. These hormones will enhance the desire for sex, make conception more viable, and promote a healthy pregnancy.

Possible Symptoms or Illnesses Which Can Be Prevented by Using This Type of Diet

There are clearly many benefits to a lifestyle built around an alkaline diet. But the benefits go even further, to impact some of the symptoms, conditions, and illnesses that plague our modern society.

Hypertension, Stroke and Heart Disease

"According to the Centers for Disease Control and Prevention, over 33 percent of adults have high blood pressure, a condition that increases the risk of heart disease and stroke. While there are a number of risk factors for high blood pressure and heart disease, including inactivity and being overweight, there is a clear and distinct link between what you eat and your risk."The average American diet contains plenty of animal-related products, and it's deficient in vegetables and fruits. This causes an acidosis metabolism and also a low urine pH, but it can also lead to hypertension and even heart disease. With high levels of magnesium and potassium, the alkaline diet contributes to healthy blood pressure. Assuring a high level of minerals through alkalizing foods decreases the risk of heart disease.

Kidney Stones

A recent study estimates that one out of ten people will have kidney stones sooner or later. This statistic is worrying, and if nothing changes in our diet, your risk of being the one increases. The acid environment is the perfect kind of environment for developing kidney stones. Unfortunately, the average diet is high in sodium, animal proteins, and sugar, which are all nutrients that the kidneys have difficulty filtering. Calcium, sodium, oxalate, phosphorus, and uric acid are some of the most common stone promoters. These substances are filtered easily by the kidney of a young person, but as we get older, the kidney doesn't function as it used to. Eliminating a kidney stone is something extremely painful, but they are avoidable. So, if there is an easy mean of prevention, it's crucial to take advantage of it and avoid the extreme discomfort of passing a kidney stone. Therefore, you will need to make sure you consume alkaline food and prevent this from happening. The alkaline cure can be even more useful than consuming beer or wine to prevent and dissolve kidney stones.

Muscle Mass

Aging and a passive lifestyle are the main causes of losing muscle mass. Every person needs a certain amount of calories to maintain muscle mass. Losing muscle means that the body will need to consume fewer calories to maintain what it still has, leading to the potential for weight gain if eating habits are not altered. Lost muscle mass also results in less energy to exercise and build back muscles. In other words, muscle loss can eventually lead to more muscle loss, which can definitely affect your mobility, not to mention that you become more vulnerable to fractures and falls. There are two approaches to prevent this from happening. The first one is an increased caloric intake to provide enough energy to work out and increase your muscle mass (protein intake is highly important). Another approach is the alkaline way. A study conducted by the American Journal of Clinical Nutrition discovered that high alkalizing food reduces the acid level and also preserves muscle mass. As a general rule of thumb, consume vegetables and fruits to get the necessary minerals and vitamins to preserve your muscle mass, mobility, and independence. By doing so, you will be less fragile and less vulnerable to falls or fractures.

Type 2 Diabetes

It is estimated that around 26 million people living in the US have type 2 diabetes and around 10% of adult Americans have this disease, according to the Center for Disease Control and Prevention. Type 2 diabetes is a metabolic disorder in which your blood sugar is higher than normal and your cells resist the process of balancing blood sugar with the hormone insulin. Luckily, this disease can be prevented if you fully understand its roots and causes.

As studies have shown, the normal high-acid diet is a factor in increasing the risk of this disease. "In a study published in Diabetologia in 2013, researchers conducted a 14-year cohort study analyzing dietary information collected from a questionnaire from almost 70,000 French women. From the responses, the researchers calculated the potential renal acid load (PRAL) and found a trend correlating a high dietary acid load to an increased risk for type 2 diabetes."

Blood sugar gets high after consuming a large number of carbs, and normally all the excess glucose should be turned into "fuel" and used as energy. Insulin is known as a hormone which turns glucose into energy, and when the body doesn't use insulin or doesn't use it well enough, glucose will remain in the blood, leading to high blood sugar. Coincidence or not, processed foods are rich in carbs, which are considered the main cause of high levels of glucose. They also have a higher acidity, which leads to the conclusion that the acidic food type favors the accumulation of glucose in greater amounts, and at some point, the glucose can't be turned into energy.

Consuming alkaline foods limits the spike in blood sugar because they have a lower concentration of carbs, and the resulting glucose can be easily processed and turned into energy, so it doesn't get stored in the blood. Obviously, this decreases blood sugar and also the risk of having type 2 diabetes.

Chapter 20: The Ideal 30-Day Meal Plan for an Alkaline Diet

The alkaline diet is focused on improving the health of your body by changing the pH level and making it more alkaline than acid. A standard diet consisting of fast food and other processed foods causes high acidity in your stomach and entire digestive system, and apparently, this state leads to most of the diseases currently troubling humanity. Therefore, everything which has high acidity has to be removed from your daily diet, and if you are wondering what you can eat, don't worry, you can see below a detailed menu of what you can eat during a 30-day meal plan on the alkaline diet. Food waste is something we're all trying to avoid, but disposing of most of the food you purchased because it's junk or too processed is something you need to do for your health. There are a few things you will need to obey when trying an alkaline diet:

- Eat more natural and less processed. Processed food has a lot of ingredients and some chemicals that humans shouldn't be consuming;
- Focus on fresh food and try to avoid preserved food, unless there are some fruits and vegetables which are out of season. You will probably need to shop more frequently;
- Have your meals at regular times, so you will need to have scheduled meals. This part is very important on any diet, as it helps your digestive system and metabolism work properly.

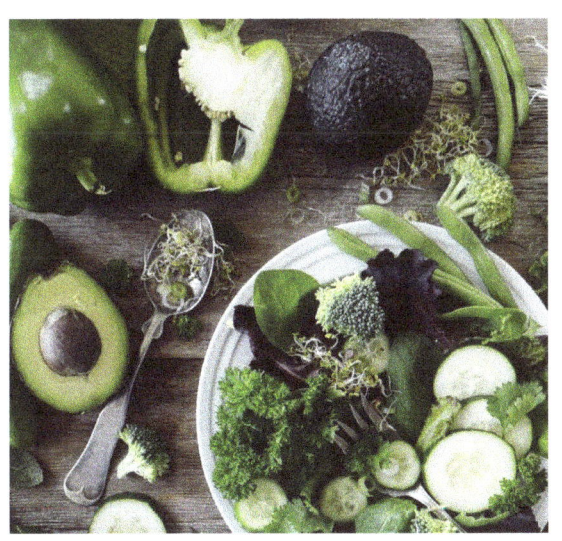

Now, that you have cleaned your refrigerator and kitchen of the junk food (and processed food) you can compile a shopping list with alkaline food. To fill up your refrigerator with alkaline food may not be very cheap, as natural food tends to be more expensive than processed food. However, just think about the money you save by preventing some medical appointments or spending money on medicine. Also, since fruits and vegetables are more perishable, you have to buy more often, which is definitely not a money saver. Still, there are some types of food which you can buy preserved or frozen so that you can buy them in higher quantities. To have a glimpse of what you need to buy, you will need to focus on your favorite fruits, vegetables, nuts or seeds, tubers, whole grains or lean proteins (usually up to 5 of them). The shopping list for the first-week plan should include brown rice, potatoes, onions, eggplants, broccoli, cauliflower, bok choy, bananas, grapefruit, tomato sauce, mushrooms, and many other ingredients.

If you are still confused about what you need to buy and eat, perhaps this detailed menu can help you.

WEEK 1

Day	Breakfast	Lunch	Dinner	Snacks
Monday	Brown Rice Porridge	Potpie Made of Vegetables	Cheesy Scalloped Potato and Onion Bake	Banana Candy Coins
Tuesday	Breakfast Fajitas	Curried Eggplant	BBB Soup	Cauliflower Popcorn
Wednesday	Baked Grapefruit	Alkaline Stuffed Peppers	Alkaline Pasta with Tomato Sauce	Herbed Crackers
Thursday	Home Fries Made of Baby Potatoes	Mushroom-Miso Soup with Wild Rice	Quinoa and Avocado Salad	Healthy Hummus
Friday	Garden Pancakes	Grilled Veggie Stack	Roasted Veggies	Cashew Butter Fudge
Saturday	Vanilla Bean and Cinnamon Granola	Alkaline Lasagna	Nori Vegetables Rolls with Avocado-Jalapeño Spread	Chocolate - Cherry Smoothie
Sunday	Salad of Summer Fruits, Mint and Lime	Layered Ratatouille	Salad of Kale and Baby Tomato	Apple Pie Crumble

Sticking to this diet may not be the easiest thing to do, as you will definitely have cravings for your favourite fast food or processed foods. Smoothest are designed to replace the processed sweets, and the other food should provide the necessary nutrients for you to make it through the day. As you can probably think, this diet is not high on calories, so it can help you with weight loss, especially if you combine it with physical exercise.

WEEK 2

Day	Breakfast	Lunch	Dinner	Snack
Monday	Strawberry Coco Chia Quinoa	Salad of Butter Lettuce, Avocado, Cucumber, Pomegranate and Pistachios	Pad Thai Salad	Cucumber Sandwiches
Tuesday	Apple Parfait with Non-Dairy Products	Avocado Wrapped in Lettuce	Warm Spinach Salad	Cauliflower Popcorn
Wednesday	Almond Butter Crunch Berry Smoothie	Kale Pesto Pasta	Summer Dinner Salad	Mushroom Pate
Thursday	Almond Butter Oats with Apple	Green Goddess Bowl with Avocado Cumin Dressing	Avocado-Caprese Salad	Eggplant Rollups
Friday	Spinach and Berries Power Smoothie	Quinoa Burrito Bowl	Curried Eggplant	Herbed Crackers
Saturday	Quinoa Porridge	Thai Quinoa Salad	Veggies Potpie	Healthy Hummus
Sunday	Alkamind Warrior Chia Breakfast	Asian Noodles with Sesame Dressing	Pad Thai Salad	Banana Candy Coins

Week 2 is about consolidating your diet, as you are already experiencing the benefits of the alkaline diet from week 1. Most likely you feel more energized, you have a better mood, and overall, you feel better about yourself. Therefore, it's important to stick to the diet and try to avoid any temptations represented by processed food (of any kind). When it comes to shopping, you must include in your list vegetables like broccoli, lettuce, spinach, cucumber, eggplant, fruits like bananas, apples, avocado, different kind of berries, almonds, strawberries, cherries, but also other ingredients like mushrooms, one special type of pasta, sesame and so on. The menu below can help you with the meals you can eat during this week and it also sticks to the 80/20 rule.

WEEK 3

Day	Breakfast	Lunch	Dinner	Snack
Monday	Baked Grapefruit	Alkaline Lasagna	BBB Soup	Apple Pie Crumble
Tuesday	Home Fries Made of Baby Potatoes	Potpie Made of Vegetables	Dinner Quinoa and Avocado Salad	Herbed Crackers
Wednesday	Brown Rice Porridge	Grilled Veggie Stack	Celery Soup	Banana Candy Coins
Thursday	Vanilla Bean and Cinnamon Granola	Alkaline Stuffed Peppers	Nori Vegetables Rolls with Avocado-Jalapeño Spread	Healthy Hummus
Friday	Breakfast Fajitas	Salad of Avocado, Quinoa, Parsley, Tomato and Pine Nuts with Olive Oil	Cheesy Scalloped Potato and Onion Bake	Snack Cauliflower Popcorn
Saturday	Herb Omelet	Curried Eggplant	Alkaline Pasta with Tomato Sauce	Cashew Butter Fudge
Sunday	Garden Pancakes	Chives, Lima Beans and Roasted Beans with Walnut Oil	Nutmeg and Spinach Soup	Chocolate - Cherry Smoothie

By week 3 you feel more energized and you should feel that this diet is worth following. Although you turn away from meat or dairy products (which happen to be some of the most acid foods), the food you are eating is consistent enough and you don't have to worry about getting hungry. Unlike other diets, the 30-day alkaline meal plan allows you to have all 3 major meals of the day, plus snacks. You would be surprised how well-balanced this alkaline diet is, as it can give you the proper nutritional ratio for your daily needs (proteins/carbohydrates/fats). In your shopping list, you will need to include broccoli, brown rice, bok choy, avocado, almonds, grapefruits, celery, eggs, bananas, quinoa, baby potatoes, cauliflower, jalapenos, onions, eggplants, tomato sauce, vanilla, cinnamon, spinach, nutmeg, limes, and beans and so on. Sounds convincing enough? Well, take a look at what week 3 has reserved for you to find out more about the ingredients you need!

WEEK 4

Day	Breakfast	Lunch	Dinner	Snack
Monday	Apple Parfait with Non-Dairy Products	Kale Pesto Pasta	Quinoa and Avocado Salad	Tarragon Crackers
Tuesday	Almond Butter Crunch Berry Smoothie	Cauliflower Soup with Roasted Garlic	Summer Dinner Salad	Cinnamon Cashews
Wednesday	Watermelon-Cherry Smoothie	Avocado Wrapped in Lettuce	Beefless "Beef" Stew	Cheesy Broccoli Bites
Thursday	Brown Rice Porridge	Potato and Broccoli Soup	Nori Vegetables Rolls with Avocado-Jalapeño Spread	Banana Candy Coins
Friday	Garden Pancakes	Quinoa Burrito Bowl	Alkaline Pasta with Tomato Sauce	Cheesy Baked Kale Chips
Saturday	Breakfast Fajitas	Curried Eggplant	Avocado-Caprese Salad	Chocolate - Cherry Smoothie
Sunday	Almond Butter Oats with Apple	Mushroom-Miso Soup with Wild Rice	Cheesy Scallop Potato and Onion Bake	Herbed Crackers

So far the diet has not been an easy task, but it takes around 30 days to get used to it. After that it becomes a habit. And the habit is reinforced by how good you feel and the good associations you have with the progress you make each time you take another step. You can feel the difference between the first day of the plan and the last day of week 3. There is increased energy; you look and feel better. You look like a flower which has been properly taken care of.

There is only one week left of the 30-day plan of the alkaline diet, so you are nearly there, and you can congratulate yourself on coming so far on this plan and also taking this diet. Every time you try something new, the beginning is harder, and the longer you practice it, the more familiar you get to it. That's why week 4 should be a walk in the park. Most of the ingredients you need for this week's menu can be found in the shopping list for the previous week. You will need apples, kale, avocado, cauliflower, cinnamon, almonds, watermelon, cherries, broccoli, lettuce, brown rice, potatoes, tomatoes, bananas, quinoa, jalapenos, caprese, eggplants, onions, etc. You can find out more about the ingredients if you check the menu below.

The alkaline diet is diverse and includes different meal types like breakfasts, snacks, salads, soups, main dishes, desserts, and smoothies. You can eat frequently enough that you won't feel hunger at all. Here you will learn how to prepare some of the most delicious and nutritious food you can consume. Some of the recipes can be found below, but if you are interested to find out everything there is to know about them, a simple internet search should be able to find them easily.

Breakfast

Some people are convinced that breakfast is the most important meal of the day. Well, the alkaline diet allows you to honor this meal in a very healthy and nutritious way. Breakfast doesn't have to be all ham and eggs or cereals with milk. There is also an alkaline alternative which is just as nutritious and possibly even healthier. As you already noticed in the 30-day meal plan, there are several meals to enjoy at breakfast. One specific dish you can enjoy during breakfast is an herb omelet.

The omelet is possibly the most popular choice when it comes to breakfast, and it's simple to prepare one. Eggs are reliable, high-protein meal, and the yolk is very alkaline. Combining this meal with fresh herbs can give the alkaline boost you are looking for. In order to prepare the herb omelet, you will need two eggs, butter, sea salt (rock salt can also be a valid substituent, but use it in moderate quantities), one-half of a bunch of chopped chives, and one-half of a bunch of chopped parsley. Try to use a non-stick frying pan and melt the butter in it, while you break the eggs into a bowl and beat them. You can fold the omelet and cook it for around one more minute.

Snacks

The basic meal plan doesn't forget about snacks at all. Everyone likes a snack once in a while, but there aren't too many healthy options out there. Chips and other highly processed snacks are caloric bombs, and they are not healthy. If you don't want to renounce the habit of eating snacks, but you want to try something healthy instead, you can try some alkaline snacks. They can help you boost your energy and feel great as well. In the 30-day meal plan, you can see some really interesting snack ideas.

Conclusion

Thank you for making it to the end. We are all just human. We aren't perfect, and messing up happens even if we have planned as much as we can. If you find that you end up giving into temptation and mess up a bit, don't simply throw in the towel and give up. The cup of coffee or that piece of chocolate doesn't mean you're a failure and does not mean you should stop your cleanse. A slip up may slow down your progress, but it does not bring it to a stop.

You are doing this cleanse for you and nobody else. If you slip, realize what happened, and then get back on track for your next meal. You may even notice that eating "off cleanse" makes you feel crappy. You may feel like your energy slumped, you develop of headache, or you may feel bloated. When this happens, simply recommit. Remind yourself of what your goal is and then remember that the next meal you have is another chance to make a different choice.

Dr Sebi's disclosures have a great deal of useful impacts. One advantage of the Dr. Sebi food routine is its tough accentuation on plant-based nourishments. The get-healthy plan advances eating a major scope of vegetables and natural products, which are inordinate in fiber, nutrients, minerals, and plant mixes.

Diets wealthy in greens and organic products were identified with diminished bothering and oxidative weight, notwithstanding security contrary to numerous sicknesses. A gander at 226 people, people who ate at least 7 servings of greens and natural products following day had a 25% and 31% reduction event of disease and heart issue, individually.

Besides, the vast majority are not ingesting adequate produce. In a 2017 report, 9.3% and 12.2% of people met the proposals for veggies and natural product, individually.

Also, the Dr. Sebi diet advances devouring fiber-rich entire grains and sound fat, comprising of nuts, seeds, and plant oils. These suppers had been associated with a lower danger of heart sickness. At last, eats less than limit very handled suppers are identified with better generally eating routine top notch.

The Dr. Sebi food routine accentuates eating supplement rich greens, natural products, whole grains, and stimulating fat, which may likewise bring down your peril of heart issue and most malignancies.

Most likely, you have experienced an alkaline dinner program someplace on the web or in some understanding materials. What is an alkaline diet, and is this diet healthy for you? This diet all began when specialists took a stab at considering the pH level of the body. In an individual's body, the earth can be acidic or alkaline. When the pH level is high, then nature is chemical. In opposite, low pH implies the environment is acidic. The body doesn't have one single pH level; slightly, it can contrast contingent upon the area. The pH level in the stomach is unique about the urinary bladder.

This diet is mainly about eating nourishments which can advance alkaline condition in the body while not eating food sources that elevate acidity to the body. What could be the purpose of this program? To begin, nourishments that can advance an alkaline situation in the body are viewed as healthy. Instances of these nourishments incorporate vegetables, organic products, soy items, nuts, vegetables, and oats. On the off chance that you have seen, these nourishments are plentiful in protein, nutrients, and minerals.

The other rule of an alkaline diet is to dodge acid nourishments because these are food sources that can make your body in danger for weight gain, heart issues, kidney, and liver diseases. Not many of the numerous acid nourishments incorporate caffeine, food sources with high additives like canned merchandise, soft drinks, fish, meat, liquor, and nourishments with high sugar content. At the point when you then again, the alkaline diet; isn't uncommon for everybody, particularly when discussing a healthy diet.

As per specialists, acidic nourishments can diminish the pH of an individual's pee. At the point when the pH is unusually low, kidney stones will appear in general structure. To check this circumstance, an individual needs to expand the pH through eating alkaline-rich nourishments, that basic.

Since an alkaline diet implies keeping away from the liquor and some other nourishments with high acidity, it likewise means that you will diminish the danger of treating diseases related to an unhealthy diet like diabetes, hypertension, and weight. Albeit no careful confirmations can demonstrate, a few scientists have expressed that the alkaline diet can lessen the danger of cancer.

On the chance that you are experiencing the herpes infection, and you have attempted current medication and different types of treatment and nothing worked, at that point, Dr. Sebi's herbs and plant-based eating regimens are what you need.

There are many Dr. Sebi affirmed supplements that, joined with the suggested nourishments, establish this eating regimen. Bowman structured this nourishment plan for individuals who wish to utilize characteristic strategies to forestall or treat their ailments. It was planned for limiting dependence on western medication and depending more on all encompassing ways to deal with bettering your wellbeing.

You can surprise yourself, your family, and your friends with new, delicious dishes, snacks, salads, desserts, or smoothies. Also, the types of foods to eat, the benefits and drawbacks of the diet, its significance to weight loss, and the supplements involved, and how it reverses medical illnesses.

I hope you have learned something!

Dr. Sebi Cure for Herpes

Table of Contents

INTRODUCTION **91**
    SIGNIFICANT FACTS ABOUT HERPES..91
    SYMPTOMS OF HERPES URINE AND DISCHARGE PROBLEMS FOR WOMEN 91
    BLISTERS INSIDE THE URETHRA 92
    FATIGUE 93
    SPINAL PAINS 93
    FLU-LIKE SYMPTOMS 93
    HEADACHES 93
    SWOLLEN LYMPH NODES 93
    BLISTERS ON THE GENITALS 93

CHAPTER 1: WHAT IS HERPES VIRUS **94**
    CAUSES OF HERPES SIMPLEX VIRUS 94
    INDICATIONS OF HERPES VIRUS 94
    TYPES OF HERPES VIRUS 96
    MANIFESTATIONS OF HERPES VIRUS 96

CHAPTER 2: WHAT ALLOPATHIC MEDICINE GIVES US **97**
    REALITIES ABOUT DR. SEBI'S HERPES CURE 97

CHAPTER 3: A NEW APPROACH TO HERPES **100**
    METHOD 1 – CURING HERPES VIA DR. SEBI'S FOOD PLAN 100
    METHOD 2 – TREATING HERPES VIA WATER FASTING 102
    METHOD 3 – VIA JUICING 103
    METHOD 4 – VAIN WATER FASTING AND JUICING 103

CHAPTER 4: DR. SEBI'S HERPES CURE IS YOUR BEST OPTION **104**
    WHY DR. SEBI CURE FOR HERPES IS THE BEST 104

CHAPTER 5: SEBI HERPES CURE EFFECTIVENESS **107**
    WHY CAN IT CURE HERPES 107
    SOME FACTS ABOUT DR. SEBI'S DIET FOR HERPES CURE 108

CHAPTER 6: DR. SEBI FINAL CURATIVE PROCESS OF HERPES VIRUS **109**
    DR. SEBI FINAL CURATIVE PROCESS OF HERPES VIRUS 109
    UNDERSTAND THE EFFICACY OF THE HERBS FOR THE CURE OF HERPES..........................110
    DANDELION ROOT EFFECTIVENESS FOR HIV/AIDS AND HERPES 111
    SCIENTIFIC PROOF OF DANDELION FOR THE TREATMENT OF HIV/AIDS AND HERPES 111
    PREPARATION OF DANDELION FOR THE REVERSING HIV/AIDS VIRUS 112

CHAPTER 7: HEALING AND RECOVERING FROM STDS **113**
    CAUSES OF STDS 113
    HERPES 114

CHAPTER 8: SEBI'S REVITALIZING HERBS FOR HERPES CURE **118**
    DANDELION 118
    ELDERBERRY 121
    LAVENDER 123

- Sage 124
- Cascara Sagrada 125
- Blue Vervain 126

CHAPTER 9: CLEANSING HERBS 128
- Mullein 128
- Sarsaparilla Root 128
- Chaparral 128
- Guaco Herb 128
- Cilantro 128
- Burdock Root 128
- Pao Pereira 128
- Pau D'arco 128
- Essential Oregano Oil 129
- Ginger Essential Oil 129
- Sea Salt Bath 129
- Holy Basil 130
- How to Extract Essential Oils for Herpes 130

CHAPTER 10: THE STRATEGIES DR. SEBI USED IN CURING HERPES SIMPLEX VIRUS 131
- Detoxification and Cleansing of the Body Organs 131
- Herbs Used for Fasting to Enable Detoxification 131
- Facts and Tips Needed While Using Dr. Sebi's Diet 132

CHAPTER 11: BENEFITS OF HERBAL MEDICINE 133
- Echinacea 133
- Ginseng 134
- Ginkgo Biloba 134
- Elderberry 135
- St. John's Wort 135
- Turmeric 136
- Ginger 136
- Valerian 137
- Chamomile 137

CHAPTER 12: DR. SEBI'S NATURAL ERECTILE DYSFUNCTIONS CURE 138
- Definition of Disease 138
- How to Cure the Root-Cause of Erectile Dysfunctions 138
- Cleansing or Detoxification 138
- How to Undergo a Cleanse 138
- The Various Types of Cleansing 139

CHAPTER 13: THE MAJOR RISK FACTORS OF SEXUALLY TRANSMITTED DISEASES ... 141
- Underlining Sexually Transmitted Infection 141
- Unhealthy Age 141
- Multiple Sexual Partners 141
- Unsafe Sex 141
- Immune Destroying Drugs 142
- Alcohol 142
- Dr. Sebi's History 142
- The Significance of Dr. Sebi's Diet 143
- Dr. Sebi's Forbidden Foods 143

CHAPTER 14: DR. SEBI'S FOODS 144
Peaches 144
Plums 144
Watercress 145
Cantaloupes 146
Wakame 146

CHAPTER 15: DIAGNOSING AND ACCEPTANCE 147
Changes in the Lifestyle 147
Risk factors for outbreaks 148

CHAPTER 16: BENEFITS OF DR. SEBI'S DIET 149
Protects Muscle Mass and Bone Density 149
Increased Muscle Mass 149
Increase Energy Levels 149
Reduce Risk of Stroke and Hypertension 150
Lowers Chronic Pain and Inflammation 150
Body Detox and Cell Cleaning 150

CHAPTER 17: DEALING WITH THE HERPES STIGMA 152
Telling Your Partner About HSV 152
Tell My Partner 153

CHAPTER 18: HIV 155

CHAPTER 19: PRECAUTIONS REGARDING PH BALANCE & THE ALKALINE DIET 157
Achieve Permanent Results 157

CHAPTER 20: HEALTHY LIFESTYLE 159
Train your mind 159
Mind focus is very important 159
Health tasks at hand 160

CHAPTER 21: ALKALINE DIET RECIPES TO GET RID OF HERPES 162

CONCLUSION 186

Introduction

Herpes fix is a typical point encompassed with such a significant number of inquiries and no reliable answer. In the event that you have herpes, your brain might be loaded with questions identified with herpes treatment. Herpes is a disease that is spreading all around the globe, a great number of individuals are influenced by herpes, but with regards to herpes fix, nobody thinks about it. The ongoing revelation of herpes treatment is Dr. Sebi's herpes fix.

This isn't just a name; however, the most anticipated comprehensive solution for herpes that can cause your fantasy about getting the chance to free of herpes work out as expected. Dr. Sebi is the author of Dr. Sebi's Inquire about Foundation. The organization that professes to fix illnesses like malignancy, AIDS., lupus, diabetes, fibroids tumor, joint inflammation, sickle cell sickliness, and now herpes as well.

Every one of these illnesses, including herpes, are the large difficulties for the human to deal with, and now it is an ideal opportunity to get an answer for every one of them. The sicknesses like herpes need more mindfulness and information on the grounds that with the assistance of these, you deal with the successive episodes of herpes as well as control the transmission up partly. You ought to know about the infection, at exactly that point you can discover your responses for the herpes treatment.

Significant Facts About Herpes

You should be eager to think about the herpes fix; however, you have to comprehend the significant actualities of herpes before that. Herpes is an explicitly transmitted ailment which can without much of a stretch spread starting with one individual then onto the next through immediate and roundabout contacts.

Herpes is by and large of two sorts—HSV1 and HSV2. At the point when the herpes infection is available on the outside of the skin of a contaminated individual, it can, without much of a stretch, give to someone else through the wet skin which lines the mouth and genital pieces of the body. Herpes can influence you in two different ways rationally and physically.

In the event that you have herpes and visit your PCP, he may recommend you antiviral herpes drugs. These drugs can give you alleviation from the irritating manifestations of herpes, but the terrible side is that they can likewise give you genuine reactions. At the point when you quit taking these pills, you are similarly inclined to episodes as much as some other patient who has never taken these antivirals.

Symptoms of Herpes Urine and Discharge Problems for Women

At the point when pee comes into contact with an open injury, stinging is a typical sensation. Ladies experience more difficulty with pee ignoring the wounds than men as a result of the shape and position of the urethra. Ladies may likewise observe an adjustment in release when the herpes infection is dynamic. Rather than white, watery, and normally unscented, the release might be thick, with a yellow tinge and a sharp smell. This is an indication of disease in the cervix.

Blisters Inside the Urethra

The urethra is the cylinder that interfaces the urinary bladder to the private parts. The people with herpes type-2 can frame difficult bruises on the inward coating of this cylinder. While peeing, an individual may feel a consuming or extremely sharp steel sensation when pee disregards these bruises. Not at all like genital or mouth bruises, the specialist may need to lead tests to affirm a herpes disease when the urethra is influenced.

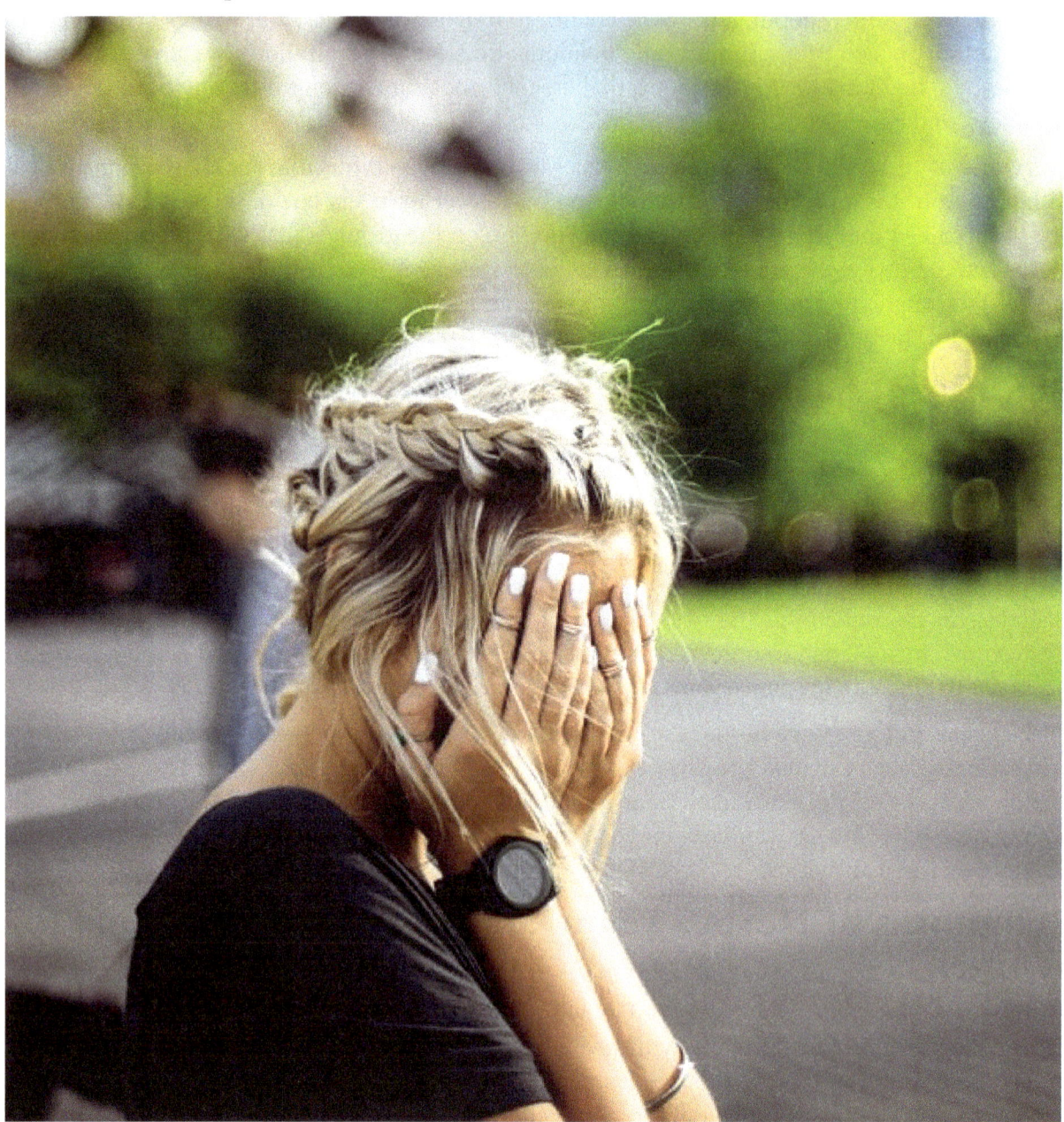

Fatigue

Individuals with a herpes infection contamination may see general sentiments of tiredness and shortcoming and an absence of vitality. Weakness may likewise discover its way into the muscles, leaving them feeling agonizing or substantial. This side effect can likewise cause brevity of breath, weight reduction, uneasiness, and gloom, and leave individuals feeling like they have to snooze as often as possible during the day.

Spinal Pains

The herpes type-2 infection can influence the lumbar and sacral nerve roots, prompting issues with the nerves and nerve endings. Individuals with herpes viral contamination can create torment in the lower back, posterior, and thighs, particularly if the disease is revolved around the privates. This sort is regularly intermittent and can be very awkward and excruciating.

Flu-Like Symptoms

Influenza-like side effects that can create alongside herpes contamination incorporate a fever with cools, an irritated throat, a diligent hack, and a runny or stuffy nose. A few people may encounter queasiness and retching or the runs. The safe framework kicks vigorously to battle the contamination, yet until it can finish its work, the herpes infection leaves a great many people feeling exhausted.

Headaches

Headaches and the herpes infection go connected at the hip when a flare-up happens. Indications of headaches incorporate general head torment, which can move from a moderate, dull yearn to an extreme, throbbing agony behind the eyes. Different side effects incorporate peevishness and affectability to sound and light. This cerebral pain may likewise cause summed up muscle throbs, inconvenience dozing or focusing, obscured vision, queasiness, and loss of craving.

Swollen Lymph Nodes

Lymph hubs are little bean-formed organs all through the body. The lymphatic framework goes about as a seepage or sifting activity, conveying lymph liquid, supplements, and waste material through the tissues and the circulation system. Generally found in the neck, the crotch, and under the arms, these hubs expand and become delicate during disease or damage. At the point when somebody has genital herpes, the organs around the genital territory will expand and might be sore.

Blisters on the Genitals

At the point when genital rankles happen, the herpes type-2 infection (HSV 2) is as often as possible suspected as a reason. It will initially begin with a comparative inclination to that of the mouth wounds, yet with greater power because of the affectability of the zone.

Chapter 1: What is Herpes Virus

Herpes infection is drawn-out contamination that is brought about by the herpes simplex virus (HSV). The genital district, the oral locale, the skin, and the butt-centric area are the areas of the body that are influenced by this infection.

This ailment is known for an extremely prolonged stretch of time, and it normally assaults people causing a few ailments; some are mellow and some are perilous.

The genital herpes is one of the most widely recognized kinds of herpes simplex infection. The genital herpes infection is an explicitly transmitted disease that affects to genital and butt-centric rankles. There might be bruises which additionally influence the mouth and face.

A few instances of the rehashed appearance of genital herpes are brought about by HVS 2. A large portion of this disease is spread from victims who don't realize they have it, and more often than not, the side effects are asymptomatic in a victim.

People can contract this contamination through a sexual relationship with a victim infected with HSV. Additionally, you can get contaminated from your sex accomplice who doesn't encounter any indications of this disease whatsoever.

Moreso, the subsequent kind can be brought about by oral-butt-centric contact or butt-centric contact with a victim. HSV 2 is the most predominant herpes infection disease that happens, yet the HSV 1 happens less ordinarily.

Causes of Herpes Simplex Virus

The reasons for herpes infection are:

- Direct contact with the liquid of the skin of a tainted individual.
- Direct contact with the liquid present in the outside of the butt and private parts.
- The utilization of a tainted individual's eyeglasses.
- A sexual relationship with numerous sex accomplices.
- An oral sexual relationship with victims with indications of bruises in the mouth.

Indications of Herpes Virus

A portion of the side effects of this disease that could be seen despite the fact that they are now and again not indicative are:

- Burning and tickling in the privates.
- Inflammation of the rear-end or rectum.
- Pains in the influenced body area.
- Uninviting vaginal release.
- Red tinge rankles on the skin.

- Cold disturbing bruises in the mouth and lips.
- Illness.
- Increased temperature
- Painful pee.
- Presence of irritation in the cervix.
- Lymph hubs become augmented.
- Itching in the influenced zone.
- Sores in the genital area.
- The presence of an ulcer and sudden irritation.
- Muscle throbs.
- Difficulty in pee.
- The blankness of the herpes virus in the sufferer's body.

Herpes simplex infections, which set up themselves in the human tangible neurons, give a procedure called inactivity.

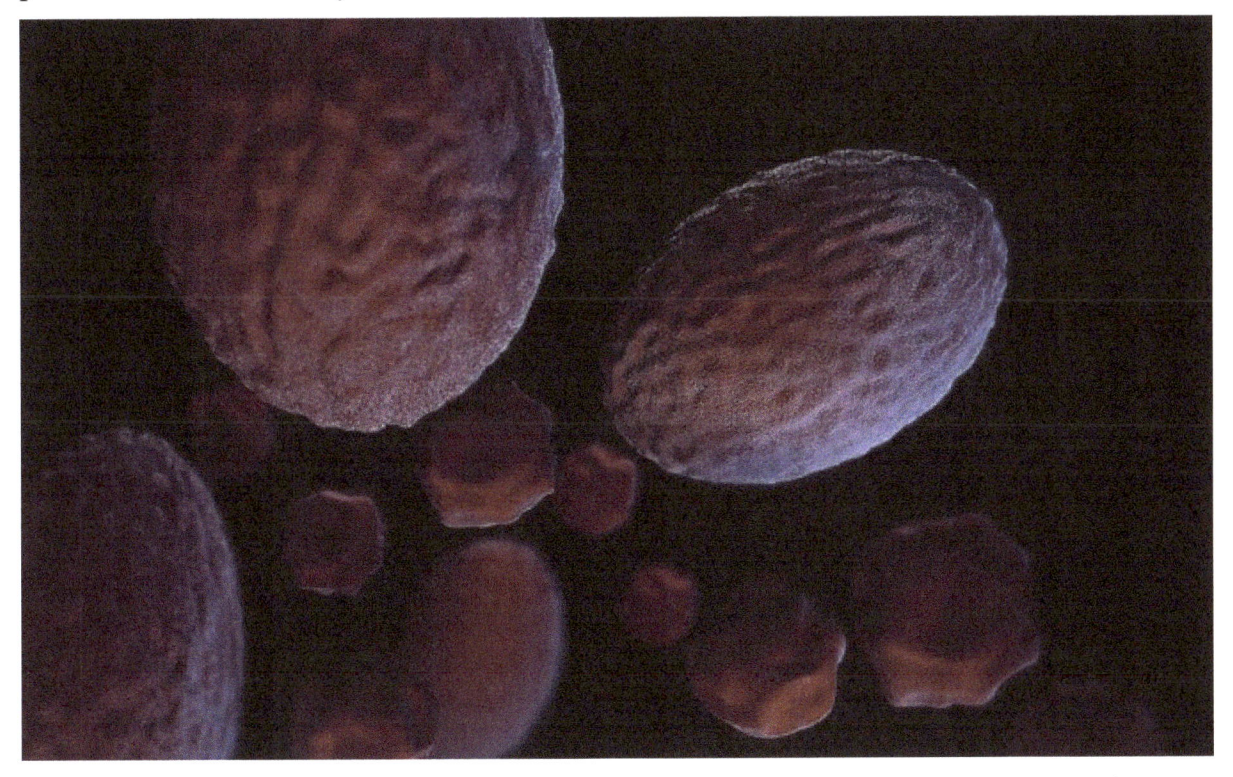

The type 1 infection causes most oral herpes contaminations, while the type 2 infection is answerable for most genital herpes. Since the tactile neurons express moderately hardly any major histocompatibility complex (MHC) 1 particle, the contaminated cells are wasteful at introducing viral antigens to circling lymphocytes.

Upgrades, for example, fever, passionate pressure, or feminine cycle, reactivate the infection and contaminations of the encompassing epithelial tissues. Initiation of the type 1 infection can result in rankles around the mouth that are incorrectly called mouth blisters.

The type 2 infections can cause genital bruises, yet individuals tainted with either type 1 or 2 infections frequently come up short on any clear indications.

Contaminations of type 2 infection, which is explicitly transmitted, represent a genuine danger to the children of tainted moms and can expand transmission of HIV, the infection that causes aids (Campbell Reece, 2008).

Types of Herpes Virus

The types of herpes infection are:

- **Herpes simplex 1 and 11**. Instances of this type of herpes infection are cold and genital wounds.
- **Varicella-zoster**. Instances of this sort of herpes infection are shingles and chickenpox.
- **Epstein-Barr infection**. Instances of this type of herpes infection are mononucleosis and Burkitt's lymphoma.

Manifestations of Herpes Virus

There are three manners by which herpes infection show:

1. This happens through the change of existing infections. RNA infections will, in general, have an uncommonly high pace of change since mistakes in recreating their RNA genomes are not rectified by editing. Some transformation changes their current infections into new hereditary assortments that can cause illness, even in individuals who are resistant to the infection.

2. Distribution of herpes infection from a little secluded human populace. For example, aids went un-named and unnoticed for a considerable length of time before it started to spread the world over. Accordingly, mechanical and social elements, including reasonable worldwide travel, blood transfusions, extramarital perversion, and the maltreatment of intravenous medications, permitted a formerly uncommon human illness to turn into a worldwide one.

3. The spread of existing infection from different creatures. Researchers evaluated that seventy-five percent of new human infections start along these lines. Creatures that hold and can transmit a specific infection however are commonly unaffected by it are said to go about as a characteristic supply for that infection (Campbell Reece, 2008).

In the following parts, we are going to open you to who Dr. Sebi is, the methodology Dr. Sebi utilized for the fix of herpes and HIV infection and the eating regimens vital for the fix them.

Chapter 2: What Allopathic Medicine Gives Us

Humans have been acquainted with various types of medicines, among which we have homeopathy, allopathy, natural medication, and a few different treatments. Homeopathy is a treatment that regards an individual all in all. Homeopathic medications are chosen after a case-investigation and individual assessment, which incorporates a clinical history check, mental and physical constitution, and so on. This implies homeopathic treatment centers around the patient as an individual just as his neurotic condition.

Allopathy, then again, is the study of rewarding maladies with variable cures, not the same as the impact of the ailment itself. This type of treatment has been the standard in past decades. Individuals wholeheartedly acknowledged this treatment without posing inquiries concerning its source, dependability, and impacts. This type of treatment keeps on flourishing because of the large number of dollars that pharmaceutical organizations spend on commercial yearly. Both of these frameworks have attempted. However, they have not been able to fix herpes infection forever on the human body. This makes them off-limits territory for herpes patients. To the extent, rewarding herpes is your primary need; all the antiviral medications you have been spending on so far will do little to nothing to help free your collection of herpes. The impacts given by these medications can be effortlessly acquired by some different methods, an elective that will free you of the side effects and the reactions.

Regular medication has given us no other option than to go to customary techniques. The equivalent conventional daily practice for a herpes fix that was watched decades back is despite everything being followed today to fix herpes patients. The far-reaching of herpes throughout the years has made discovering its fix a worldwide concern. As the infection keeps on plaguing millions all around, another settled has been reached, that is, to go to the customary remedy for herpes over traditional medication. It required some investment and contemplations, yet in the long run, everybody is beginning to see the recuperating force and excellence of natural herpes fix, which was unfathomably utilized by Dr. Sebi to fix a huge number of herpes patients.

Realities About Dr. Sebi's Herpes Cure

In contrast to customary specialists, Dr. Sebi didn't see maladies and sicknesses as a result of germs intrusion, bacterial contamination, or an infection. To him, it is all a matter of where and when the mucous film has been undermined. Contingent upon the sight, the illnesses can be effortlessly arranged. Dr. Sebi is famous for restoring the most feared illnesses like notorious malignancy, herpes infection, hypertension, diabetes, and numerous different ailments.

Alongside his other treatment strategies, Dr. Sebi's herpes fix is about what to eat and what not to eat on the off chance that you are tainted with the herpes infection. This treatment is to prepare for the ingestion of hurtful and costly medications, which never really direct the recurrence of episodes. Rather than these toxic pills, one can essentially select the characteristic fix.

Each and every other malady that has been known to be hopeless by specialists everywhere throughout the world can be relieved by Dr. Sebi's herpes fix. You're eating routine will be as per what your invulnerable framework cherishes and what the infection despises. The food will, for the most part, contain each supplement your body needs to remain dynamic.

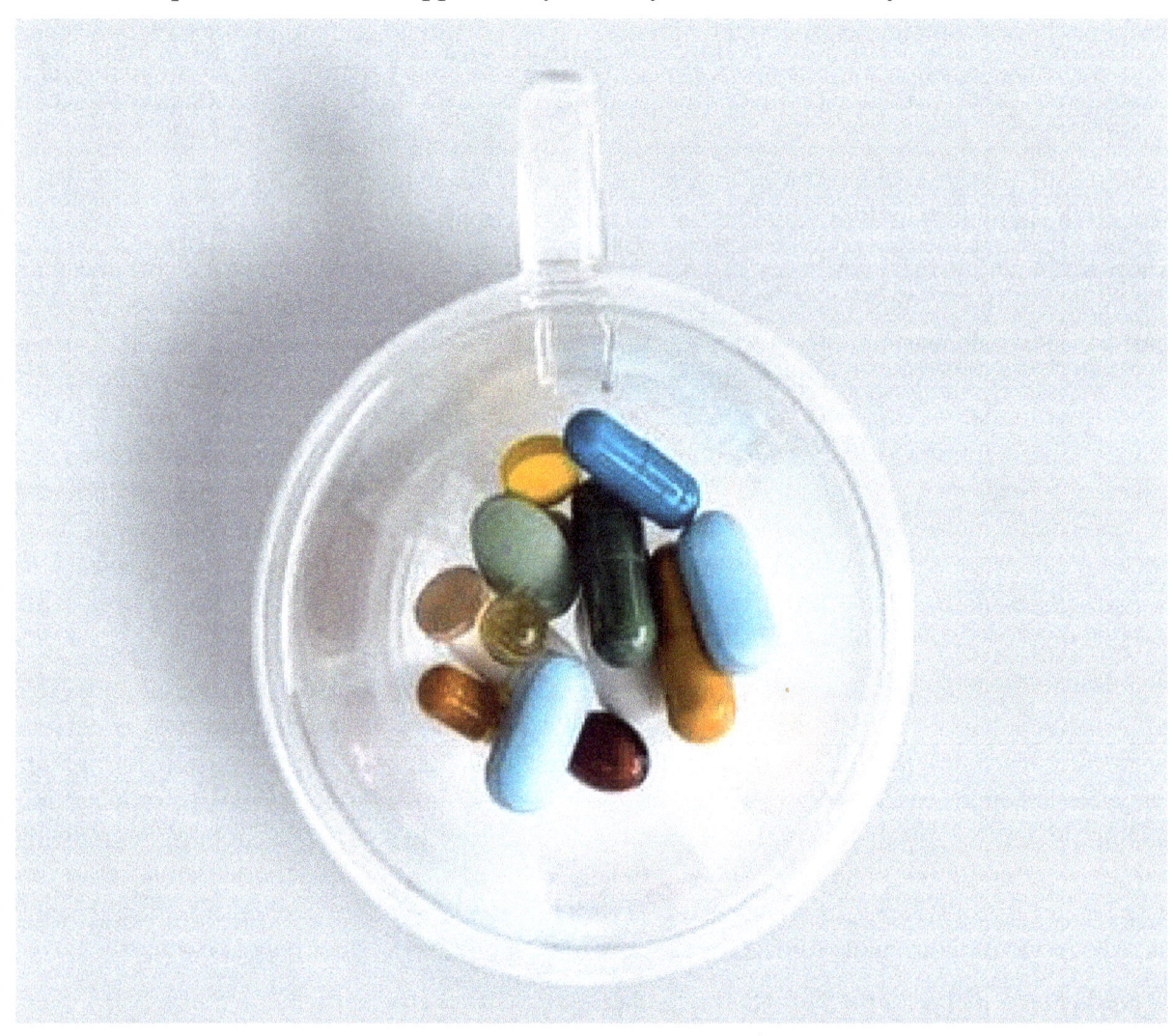

Eat a greater amount of Dr. Sebi's suggested products of the soil, sodas, sweet, and greasy nourishments. Eat less of the accompanying or thoroughly avoid them during flare-ups:

- Almonds
- Cashews
- Corn
- Meat
- Nuts (with the exception of the ones suggested by dr. Sebi)

- Barley
- Cereals
- Chicken
- Oats and peanuts

The mentioned contain l-arginine, an amino corrosive that stifles l-lysine, the amino corrosive that is answerable for hindering the development pace of the infection. Attempt, however much as could be expected to keep away from these during your disease stage and after. There is a particular basic eating routine that was exclusively roused by Dr. Sebi, and it is pointed towards giving the body alkalizing nourishments that decline bodily fluid with the assistance of Dr. Sebi herpes fix. The rationale behind this fix is the formation of a situation that is poisonous to the herpes infection, one in which it thinks that it's hard to develop. For this to occur, you have to eat nourishments that are toxic to the infection. This motivating force involves taking spices and Dr. Sebi's homegrown oil, a superior option in contrast to taking the toxic antivirals, which are just fit for harming the body. Dr. Sebi's herpes fix is explicitly intended to assault the cell structure of the herpes simplex infection, in this way giving you a herpes free life.

The indications for herpes disease are now and then "trickish" and unnoticeable, which makes herpes patients not to realize they have to see a specialist; for other people, the manifestations are extreme. They generally show inside possibly 14 days of interacting with the infection. Once in a while, the side effects would disappear in a couple of days, while on different occasions, the manifestations continue for up to a month. Herpes victims can identify with this experience.

On account of antivirals, you have to see a specialist, get solutions, and invest a portion of your well-deserved bucks on the most generally utilized pills for herpes treatment. Famicyclovir, Valtrex, and acyclovir are the most mainstream antiviral medications. They are utilized to treat particular sorts of infections. These medications altogether diminish the recurrence of flare-ups, and they are additionally helpful in rewarding mouth blisters. The drawback to these antiviral medications is the way that there will consistently be an episode now and again. This circumstance can be overwhelming just as disappointing as during the flare-up; your development gets restricted as most would not need individuals around them to see the rankles on their countenances. Dr. Sebi's herpes cure is the best regular approach to treat herpes.

In the event that you are one of those endless herpes casualties who have spent such a lot of cash on antivirals, it is time you give Dr. Sebi's common cure an attempt. Conflicting with the standard and looking for help in every conceivable spot is the best way to deal with the herpes infection. Herpes casualties have depended such a great amount on antivirals in the past years that they don't understand how much harm it has done to them. Herpes victims take these pills consistently without disapproving of the impacts the extent that the episode is kept under control. With the various revelations about the destructiveness of current medication, nobody would need to check out that once more. The requirement for another bearing in handling the herpes infection drove Dr. Sebi's exploration establishment to the advancement that is being praised today.

Chapter 3: A New Approach to Herpes

Method 1 – Curing Herpes via Dr. Sebi's Food Plan

Dr. Sebi frequently referred to that so one can heal the frame, one has first to cleanse the body, then feed it the nutrients it wishes. Dr. Sebi contends that "diseases" cannot live in an alkaline frame and so it's far vital to cleanse and alkalize the body to carry it to a more fit state.

Step 1: Smooth up the Machine

Detoxifying the gadget is pivotal to freeing the edge of ailments. To start with, we start with the guide of purging out the colon (entrails).

Colon cleanse

Use the chelation 2 for this. You can make your own if you can't buy it. There also are other techniques for cleaning the colon and cleansing out the bowel. Any appropriate colon cleanses recipe needs to assist.

Apple Onion Colon Cleanse Recipe

Preparation time: 10 Minutes

Cooking time: 5 Minutes

Serving: Devour approximately three to 4 ounces within the morning.

Ingredients:

- 1 Apple
- A trickle of pectin (the white part of the citrus. Whilst you peel an orange or lime, that white component you see)
- 1 Big onion

Direction:

1. Mix or blend together with water.

Nutrition:

- Calories 138
- Protein 2.1g
- Carbohydrate 35.3g
- Sugar 23.2g
- Fiber 5.7g
- Fat 0.1g

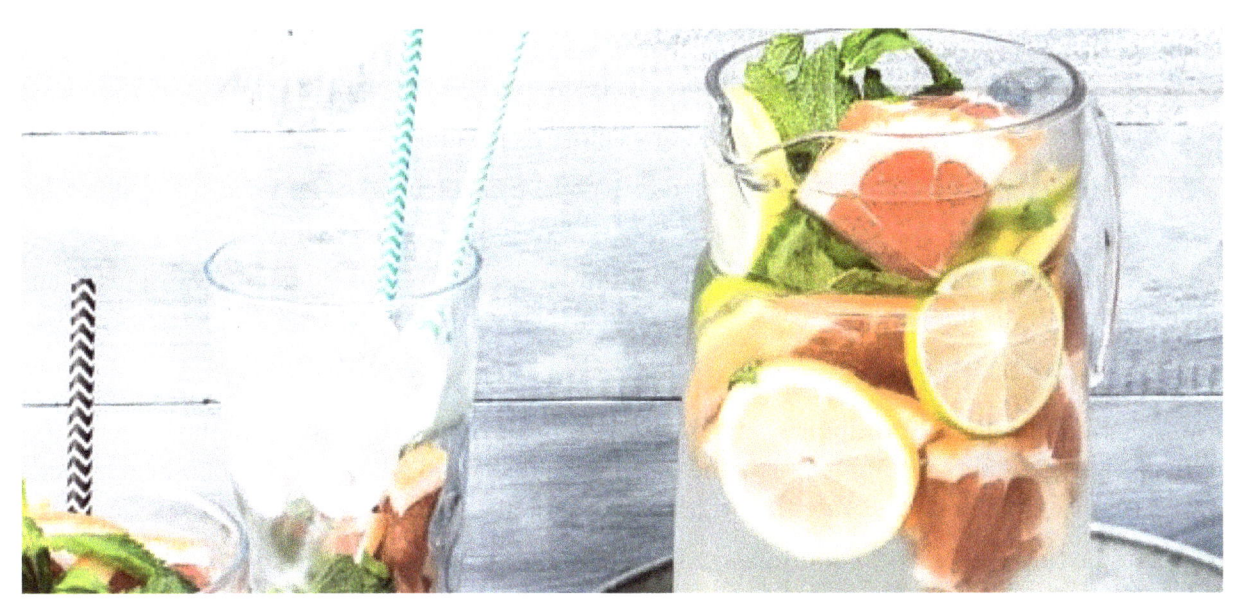

Step 2: Cleanse More to the Organs of the Body

The Viento is blanketed in Dr. Sebi's small cleaning package deal as it allows you to clean the frame at a mobile stage. You can make your very own Viento system. You can actually but cross instantly to step three.

Step 3: Easy and Nourish the Blood

The iron plus and bio Ferro will assist to cleanse the blood, enhance move to the frame, and nourish the cells. As stated, you can purchase or make your very own—it's far very smooth to do that.

Dose: Take the spices as coordinated on the true framework.

Throughout this technique, the weight loss plan should be very mild, along with only alkalizing meals, often fruits and greens. Follow Dr. Sebi's nutritional manual, however, some items on the listing ought to no longer be fed on while one is trying to reverse extreme health conditions.

Matters on the listing to eat: Culmination, greens together with lettuce, lambs sector, dandelion greens, mustard vegetables, amaranth vegetables and lettuce, mushrooms, vegetables, coconut (water and jelly) natural teas, inexperienced juices, and smoothies.

Matters at the listing to avoid: Oils, chickpeas, avocados, nuts (all), and grains (all).

Notice: Other than the teas, the entire thing else you eat up should be all uncooked, for example uncooked. Purchase characteristic if suitable, if not, does the quality you can, and make certain suppers are washed appropriately before use.

Hydration: Drink plenty of water to flush the system.

Bladderwrack/sea moss: Add the bladderwrack/sea moss aggregate to smoothies and have it in teas.

If cash is a huge issue, in phrases of being capable of affording the herbs, then move a chunk lighter at the herbs.

Begin by cleaning the bowel and changing the eating regimen to predominantly end result and greens, preferably one hundred% uncooked or as close as feasible.

Use the bromide powder (sea moss and bladderwrack) to make shakes and feature teas day by day.

Further, add the elderflower, burdock, dandelion, sarsaparilla, and ginger to your regimen. Integrate them to make teas.

Method 2 – Treating Herpes Via Water Fasting

Water fasting may be extraordinarily effective. It might be one of the easiest methods to rid the body of pathogens and pollutants, raise the immune gadget, and allow the frame to heal. It isn't always really helpful to begin water fasting rapidly without a preceding fasting incursion.

There are fasting clinics one ought to visit. I am aware that the numbers are increasing, lengthy status centers with suitable reputations are tangle wood wellbeing middle and true north wellness center (U.S. Based). It's not a reasonably-priced venture, such a lot of humans won't be able to come up with the money for the ride to a center.

But one doesn't need to go to a fasting center with the intention of rapid. If there are not any other extreme underlining health conditions, you could build up to a fast through preparing the frame (so to reduce the consequences of detox signs). Make sure you have a guide around you, together with a partner or buddy, and additionally, preferably someone with the revel in of fasting

Constructing up to Water Fast

- Start with three days of bowel cleanse.
- Consume a complete plant-based total food regimen for seven days.
- Do another effective 3-day bowel cleanse consuming uncooked culmination and greens for the duration of this period.
- Do a seven days mono-rapid ideally on grapes, mango, melon, or apples.
- Follow up with a 3-day juice fast, mainly inexperienced juices and the juices of citrus culmination.
- Begin your water fast.

Reminder: It's far most popular for lengthy fasting tries to go to a fasting health center where you may have the understanding of individuals who can help you thru the difficult days beforehand. In case you aren't capable of going to a fasting health facility, then it might be vital to have help round you. If fasting on one's very own, it isn't advisable to move past 7-10 days.

Who Ought not to Fast

It isn't always recommended that some people go on a water fast, these encompass:

- Pregnant ladies.
- Those are handling anorexia.
- People laid low with debilitating diseases and have little energy.
- Those in advanced stages of diseases e.g. Cancers.
- Individuals who are affected by intense intellectual disorders that require professional treatment. If you are tormented by a less severe mental ailment, it's far essential to have support around you.

It is vital that the fast is broken successfully.

- Start with the handy juices, vegetable juices, non-sweet fruit juices. Have them for three consecutive days (assuming a 7 to ten days water rapid. The longer the water fasts, the slower and longer the re-feeding length).
- Have raw culmination for some other two days.
- Introduce mild raw salads.
- Slowly introduce other foods.

Note: Eat small food as wished, chunk foods well, pay attention to the frame's signals.

Method 3 – Via Juicing

After the initial bowel clean of at least three days, have handy juices and teas. This consists of inexperienced or vegetable juices specifically, you will have more of those at the start, then add fruit juices (citruses and melons).

- Constructing as much as a juice speedy
- Three days of colon cleanse.
- Seven days all raw culmination and greens.
- Begin juicing.
- Examine constipation.

The duration varies; set a minimum goal of 21 days. Take natural teas, such as those mentioned above, further growth water intake.

Tip: Gracefully taste your juices within the mouth earlier than swallowing.

Method 4 – Vain Water Fasting and Juicing

This is where water fasting and juicing are combined. With this approach, a deliberate sample is created consuming a balance of fruit juices and water.

- Blended water and juice plan
- Juice in the mornings
- Water within the days
- Juice at night

Chapter 4: Dr. Sebi's Herpes Cure Is Your Best Option

You presumably know at this point what really Dr. Sebi herpes fix is. Truly, Dr. Sebi's solution for herpes is continuously arriving at each side of the world. The purpose of it picking up prevalence so brisk isn't a large number of dollars spent on commercials. Nor is it well known in light of the fact that some big-name is embracing it. It is dazzling the hearts of herpes patients in such a case that its adequacy.

Basic on the grounds that the recuperating standards of this incredible cultivator are successful, the present reality is discussing him. Everybody today knows him as a man who helped millions conquer the illnesses wherein allopathy helped less. Notwithstanding, later on, it was understood that Dr. Sebi's standards were extraordinary in all the wellbeing inconveniences. Today, we won't just discuss what Dr. Sebi's herpes fix is about, yet we will reveal to you why Dr. Sebi herpes fix is the best alternative you ought to go for.

Dr. Sebi was a famous herbalist who mended numerous patients when allopathic specialists couldn't give any assistance. He identified the enchantment that herbs conveyed, and utilizing that supernatural made numerous lives excellent and malady free. Similar standards of mending, when applied to herpes, gave sudden and incomprehensible outcomes. What the allopathic specialists couldn't reply, what the researchers couldn't stop can be fixed with the assistance of Dr. Sebi's remedy for herpes.

There was nothing taking a shot at mouth blisters and different manifestations of herpes, yet this botanist had at the top of the priority list some marvel herbs that can really give another opportunity for herpes patients to live. In spite of the fact that it is likewise critical to perceive how it is done, at the same time, before that, let us see why Dr. Sebi herpes fix is the best accessible option for you. When you know why you ought to go for Dr. Sebi's herpes fix and what makes it best, we will likewise expand how it functions and what Dr. Sebi's remedy for herpes is comprised of.

Why Dr. Sebi Cure for Herpes Is the Best

Sebi herpes fix is the best since it works in herpes: Dr. Sebi herpes fix is the best basic since it is successful. Truly, we truly don't have a great stock of powerful medications for herpes. There are antiviral medications that aren't really viable. They simply control the indications and simply make you feel great when nothing is well inside your body. The herpes simplex infection repeats the manner in which it needs to, and no antiviral can take care of business. For simply spoiling the manifestations as well, they prompt a great number of reactions. Along these lines, it is an absolute penance of wellbeing to pick antiviral treatment for herpes.

There are a couple of different herbs that are sheltered; however, they don't give escalated results as required by the human body to battle against herpes. Along these lines, Dr. Sebi's herpes fix is actually what you need, and in light of the fact that we don't generally have something successful against herpes, it is consequently the best.

Sebi herpes fix is the best alternative since it is the main safe choice: Dr. Sebi's solution for herpes has comprised all things considered and characteristic items and subsequently, you can make certain of wellbeing. Herbs have consistently been with the people, and the explanation they are favored even today is positively no symptoms.

Since Dr. Sebi's herpes fix is likewise comprised of herbs, you don't need to bargain with your present and future wellbeing. Truth be told, these herbs demonstration like enchantment in destroying the herpes simplex infection, yet additionally in improving your wellbeing consistently.

The individuals who have utilized Dr. Sebi's remedy for herpes have revealed that they felt increasingly vigorous and sound not long after subsequent to beginning the course. Along these lines, in light of the fact that Dr. Sebi's solution for herpes is sheltered, free from symptoms, and furthermore is gainful for your future wellbeing, it is the best elective you have for herpes.

Sebi solution for herpes is best since it is savvy as well: unlike antiviral medications, you need no remedy each time you purchase Dr. Sebi herpes fix. This sets aside a great deal of cash that goes into the conferences.

It is best since it is guaranteed by researchers: several examination discoveries have concurred that the herbs utilized in Dr. Sebi herpes fix are powerful against herpes. A few investigations have demonstrated that the herbs have strong antiviral properties. Characteristic antiviral capacities can kill the herpes simplex infection from the human body.

Notwithstanding the antiviral capacities, tests have additionally recommended that the herbs utilized in Dr. Sebi's remedy for herpes are invulnerable modulatory in nature. This implies that all of them impact your ailment battling component. With a more grounded insusceptible framework, you can basically control the replication of herpes simplex infection and this is the way to carry on with a herpes free life. Every one of these investigations testing the security and viability of Dr. Sebi herpes fix makes it the best choice you have for herpes.

Dr. Sebi's herpes fix is the best since it gives you herpes free life: one of the straightforward purposes for Dr. Sebi's herpes fix being the best is the final products it conveys. No other treatment accessible can give you herpes free life, but Dr. Sebi's herpes fix can. In this way, for a herpes free life, you simply need to trust Dr. Sebi's herpes fix and life is going to change drastically. Indeed, you can consider it a mysterious wand, or god's assistance or something different. Be that as it may, it is best since it can assist you with disposing of the irritation herpes is making in your brain just as in your body.

These were the reasons that make Dr. Sebi's solution for herpes the best one we have. Presently, in the event that you truly think you need to give this stunning fix an opportunity, you ought to likewise comprehend what this fix contains. The first element of Dr. Sebi's herpes fix is Tinospora cordifolia. Tinospora cordifolia picked up a notoriety for its antipyretic properties identical to some other anti-microbial accessible in the showcase.

Later on, researchers found the agony mitigating activity and invulnerability upgrading advantages of the herb. Along these lines, the integrity of Tinospora cordifolia makes Dr. Sebi herpes fix a sound method for managing the dreadful infection. Next are ayurvedically herbs purged powder of zinc and silver. These two fixings are sufficiently able to murder any intruder.

They are elements of numerous ayurvedic meds utilized for treating ceaseless hazardous sicknesses like malignancy. Presently you can consider what they can do to herpes simplex infection. You can see these two powders as a wellspring of solidarity required by the human body to execute herpes simplex infection.

Aside from the decontaminated types of minerals and the natural fixing Tinospora cordifolia, Dr. Sebi herpes fix additionally have some natural plans like punarnavadi mandoor and triphala. These ayurvedic prescriptions are recommended for the appropriate working of the kidney, liver, and a few other fundamental organs of the human body. Along these lines, in Dr. Sebi's remedy for herpes, there are herbs, there are minerals in filtered for, and thus there are some incredibly amazing and sound ayurvedic drugs.

Triphala is exceptionally nutritious, containing fundamental nutrients, minerals, and proteins; this aide the ayurvedic definition in raising human resistance. With a solid and safe framework, your body will remain safe from sometime in the future today contaminations, just as numerous incessant ailments. There are numerous individuals who know these advantages of Triphala and take the homegrown blend normally to support their resistance. Dr. Sebi's solution for herpes depends significantly on these fixings.

In the wake of taking a gander at the fixings, it is by all accounts all the more encouraging solution for herpes, isn't that so? Indeed, it has the ability to murder the herpes simplex infection. It has everything that is expected to help herpes patients carry on with a herpes free life. You may be on antiviral medications at the present time and can remain on the equivalent in the future too. Only for a couple of days, give this supernatural item a possibility and you will never need to glance back at some other herpes treatment.

Chapter 5: Sebi Herpes Cure Effectiveness

Why Can It Cure Herpes

An alkaline-rich diet that is rich in essential nutrients will help to rid your body of the herpes virus. This can be achieved by creating an environment that can't support the growth of diseases causing substances.

The cells in your body require oxygen to perform to their optimum capacity, but the chemicals and substances found in some medicines and foods rob your cells the much-needed oxygen to thrive.

Curing the herpes virus requires adequate cleansing of your body, and Dr. Sebi's plant-based alkaline diet does just that.

It is essential to know that curing herpes depends on the types of food eat and what you feed your body with.

You should avoid eating sweets and starchy foods. Eat foods that are bitter instead of sweet.

Eat more healthy vegetables such as zucchini, mushrooms, squash, cactus leaf or cactus plant flowers, and sea vegetables. Plant-based iron, such as dandelion, burdock, and yellow dock is also very helpful.

Dr. Sebi also emphasizes to practice fasting because fasting helps you to eat less and heal fast. Another good reason why Dr. Sebi diet can cure herpes is that it gets rid of mucus in your body. This is because once your mucus membrane is compromised, your immune system becomes weak, and you become to disease.

Your mucus membrane needs to remain healthy for you to be healthy because it is your mucus membrane that is in charge of protecting the cells in your body.

The plant-based diets and herbs that are the main constituents of Dr. Sebi's alkaline cell foods are very effective for curing herpes.

Dr. Sebi was able to cure herpes by detoxifying the body and effectively nourishing the body.

The following steps were what Dr. Sebi used to cure herpes:

- Put an end to consuming acid foods. Ensure your body is not fed with acidic foods.
- Clean your body of acids and toxin, and start eating alkaline diets and herbs that increase the level of oxygen in your cells.
- Feeding your body with the needed nutrients that can repair, rebuild, and completely strengthen your body at the cellular level.
- Practice fasting. Take herbs and water only during fasting. You can add green juice if the fasting becomes too difficult for you.

- Eat vegetables and fruits immediately after fasting.

Endeavor to eat foods from Dr. Sebi's nutritional guide after your body has been cured of herpes. Detoxification is at the heart of ridding the body of the herpes virus-there is no other way that will bring the necessary results."

Some Facts About Dr. Sebi's Diet for Herpes Cure

Dr. Sebi's diet herpes cure is anchored on some facts. Let us look at some of those facts that made Dr. Sebi's diet for herpes cure so effective.

- Dr. Sebi's diet is a plant-based alkaline diet is designed to eradicate acidity from the body and is effective in purifying and detoxifying the body.
- Dr. Sebi's diet helps to strengthen the immune system and prime the body to fight off diseases such as the herpes virus.
- Dr. Sebi's diet helps to eliminate mucus, heal an already compromised mucus membrane, and empowers your body to heal itself of diseases such as herpes.

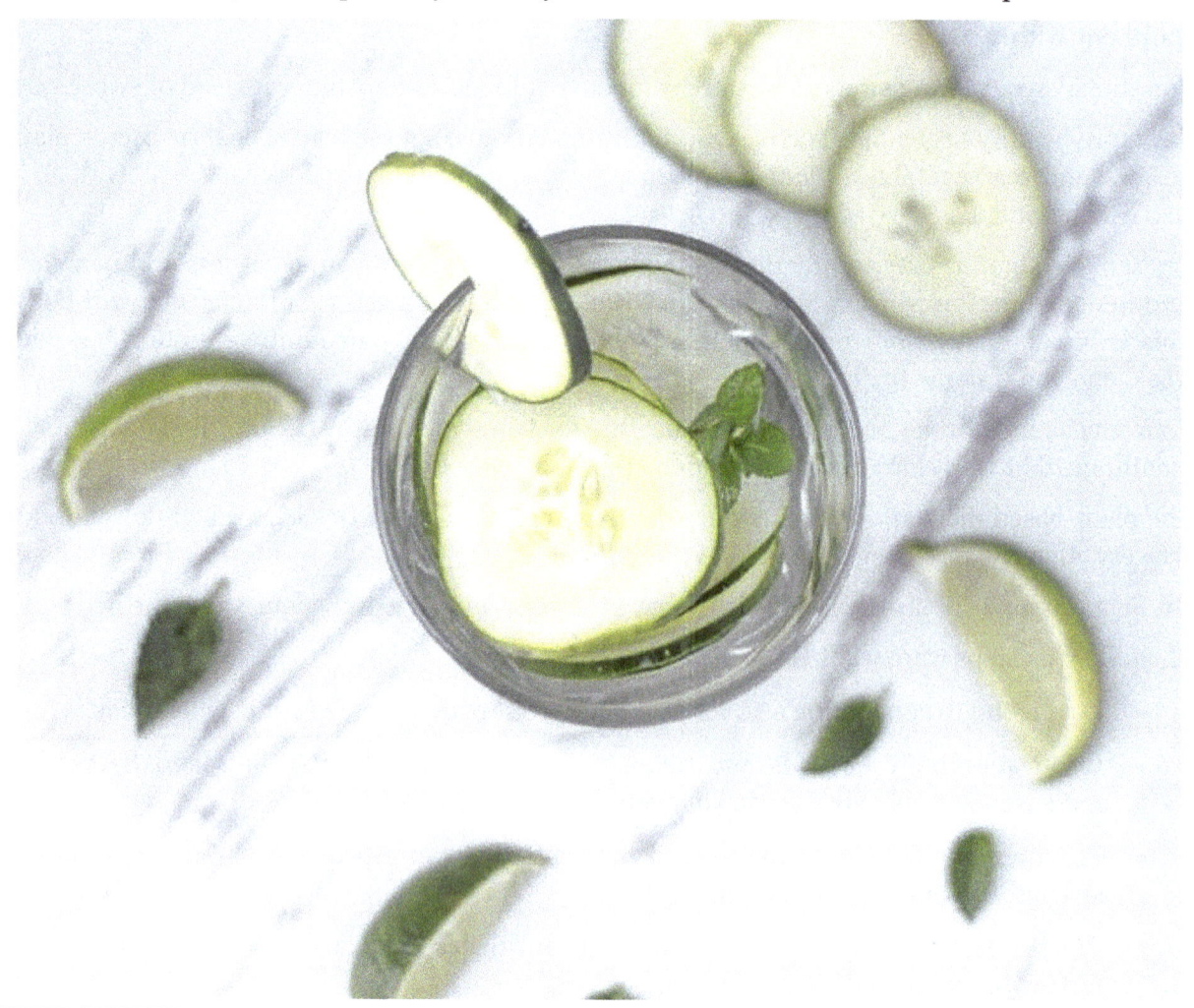

Chapter 6: Dr. Sebi Final Curative Process of Herpes Virus

Dr. Sebi Final Curative Process of Herpes Virus

After you are done with the detoxification process, you are going to start with the use of curative herbs, which are loaded with high iron contents.

Dr. Sebi recommended some of his products for the cure of the herpes virus. The product names are bromide plus powder, iron plus, bio ferro. You can use this product by following the directions: written on it by Dr. Sebi. He also recommended certain herbs you can prepare yourself at home if you cannot buy the product.

There are about eleven (11) types of herbs Dr. Sebi used for the cure of herpes. All the plants contain a rich source of potassium phosphate and iron. These herbs are listed below:

- Sarsaparilla.
- Sarsil berry.
- Guaco.
- Conconsa.
- Purslane.
- Kale.
- Dandelion.
- Lamb's quarters.
- Burdock.
- Blue vervain.
- Yellow dock

Preparation of the herbs

- Ensure the plants are well dried and preserve in a dry and clean container.
- Grind the herbs into powder form.
- Collect one tablespoon of each of the above plants and add four cups of spring water.
- Place it in a source of heat and allow boiling.
- The boiling should be done within 3 minutes or until you observe that the extracts of the plants are coming out and the color of the water changed.

- Bring it out of the heat source and leave it for a few minutes to get cool before consumption, although, herbs are best taken when hot because the bitterness will be reduced.
- Take these herbs two times daily with a glass cup until your required result is achieved.

Understand the Efficacy of the Herbs for the Cure of Herpes

Blue vervain

This plant is rich in iron, which is very good to prevent short of blood (anemia) in the body.

Sarsil berry

This plant contains iron content because it is a berry from the plant of sarsaparilla. Dr. Sebi spoke extensively on this plant and stressed on its effectiveness for the cure of herpes.

Guaco plant

This plant contains a high content of iron, strengthens the immune system, and also contains potassium phosphate that makes it effective against the herpes virus.

Sarsaparilla

This plant contains the highest iron component and it is employed for the treatment of herpes simplex and genital herpes.

Researchers suggested that sarsaparilla has mechanisms that help to treat syphilis, herpes, rheumatic affections, passive general dropsy, and gonorrheal rheumatism.

The active ingredients present in this plant that makes it effective against herpes are triterpenes, sarsaparilloside, parillin, smitilbin, and phenolic compounds.

Conconsa

This plant is an African plant. The highest concentration of potassium phosphate is embedded in it, which fights against the herpes virus.

Purslane

Purslane contains a rich amount of iron content. The herbalist has stated that this plant is effective for treating herpes simplex.

Kale plant

This plant is rich in iron antioxidants. It also contains more lysine, an amino acid ratio that's important to suppress the herpes virus. The amino acid lysine helps to inhibit the multiplication of herpes viral cells in the body.

Yellow dock
This plant is rich in iron.

Lamb's quarters
This plant is rich in iron.

Dandelion Root Effectiveness for HIV/AIDS and Herpes

This plant is rich in iron and potassium. It is one of the most popular herbs that are essential for the healing of different illnesses. It has been used for the treatment of wounds on the skin. This plant is also an essential tool used for the treatment of liver abnormalities, which helps the cleansing and detoxification of toxic substances in the body.

Moreso, dandelion helps in the removal of stones in the kidney and the bladder. It helps in the lowering of high blood pressure levels.

This plant has been extensively used in alternative medicine for the treatment of hypertension, herpes, HIV/aids, urinary tract infection, breast cancer, skin infection, and hypoglycemia in many patients.

The active ingredients present in this plant are:

- Carotenoids.
- Taraxsterol.
- Asparagine.
- Choline.
- Tannins.
- Sterols.
- Araxacin.
- Triterpenes.
- Taraxol

Scientific Proof of Dandelion for the treatment of HIV/AIDS and Herpes

Hiv/aids

Exploration uncovered from a Chinese academy of sciences builds up that dandelion upsets the replication and duplication of the human immunodeficiency virus (HIV) (hand et al. 2011). HIV replication is liable for the headway to acquired immunodeficiency syndrome.

Herpes

An exploration was completed at the Jiangxi medical college. They screened a few restorative spices against the sort 1 herpes simplex infection. After rehashed screens, dandelion was incorporated among the spices that are compelling against herpes.

Preparation of Dandelion for the Reversing Hiv/Aids Virus

- Collect the healthy root of the dandelion.
- Dry the plant with the use of direct sunlight. This should be done after you have perfectly rinsed the root.
- Grind the root into powder form.
- Collect 2 tbsp of the powder and boil in one cup of water.
- Drink this tea twice daily.

Note

Before you begin the use of this plant for HIV and aids treatment, ensure you have initially undergone the 30 days detox process to enable you to clean the body at the intercellular and intracellular level.

The detoxing process will help clean the mucus membrane, which is found in the skin and the lymphatic system. This membrane protects the cells in the body.

Also, there are several products recommended by Dr. Sebi for the treatment of HIV/aids if you do not want to use dandelion root. The products can be used together as instructed by Dr. Sebi.

Chapter 7: Healing and Recovering from STDs

STDs, which stands for sexually transmitted diseases, are still fairly prevalent even though there are well-known ways to prevent them. There are several diseases that fall into the category of STDs and are spread by sexual intercourse, but can be spread through other manners. The most common STDs are trichomoniasis, syphilis, some types of hepatitis, gonorrhea, genital warts, genital herpes, Chlamydia, and HIV.

At one time, STDs were referred to as venereal diseases. They are some of the most common contagious infections. About 65 million Americans have been diagnosed with an incurable STD. Every year, 20 million new cases occur, and about half of these are in people aged 15 to 24. All of these can have long-term implications.

These are serious illnesses that need to be treated. Some of them are considered incurable and can be deadly, such as HIV. Learning more about these diseases can provide you with knowledge on how to protect yourself.

STDs can be spread through oral, vaginal, and anal sex. Trichomoniasis is able to be contracted through contact with a moist or damp object, like toilet seats, wet clothing, or towels, although it is mostly spread through sexual contact. People who are at a higher risk of STDs include:

- Those who have more than one sexual partner.
- Those who trade sex for drugs or money.
- Those who share needles for drug use.
- Those who don't use condoms during sex.
- Those who have sex with a person who has had several partners.

Herpes and HIV are the two STDs that are chronic conditions that modern medicine can cure, but can only manage. Hepatitis B can sometimes become chronic. Unfortunately, you sometimes don't find out that you have an STD until it has damaged your reproductive organs, heart, vision, or other organs. STDs can also weaken the immune system, which leaves you vulnerable to contracting other diseases. Chlamydia and gonorrhea can cause pelvic inflammatory disease, and this can leave women unable to conceive. It is also able to kill you. If an STD is passed onto a newborn, the baby could face permanent damage, or it could kill him.

Causes of STDs

In terms of modern medicine, STDs are caused by all types of infection. Syphilis, gonorrhea, and Chlamydia are bacteria. Hepatitis B, genital warts, genital herpes, and HIV are all viral. Parasites cause trichomoniasis.

The STD germs live within vaginal secretions, blood, semen, and, in some cases, saliva. The majority of the organisms will be spread through oral, anal, or vaginal sex, but some, like with genital warts and genital herpes, can be spread simply through skin-to-skin contact. Hepatitis B is able to be spread through sharing personal items, like razors or toothbrushes.

Prevention

The most obvious step in healing for STDs is to not get one in the first place. The first tip people give in preventing STDs is to not have sex, or at least avoid sex with people who have genital discharge, rash, sores, or other symptoms. The only time you should have unprotected sex is if you and your partner are only having sex with one another, and you have both tests negative for STDs in the last six months.

Otherwise, you need to make sure you:

- Use condoms whenever you have sex. If you need a lubricant, make sure that it is one that is water-based. Condoms should be used for the entire act of sex. Keep in mind; condoms aren't 100% effective when it comes to preventing pregnancy or disease. However, they are very effective if you use them the right way.
- Avoid sharing underclothing or towels.
- Bathe after and before you have sex.
- If you are okay with vaccination, you can get vaccines for a lot of STDs, specifically Hep B and HPV.
- Make sure you are tested for HIV.
- If you abuse alcohol or drugs, please seek help. It is more common for people who are under the influence to have unsafe sex.
- Lastly, abstaining completely from sex is the only 100% effective way to prevent STDs.

There was a time when it was believed that using a condom with nonoxynol-9 would prevent STDs by killing the organisms that caused them. There has been new research that has found that this can end up irritating the woman's cervix and vagina and could increase her risk of an STD. It is recommended that you avoid condoms with nonoxynol-9.

Herpes

The most common symptoms of herpes are vaginal discharge, cold sores, pain during urination, ulcers, and blisters. There is modern medicine that can help with herpes, but none of them can cure it.

There are two forms of the HSV virus: simplex one and two. Simplex one is considered oral herpes, and simplex two is genital herpes. Over 50% of the people in the US have simplex one. In the US, about 15.5% of people aged 14 to 49 have simplex two.

If you receive oral sex from a person who has a current outbreak of cold sores around the mount ups your risk of being infected. You cannot contract genital herpes from a toilet seat.

The majority of people who have been infected with herpes won't experience any symptoms for months or years. Those who do end up having an outbreak during this initial period will have it within four days of exposure, but it can range from two to 12 days.

Most people who are infected with HSV will have recurring outbreaks. When a person has first been infected with herpes, they will have recurrences more frequently. With time, though, the remission phases will get longer, and recurrences won't be as severe.

The primary infection is the outbreak of genital herpes that happens after a person has just been infected.

The symptoms of the first outbreak tend to be very severe and could involve:

- Red blisters on the skin
- Cold sores on or around the mouth
- Malaise
- High temperature
- Pain during urination
- Enlarged, tender lymph nodes
- Itching and pain
- Vaginal discharge
- Ulceration and blisters on the external genitalia, on the cervix, or in the vagina

Most of the time, those sores will heal up, and there won't be any noticeable scarring. In outbreaks after the primary outbreak, the symptoms aren't as severe and don't last as long.

Most of the time, symptoms don't last longer than ten days and will often include:

- Red blisters
- Cold sores on or around the mouth
- Women could have ulcers or blisters on the cervix
- Tingling or burning around the genitals before the blisters show up

If HSV is present on the skin of a person infected with it, it can be given to another person through the moist skin in the genitals, anus, and mouth. The virus can also spread to other people through contact with other areas of the skin, including the eyes.

You cannot catch HSV by touching a towel, sink, work surface, or object that was touched by the infected person.

An infection will most often occur in one of the following ways:

- Having genital contact with a person who is infected.
- Sharing sex toys.
- Having oral sex from a person with current cold sores.
- Having unprotected anal or vaginal sex.

It is most common for the virus to be passed on right before the blisters appear, while visible, and until the blisters have completely gone away. HSV is also able to be passed on to another person even if there aren't any signs of a current outbreak, but it isn't that likely.

It is possible for a baby to get herpes from its mother if she has an active outbreak at the time she gives birth.

As far as modern medicine goes, there are various treatment options, most of which are home remedies.

Home remedies for herpes include:

- Painkillers, like ibuprofen or acetaminophen
- Bathing in an Epsom salt bath to help relieve symptoms
- Soaking in a sitz bath
- Using petroleum jelly on the affected skin
- Avoiding tight clothing
- Washing hands well, especially when you have touched an affected area
- Abstaining from sex until the symptoms have past
- If urinating hurts, rub some lidocaine lotion or cream to the urethra

There are some people who like to apply ice packs to the affected area.

There aren't any drugs that can get rid of herpes. Doctors will sometimes prescribe antivirals, like acyclovir, which can help prevent the virus from spreading. They can also help an outbreak to clear up quicker and can help to reduce symptom severity.

Doctors will normally only prescribe antivirals the first time a person has an outbreak. Subsequent outbreaks tend to be mild, so treatment isn't normally needed.

There is also an episodic treatment option, which is used on people who have less than six outbreaks in a single year. Whenever an outbreak occurs, a doctor will prescribe a five-day course of antivirals.

If a person has more than six outbreaks in a single year, a doctor may prescribe a suppressive treatment. There are some cases where a doctor could recommend that a person takes an antiviral each day for the rest of your life. The point of this is to try and prevent any more outbreaks. While this suppressive treatment is able to significantly reduce your risk of passing herpes onto your partner, there is still a small chance that you can.

To prevent herpes, you should follow the same prevent rules that were listed above, plus avoid kissing anybody if they have a cold sore. For most people, there are types of triggers that will cause an outbreak. These triggers could be sunbathing, friction against the skin, illness, being tired, and stress. Figuring out triggers can help to lower a person's chance of an outbreak.

Now, you can do the above, or you can try Dr. Sebi's cure. The goal of following Dr. Sebi's treatment is to create an environment where herpes can't live. Cells need to receive oxygen. Then chemicals in regular medications for herpes remove oxygen from and cells, and, most of the time, will also introduce herpes. It will take some time to help cleanse your body of herpes, but you'll do it with iron-rich plant-based items. You should start out by taking Bio Ferro and Iron Plus. Then you will need to start eating foods high in iron, which include:

- Yellow dock
- Blue vervain
- Burdock
- Lams quarters
- Dandelion
- Kale
- Purslane
- Conconsa
- Guaco
- Sarsil berry
- Sarsaparilla

Then you will want to have some bromide plus powder. The iron you are consuming is boosting your immune system, but you need to get mineral nutrition, and that's where the bromide plus powder comes in. All you have to do for this is to mix a teaspoon into a cup of boiling water. You should consume this at least two times a day.

More important than what you should consume is what you shouldn't consume. It is important that you avoid sweets and starches. You can have small amounts of sweet plant food or fruits. It is best to choose bitter foods rather than sweet. When it comes to herpes, you will want to stay away from quinoa, avocados, and chickpeas, and try to consume cactus plants, mushrooms, squash, and zucchini, as well as sea vegetables.

You can make teas out of plants like yellow dock, dandelion, and burdock. These should be consumed several times throughout the day for at least ten days. Depending on where you live, you may have to order these herbs online. You should also practice fasting. The more you are able to fast, the quicker your body will heal from herpes. If, while fasting, you start to feel weak, you can eat some dates. They may be sweet, but they won't affect your cells. Make sure you only eat them if you feel weak.

You should also eat plenty of salads. As a rule of thumb, eat salad as if you were eating a bag of potato chips, but don't eat iceberg.

Chapter 8: Sebi's Revitalizing Herbs for Herpes Cure

Dandelion

Dandelion is a flowering plant, also known as; taraxacum officinale, lentodon taraxacum, cankerwort, clockflower, common dandelion, yellow gowan, piss-in-bed, priest's crown, pissinlit, puffball, swine's snout, bitterwort, Irish daisy, tell-time, lion's tooth, blow-ball, etc. This plant is a native to Eurasia, and today, it is common in over 60 countries all over the world in the mild climates of the northern hemisphere. For centuries, these flowering plants have been used for the treatment of swelling (inflammation) of the pancreas, relieve pains that are caused by inflammation, treat and prevent cancer, tonsils (tonsillitis), skin disorder, bladder or urethra disorder, digestive and liver problems and enhance the general health of the liver and digestive system.

How Dandelion Works

Because of the chemicals compositions and nutrients like; vitamin-a, b, c, e, and k, minerals like; calcium, iron, magnesium, potassium, and other compounds like; chicoric, chlorogenic acid, and polyphenols that dandelion contains, researchers proved that it is a very effective cleansing or detoxification herbs that can detoxify or cleanse; gallbladder, kidney and purifies the blood by eliminating of heavy metals in the bloodstream and increase the rate of urine production which will lead to the cleansing of the urinary tract and inhibit crystals from forming in the urine, dissolves kidney stones and enhance kidney's health, treat and prevent diabetes by regulating blood sugar level, relief liver, and urinary disorder by enhancing the healthiness of the liver. All the above reasons are why late Dr. Sebi added dandelion as part of the cleansing herb for herpes.

Benefits of Using/Consuming Dandelion

Because of how I explained more about how dandelion works, I will just itemize the benefits of using/consuming dandelion.

These benefits include:

- It is an effective detoxifying herb that helps to detoxify or cleanse the liver and the kidney.
- It helps to treat and prevent diabetes by regulating blood sugar levels.
- It helps to fight against and relieve pains that are caused by inflammation.
- It helps to deactivate and inhibit the negative effects of free radicals in the body which is because of it anti-oxidant properties.
- It helps to reduce the level of cholesterol.
- It helps to lower blood pressure by getting rid of excess fluid in the body.

- It helps to naturally shed excess weight gain by improving the metabolism of carbohydrates.
- It helps to prevent and treat cancer by inhibiting the growth and cancer cell mutation.
- It helps to boost the immune system through the activities of the anti-microbial and anti-viral properties which in turn helps the body to fight various infections and boost the immune system. Don't forget that a herpes outbreak is severe when the immune system is weak.
- It helps to keep the skin healthy and treat and prevent skin diseases.

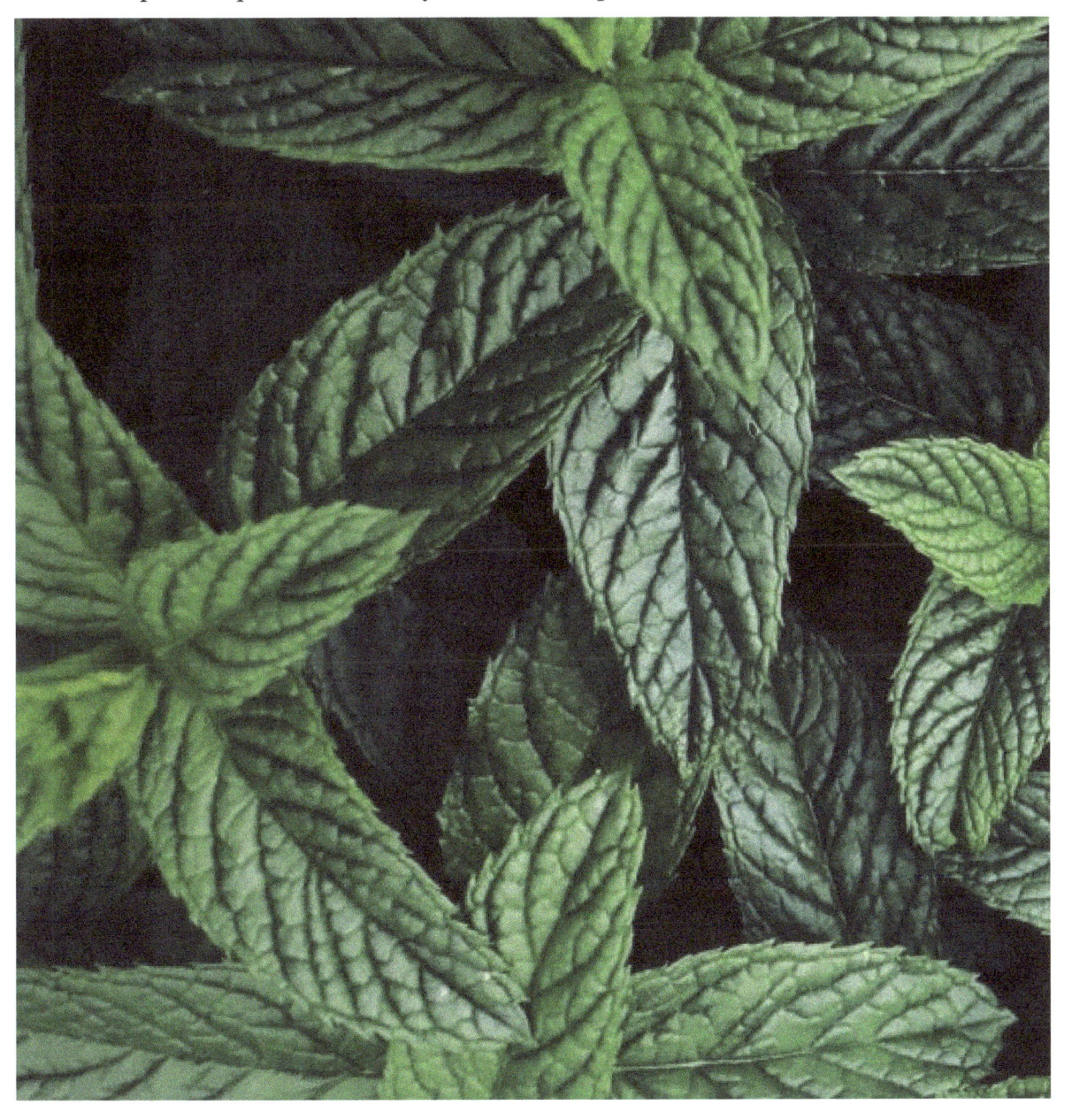

The Side Effects of Using or Consuming Dandelion

Till at the time of writing this book, consuming dandelion orally is 100% safe.

Consuming an overdose of dandelion can result in some side effects like:

- Diarrhea
- Experiencing stomach upset or irritation
- Allergic reactions
- Sometimes heartburn, but it's not common.

The notable precautions before using/consuming dandelions are:

- Pregnant and breast-feeding mothers should stay off dandelion as there is no research to know if it is harmful to them or not.
- If you are suffering from eczema, stays off dandelion as more than 85% of people with eczema suffer an allergic reaction to dandelion.
- Since dandelion slows down blood clotting, people that have any history of bleeding disorders should stay of dandelion as it might increase the risk of bleeding and bruising.
- If you are allergic to other related plants from the same family like; marigolds, ragweed, chrysanthemums, or daisies, you should stay of dandelion.
- If you have a history of any kind of kidney disorder or failure, stay off dandelion.

Medications that Interact With the Dandelion

Because of the potency of dandelion, there are medications that interact with it.

All antibiotics. Examples of antibiotic are:

- Quinolone
- Grepafloxacin (raxar)
- Ciprofloxacin (cipro)
- Trovafloxacin (trovan)
- Norfloxacin (chibroxin or noroxin)
- Parfloxacin (zagam)
- Enoxacin (penetrex) etc.

Lithium: Just like sarsaparilla, dandelion also has water pill or "diuretic" effects, and so, consuming both medications will lead to a decrease in the rate at which the body gets rid of lithium.

Medications that are processed by the liver: Any medications that can be changed by the liver will interact with dandelion. Such medications are:

- Amitriptyline (elavil)
- Atorvastatin (lipitor)
- Diazepam (valium)
- Digoxin
- Entacapone (comtan)
- Haloperidol (haldol)
- Irinotecan (camptosar)
- Lamotrigine (lamictal)
- Propranolol (inderal)
- Theophylline
- Verapamil (calan/isoptin) etc.

For dosage and preparation of dandelion tea/infusion, kindly take the following steps:
- Get some fresh leaves of dandelion and washed it under running water to remove all the dirt.
- After washing it, pour ½ - 1 cup of the washed dandelion in your saucepan.
- You should boil 4-5 cups of water and pour the boiled water inside the saucepan where you pour the dandelion and cover it for 4-5 hours or throughout the night (overnight) for it to get infused properly.
- By the next day, strain out the dandelion leaves, and you will be left with the dandelion tea/infusion.
- For the dosage, take ½ tablespoon of dandelion per ¾ cup of water three times daily. And if you ordered your dandelion online, you can take 4-10 grams of dry leaf of dandelion three times daily.

Elderberry

Elderberry is a dark purple berry from the elder tree also known as elderberries, European black elderberry, European elder fruit, European elderberry, Sambucus baccae, black elder, Arbre de judas, black-berried alder, black elderberry, boor tree, bounty, elderberry fruit, Gellhorn, common elder, fruit de sureau, hautbois, ellanwood, holunderbeeren, sambu, sambugo, schwarzer holunder, sureau, sureau noir, sussier etc. And the plant is a flowering plant from the family of adoxaceae and native to Europe. Both the leaves and fruit (berries) of elderberry have been used for centuries now for the treatment of pain and swelling arising from inflammation, help to stimulate urine production, and induce sweat to detoxify the body system.

Furthermore, the bark of the plant also serves as a laxative, diuretic, and also induces vomiting.

For the purpose of this book, I will be looking at the berries which people have been using it for centuries as a traditional medicine to treat and prevent various types of infectious diseases, influenza, headaches, sciatica, remove mucus from the upper respiratory system, and the lungs and also help in relieving nerve and heart pain.

How Elderberry Works

Elderberry is very rich, with various compounds and nutrients contained like vitamin-c, dietary fiber, phenolic acids which is a great and powerful anti-oxidants that helps to prevent and decrease the damage that is caused by oxidative stress in the body, it also contains some compound like flavonols such as kaempferol, quercetin, isorhamnetin and anthocyanins which gives the fruit the black-purple color and makes it a strong anti-oxidant that and anti-inflammation agent. Elderberry also contains some nutrients like; calories, carbs, a minute amount of protein, fat, and anthocyanins, which makes the plant to be a strong and effective antioxidant with anti-inflammatory properties.

Benefits of using/consuming elderberry

- To cleanse and detoxify the lungs and respiratory system by eliminating mucus from the upper respiratory system and the lungs.
- To treat and prevent cancer by inhibiting cancer cells mutation, and destroying the cancerous cells in the body.
- It helps to treat constipation.
- It helps to treat flu and cold in less than 24hours.
- To combat harmful bacteria in the body by preventing the growth of bacterial through its anti-bacterial properties.
- To boost and support the immune defense system by increasing white blood cell production.
- To protect and keep the skin healthy.
- Relief chronic fatigue syndrome and depression etc.

Possible Side Effects of Using/Consuming Elderberry

Till at the time of writing this book, there is no record of any side effects from researchers and people who have used elderberry, but because of the compound that are presents in elderberry, it will be wise to use it for not more than 12weeks and take a break for at least a week before using it again.

The notable precautions before using elderberry include:

- Make sure you don't allow your ward below 12 years to use/consume elderberry and those that are above 12 years should not use it for more than 10 days.
- Since there is no reliable information to know if elderberry is safe or not for pregnant and breastfeeding mothers, I strongly advise that they should stay off elderberry.

- People that have a history of suffering from an auto-immune disease like; multiple sclerosis, lupus, rheumatoid arthritis, etc. Should stay off elderberry as it has the potency to boost the immune system to become more active, which could worsen their situation.

Medications that Interact With Elderberry.

Since the elderberry has the potency to increase or boost the immune defense system, any medications that are designed to decrease the function of the immune system will certainly interact with the elderberry. Such medications include:

- Azathioprine (imuran)
- Sirolimus (rapamune)
- Basiliximab (simulect)
- Mycophenolate (cellcept)
- Corticosteroids (glucocorticoids)
- Prednisone (deltasone, orasone)
- Daclizumab (zenapax)
- Muromonab-cd3 (orthoclone okt3, okt3) etc.

Dosage and how to preparation of elderberry tea/infusion

For the dosage and how to prepare elderberry tea/infusion, kindly take the steps below:

- Boil 8-12oz of water in your saucepan.
- Once the water is boiling, measure 1 tablespoon of dried elderberries and add it to the boiling water.
- Reduce your gas and allow it to boil for at least 15 minutes.
- After the 15 minutes timing, allow it to get cold and strain it using a strainer.
- For the dosage, consume 3-4 cups daily.

Lavender
Overview

Lavender is the name given to almost the 40 herbs in the mint family. Nevertheless, the most popular form, which has enormous health benefits, is Lavandula angustifolia. This type of lavender is obtainable in almost every region of the world. And that may be the reason why it is widely used. Because of its powerful effects on the human body, herbalists from all walks of life, including Dr. Sebi use it. They use their stems, flowers, and leaves in treating numerous diseases.

Identifying lavender is an effortless task. It is needle-like and its foliage smells like balsam which is either in gray or in bluish-green color. It does indeed have the nuances of these two colors. Also, the total height of this herb is about three ft., if the growing conditions are favorable.

Properties

The constituents that make lavender an essential herb in the medical industry include the following:

- Cineole
- Terpineol
- Borneo
- Flavonoids
- Camphor
- Rosmarinic acid
- Triterpenoids
- Linabol

Health Benefits of Lavender

In addition to the above-stated facts about the lavender herb, there are many other health benefits of lavender on the medical side. For instance, if you have chronic migraines or headaches, it can act as an essential oil or head balm to relieve your pain. At the first sign of a headache, all you need to do is to rub it on the temples. Lavender also promotes deep sleep because of its sedative scent. People with sleeping disorders can creep into the land of dreams while enjoying the scents.

Apart from that, you can pour it in water and use it on your skin if you have skin problems like rashes or acne. Its antiseptic properties will clear all the problems of acne and rashes within a few days when you bath with the water. When used as a cooling remedy, it helps to heal bruises and scratches. Store the water bottle that contains the lavender in the refrigerator for a few minutes before you apply it to the scars or fresh bruises.

Other benefits include the following:

- Reduces headache
- Promotes sleep
- Protects the health of the heart
- Treats chronic migraine issues
- Heals bruises and scars
- Lessens anxiety and stress
- Assists in curing skin diseases
- Possesses anti-inflammatory qualities
- Improves the quality of hair
- It is also aromatic, insect repellent, and sedative

Sage
Overview

The ancient Greeks and Egyptians use sage to treat sprains, ulcers, bleeding, and swelling. Sage is credited with extraordinary healing properties. This is also confirmed by the modern medical experts of the 21st century. According to these experts, sage has tremendous nutritional value, which has shown promising signs in the treatment of several diseases.

This herb is native to the Mediterranean region and southern Europe. Nevertheless, it can be found in other warmer climates like in North America. In fact, it is a perennial woody herb that has an incredible impact on human health. It has blue to purplish flowers as well as grayish leaves. Sage is also known as garden save, salvia officinalis, and sage culinary among the professional herbalists like Dr. Sebi.

Uses of the sage herb

This herb is most commonly used in the form of tea. The herb can be sprinkled over salads and sandwiches or be added to the food while cooking. What Dr. Sebi recommends is only 400 mg of sage extract per day because high doses can be very toxic.

In addition, this herb can also be used to treat many skin conditions like psoriasis, eczema, and acne. You only have to regularly apply its extracts to the affected area.

Health Benefits of Sage

The tremendous nutritional value of sage has been confirmed by Dr. Sebi plus several lab tests. One tablespoon of sage contains 43% vitamin k, and that it is just the exact amount our body needs to function correctly. It is also found that sage contains b-vitamins such as riboflavin. Besides, they play an essential role in sustaining our body as a well-aligned machine.

The latest research shows that this particular herb is not only suitable for wound treatment. When its right dosage is consumed, it can facilitate the treatment of inflammation, boosting female fertility, increasing memory retention, neutralizing free radicals, preventing gastric spasms, strengthening of the immune system, preventing Alzheimer's disease, improving bone health, curing issues like arthritis and gout, managing diabetes and treatment of snake bites.

Other health benefits of sage herb

- Sage is antiseptic, antioxidant, and antibacterial.
- It also treats conditions such as weak immune system, arthritis, Alzheimer, inflammation, and diabetes.

Cascara Sagrada

Overview

Cascara sagrada is a natural herb that is highly potent. It is extracted from the bark of a tree known as the rhamnus purshiana tree. It naturally grows along the pacific coast of North America. Cascara Sagrada's other common names include sacred bark, bitter bark, sea buckthorn, and chitem bark.

Health system experts at the University of Michigan believe that this herb was used by the native Americans as early as the 15th century, specifically when they introduced it as a cure to the Spanish explorers. It is believed to be used as a laxative to treat constipation back then. It soothes the muscle cells in the colon. Up till this day, over 20% of the national laxative market in the US depends on it. That's about $ 100 million a year.

Cascara Sagrada's leaves are simple, deciduous, and cluster towards the end of the branches. The leaves are shinier green at the top and paler green underneath. They are about 15 cm long,

2-5 cm broad and are oval-shaped.

These days, it is not easy to locate cascara sagrada as their numbers have declined significantly due to strong market demand and overharvesting. Look for them at the streamside and in the moist forest if you don't see them in their native land but need them.

Health Benefits of Cascara Sagrada

Dr. Sebi discovered many additional health benefits of cascara sagrada. He believes that this herbal remedy can challenge over-the-counter pills. Cascara sagrada is known to possess the ability to treat many health problems such as muscle and joint pain, digestive problems, hemorrhoids, and anxiety. In addition, it is also very effective against many significant diseases, especially cancer—a life-threatening disease. Dr. Sebi investigated its use in the treatment of cancer and discovered that through a precise mechanism, its active component, emodin, can inhibit cancer growth.

Apart from that, the same active ingredient, emodin, possesses antimicrobial and anti-inflammatory properties. This herb is usually taken in a tablet/capsule or a liquid extract form.

Other health benefits of cascara sagrada include:

- It is anti-inflammatory
- Treats constipation
- Prevents cancer
- Anti-fungal
- Cures anxiety
- Antimicrobial
- Wanes the existence of hemorrhoids
- Improves emotional well-being
- Protects against liver diseases
- Protects against amnesia

Blue Vervain

Overview

Blue vervain is a thin, straight perennial herb that is widespread in North America. Blue vervain has green to reddish stems coupled with toothy leaves. The height of this herb is 5 feet and has 6 inches leaves with double-serrate margins in the opposite direction. This herb is also known as American vervain and vervain hastata.

Blue vervain's flower is purple-colored and usually appears in the summer. The herb is densely populated with many blue-violet flowers. However, the actual flowering time of this herb lies between the middle-late summer, and it usually lasts 30 to 45 days. This flowering time gives the flowers a flory scent.

Uses of Blue Vervain Herb

Blue vervain is not known to most people. It is undoubtedly the herbal remedy that is least known. But as far as its medicinal properties are concerned, it possesses magical powers. Several research works conducted have shown its leaves and flowers containing many active ingredients. They have antipyretic, diuretic, and antispasmodic properties. In addition, it also helps calm the nervous system, detoxifies the body, reduces inflammation, and relieves chest congestion.

Romans and Greeks considered it a sacred herb because of the extraordinary qualities mentioned above. Dr. Sebi, a well-known traditional physician, often recommended this herb for almost all types of plague and fever. In addition, some historians believe that blue vervain was applied to the wound of Jesus after his removal from the cross.

Though this herb can be consumed in several forms, using it as tea is what Dr. Sebi recommended. According to him, it has effects that are described as fast-acting and potent with a unique composition of phytochemicals and acids, and that's why it's best to combine it with tea. All that is needed is to infuse the herb's flower, root, and leaves into warm water and enjoy them.

Health Benefits of Blue Vervain Herb

- Treats respiratory disorder
- Detoxifies the body
- Antimicrobial
- Boosts gum health
- Cardioprotective
- Antibacterial
- Anti-anxiety relaxant
- Keeps the nervous system healthy
- Anti-inflammatory and reduces swelling
- Relieves depression
- Eases menstrual pain

Precaution

Keep in mind that Dr. Sebi recommends blue vervain in small doses. High doses can cause diarrhea or vomiting due to its potency. If you are, however, pregnant or a breastfeeding mother, talk to your doctor first because this herb also affects your blood pressure.

Chapter 9: Cleansing Herbs

Mullein

Mullein helps to cleanse the lung and also helps to activate lymph circulation in your neck and chest.

Sarsaparilla Root

Sarsaparilla root helps to purify the blood and target herpes. Jamaican sarsaparilla roots are highly recommended because it is a great source of iron, and it is good for healing.

Chaparral

Chaparral helps to cleanse harmful heavy metals from your gallbladder and blood and also cleanse the lymphatic system.

Guaco Herb

Guaco heals wounds, cleanses the blood,

Promotes perspiration, increases urination, keeps your respiratory system healthy, and improves digestion.

The leaves of guaco can be used to relieve pain, treat some types of venereal disease, expel phlegm, reduce inflammation, thin the blood, and kill bacteria. You have to drink a lot of water when using the guaco herb.

Cilantro

Cilantro helps to remove heavy and harmful metals from your cells, and this is essential for the healing of herpes because the herpes virus hides behind your cell walls.

Burdock Root

Burdock root helps to cleanse the lymphatic system and the liver.

Pao Pereira

Pao Pereira effectively helps to subdue the herpes virus, and it also inhibits the duplication of the herpes virus genome.

This herb is an awesome herb to help to fight the herpes virus.

Pau D'arco

The chemical constituents contained in pau d'arco have shown in vitro anti-viral properties against HSV-1 and HSV-2, and other viruses such as poliovirus, influenza, and vesicular stomatitis virus.

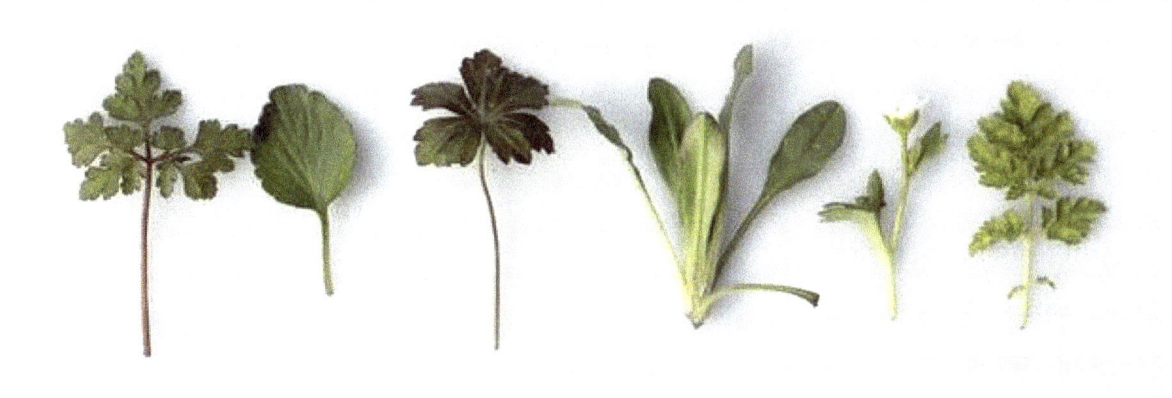

Essential Oregano Oil

Essential Oregano oil is a great anti-viral that can suppress the herpes virus. It works best at ninety percent concentration.

Apply essential oregano oil to your lower spine because your lower spine is the point where HSV-2 is dormant.

You can also apply it to your genital area and under your tongue.

Ginger Essential Oil

The ginger essential oil can kill the herpes virus on contact. But you should dilute the ginger essential oil with a carrier oil be used.

The ginger essential oil has the same effect as essential oregano oil.

Sea Salt Bath

Sea salt helps to absorb electrolysis through your skin and reliefs your skin during a herpes virus outbreak. To achieve this, you need to add a cup or half a cup of sea salt into a tub filled with warm water and soak your skin in it for some time.

Ensure that the sea salt dissolves completely.

Holy Basil

Stress is one of the factors that can trigger a herpes outbreak through adrenal fatigue. Holy basil is an adaptogen that relieves adrenal fatigue and prevents the outbreak of herpes through stress.

How to Extract Essential Oils for Herpes

There are numerous oils for herpes, and the one thing that we have to take into consideration is the extraction process.

The proper extraction of these oils from their natural sources is a delicate process that requires a lot of experience as well as the right materials.

There are numerous methods of extracting essential oils, but we are going to cover the two most important techniques, which are:

- Steam distillation
- Cold press

Steam distillation

The process of steam distillation makes use of steam and pressure for the extraction process. This process is a simple one, but without the right expertise, it can definitely go wrong.

The raw materials are placed inside a cooking chamber made of stainless steel, and when the material is steamed, it is broken down, removing the volatile materials behind.

When the steam is freed from the plant, it moves up the chamber in gaseous form through the connecting pipe, which goes into the condenser.

Once the condenser is cool, the gas goes back into liquid form, and this is the essential oil that can be collected from the surface of the water.

Cold pressing

The cold press process extracts oils from the rind of the citrus as well as the seeds oil the carrier oil. This process requires heat but not as much heat as the steam distillation process with a maximum temperature of 120F for the process to go as planned.

The material which is heated is placed in a container where it is punctured by a device which rotates with thorns. Once the process of puncturing is complete, the essential oils are released into a container below the puncturing region. These machines then make use of centrifugal force to separate the essential oil from the juice.

Both processes are essential, and it has to be done properly with the right level of information from experts who know a lot about the process, if not extremely harmful situations can occur rather than good results.

Chapter 10: The Strategies Dr. Sebi Used In Curing Herpes Simplex Virus

The herbs Dr. Sebi used for the treatment of herpes are very effective, and the formulations are produced to improve the immune system in the body system.

The individuals that must use Dr. Sebi's herb for the treatment of herpes simplex virus must learn how to eat plant-based foods, which are strong alkaline diet responsible for the cure of this disease.

Dr. Sebi used several strategies for the treatment of this ailment. The treatment ranges from the consideration of his fast therapy, which helps in the detoxification of the body's organs, and the use of herbs that are responsible for reenergizing/revitalizing the body.

All of the herbs Dr. Sebi used are important in improving the immune system in the body and subsequently fight the viral cell.

One of his strategies is the engagement in fast that enables detoxification and cleansing. The other strategy he used was the use of curative herbs that helps in revitalizing the body and bringing it to its normal state.

Detoxification and Cleansing of the Body Organs

Dr. Sebi made use of certain numbers of herbs for the detoxification of the body organs. The herbs detoxify organs such as the liver, kidney, lungs, lymph gland, bladder, and many organs.

He detoxified the body through the intracellular and intracellular levels. This will help in the removal of excess mucus and toxins thereby, flushing out the viral cells in the body.

When you undergo detoxification of the body, you are at the point of eliminating the herpes virus in your body. The virus affects the immune system and the central nervous system (CNS). Hence, your body must undergo detoxification to activate and flush them out before you could declare that you are free from this virus. He encourages 15 days of fasting plans in order to hasten the detoxification process.

Herbs Used for Fasting to Enable Detoxification

The fasting program should be done for good consecutive 15 days without the consumption of the foods you were eating before.

The detoxification herbs Dr. Sebi used are listed below:

- Nopal plant
- Stinging nettle root.
- Elderberry.
- Linden leaf.

- Sea moss plant.
- Burdock root

Facts and Tips Needed While Using Dr. Sebi's Diet

- Avoid consumption of oily foods such as vegetable oil.
- Drink only alkaline water, not tap water.
- Do not eat deep-fried foods.
- Drink one gallon of spring or alkaline water every day.
- Eat fruits, vegetables, and all foods designed by Dr. Sebi.
- Take all meals on or before 6-7 pm every day before going to bed.
- Junk food should be avoided.
- Avoid foods prepared in the restaurant.
- Canned or bottled juice must be shunned.
- Consume only raw and organic nuts and seeds.
- Consume only organic sea salt.
- Avoid the use of non-organic sweeteners.
- Do not consume microwaved food.
- Use all plates and cups for food intake except plastics.
- Shun the consumption of sodas.
- Refined foods must be shunned.
- Do not eat grains that are not listed in Dr. Sebi's diet.
- Eat only organic foods.

The significance of these detoxifying herbs is below:

- Provide the body with irons, which is very important for the herpes virus cure.
- Remove toxic waste from the body.
- Multiply cells in the body.
- Cleanses and promotes blood.
- Provides energy for the body.
- Revitalize the body.

Chapter 11: Benefits of Herbal Medicine

Numerous homegrown arrangements may have benefits. Others may have no conspicuous or demonstrated advantage, and a few, truth be told, can be hurtful. For a large portion of the over-the-counter spices you can purchase, there is likely little danger of having a terrible response in the event that you follow the bearings. For instance, you may drink some peppermint tea to settle your stomach. Even under the least favorable conditions, it can support your furious stomach, best-case scenario, it can taste decent, warm you up, and not have any negative symptoms! As another model, certain echinacea types are acknowledged in certain nations for the treatment of colds and cold side effects. While, by far, most of the spices don't have any noteworthy symptoms, be that as it may, alert ought to be utilized on the off chance that you are thinking about including natural enhancements throughout your life.

For a considerable length of time, societies around the globe have depended on conventional homegrown medication to meet their medicinal service's needs.

In spite of clinical and innovative progressions of the cutting edge period, the worldwide interest for homegrown cures is on the ascent. Truth be told, it's evaluated that this industry earns about $60 billion every year.

Some common cures might be more moderate and open than regular medications, and numerous individuals incline toward utilizing them since they line up with their own wellbeing belief systems.

No different, you may ponder whether natural choices are successful.

Here are 9 of the world's most mainstream natural prescriptions, including their principle advantages, utilizes, and important security data...

Echinacea

Echinacea, or coneflower, is a blooming plant and a famous natural cure.

Initially from North America, it has, for some time, been utilized in native American practices to treat an assortment of infirmities, including wounds, consumes, toothaches, sore throat, and agitated stomach. Most pieces of the plant, including the leaves, petals, and roots, can be utilized therapeutically—however, numerous individuals accept the roots have the most grounded impact. Echinacea is normally taken as a tea or enhances yet can likewise be applied topically.

Today, it's fundamentally used to treat or forestall the regular cold; however, the science behind this isn't especially solid.

One survey in more than 4,000 individuals found a potential 10–20% diminished danger of colds from taking echinacea; however, there's almost no proof that it treats the cold after you have gotten it.

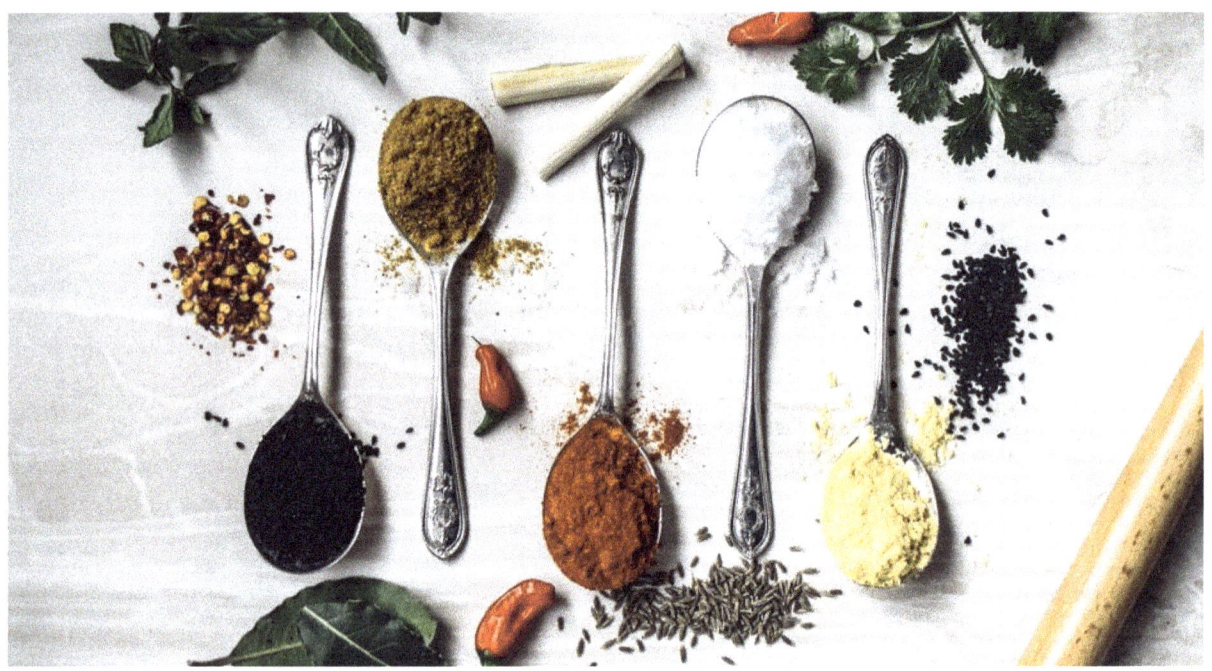

Despite the fact that inadequate information exists to assess the drawn-out impacts of this spice, transient use is commonly viewed as sheltered. All things considered, symptoms like sickness, stomach torment, and skin rash have sometimes been accounted for.

Ginseng

Ginseng is a restorative plant whose roots are normally soaked to make a tea or dried to make a powder.

It's every now and again used in conventional Chinese medication to diminish aggravation and lift invulnerability, cerebrum capacity, and vitality levels.

A few assortments exist; however, the two most well-known are the Asian and American sorts—Panax ginseng and Panax quinquefolius, individually. American ginseng is thought to develop unwinding, while Asian ginseng is viewed as additionally animating, in spite of the fact that ginseng has been utilized for a considerable length of time, current exploration supporting its viability is inadequate.

A few test-cylinder and creature templates propose that it's one of a kind mixes, called ginsenosides, gloat neuroprotective, anticancer, antidiabetic, and safe supporting properties. Regardless, human exploration is required.

Transient use is viewed as generally protected; however, ginseng's drawn-out wellbeing stays indistinct. Potential reactions incorporate cerebral pains, helpless rest, and stomach related problems.

Ginkgo Biloba

Ginkgo biloba, likewise referred to just as ginkgo, is a homegrown medication obtained from the maidenhair tree.

Local to china, ginkgo has been utilized in customary Chinese medication for a great many years and stays a top-selling homegrown enhancement today. It contains an assortment of powerful cancer prevention agents that are thought to give a few advantages (trusted source).

The seeds and leaves are customarily used to make teas and colors; however, most present-day applications use leaf extricate.

A few people likewise appreciate eating the crude foods grown from the ground seeds. Nonetheless, the seeds are somewhat harmful and should just be eaten in little amounts, if by any means.

Ginkgo is said to treat a wide scope of sicknesses, including coronary illness, dementia, mental troubles, and sexual brokenness. However, considers have not demonstrated it compelling for any of these conditions.

In spite of the fact that it's very much endured by the vast majority, conceivable symptoms incorporate cerebral pain, heart palpitations, stomach related problems, skin responses, and an expanded danger of dying.

Elderberry

Elderberry is an old homegrown medication commonly produced using the cooked product of the Sambucus nigra plant. It has, for quite some time, been utilized to assuage cerebral pains, nerve torment, toothaches, colds, viral diseases, and blockage.

Today, it's essentially showcased as a treatment for side effects related to this season's flu virus and regular virus.

Elderberry is accessible as a syrup or tablet, in spite of the fact that there's no standard measurement. A few people like to make their own syrup or tea by cooking elderberries with different fixings, for example, nectar and ginger.

Test-tube examines show that its plant mixes have cell reinforcement, antimicrobial, and antiviral properties; however, human exploration is inadequate.

While a couple of little human investigations demonstrate that elderberry abbreviates the length of influenza contaminations, bigger examinations are expected to decide whether it's any more successful than regular antiviral treatments.

Momentary use is viewed as protected, yet the unripe or crude natural product is poisonous and may cause manifestations like queasiness, regurgitating, and looseness of the bowels.

St. John's Wort

St. John's wort (SJW) is a homegrown medication obtained from the blossoming plant Hypericum perforatum. Its little, yellow blossoms are ordinarily used to make teas, cases, or concentrates.

Its utilization can be followed back to old Greece, and SJW is still much of the time recommended by clinical experts in parts of Europe.

Generally, it was used to help wound mending and reduce a sleeping disorder, wretchedness, and different kidney and lung infections. Today, it's, to a great extent, recommended to get gentle moderate despondency.

Numerous examinations note that transient utilization of SJW is as successful as some ordinary antidepressants. Be that as it may, there's restricted information on long haul wellbeing or viability for those with serious despondency or self-destructive musings.

SJW has moderately barely any symptoms yet may cause unfavorably susceptible responses, dazedness, disarray, dry mouth, and expanded light affectability.

It additionally meddles with various prescriptions, including antidepressants, contraception, blood thinners, certain agony meds, and a few kinds of malignant growth medicines.

Specific medication connections could be deadly, so on the off chance that you take any doctor prescribed prescriptions, counsel your medicinal services supplier preceding utilizing SJW.

Turmeric

Turmeric (Curcuma longa) is a spice that has a place with the ginger family.

Utilized for a great many years in cooking and medication the same, it has as of late accumulated consideration for its strong calming properties.

Curcumin is a significant dynamic compound in turmeric. It might treat a large group of conditions, including constant aggravation, torment, metabolic disorder, and tension.

Specifically, various investigations uncover that supplemental dosages of curcumin are as powerful for easing joint inflammation torment as some regular mitigating prescriptions, for example, ibuprofen.

Both turmeric and curcumin supplements are broadly viewed as sheltered. However extremely high portions may prompt looseness of the bowels, cerebral pain, or skin disturbance.

You can likewise utilize new or dried turmeric in dishes like curries, in spite of the fact that the sum you commonly eat in food isn't probably going to have a critical restorative impact.

Ginger

Ginger is an ordinary fixing and natural medication. You can eat it new or dried; however, its fundamental restorative structures are as a tea or case. Much like turmeric, ginger is a rhizome or stem that develops underground. It contains an assortment of gainful mixes and has, for some time, been utilized in customary and people practices to treat colds, sickness, headaches, and hypertension.

Its best-settled current use is for assuaging sickness related to pregnancy, chemotherapy, and clinical tasks.

Besides, test-cylinder and creature research uncovers expected advantages for rewarding and forestalling ailments like coronary illness and disease, despite the fact that the proof is blended.

Some little human examinations suggest that this root may lessen your danger of blood clump development, despite the fact that it hasn't been demonstrated any more compelling than traditional treatments

Ginger is all around endured. Negative reactions are uncommon, yet huge portions may cause a gentle instance of indigestion or looseness of the bowels.

Valerian

At times alluded to as "nature's valium," valerian is a blooming plant whose roots are thought to instigate serenity and a feeling of quiet.

Valerian root might be dried and expended in a container structure or soaks to make tea.

Its utilization can be followed back to old Greece and Rome, where it was taken to calm fretfulness, tremors, cerebral pains, and heart palpitations. Today, it's frequently used to treat a sleeping disorder and nervousness.

All things considered, proof supporting these utilizations isn't especially solid.

One audit saw valerian as to some degree viable for inciting rest, yet a considerable lot of the investigation results depended on emotional reports from members.

Valerian is generally protected; however, it might cause gentle reactions like cerebral pains and stomach related problems. You shouldn't take it in case you're on some other narcotics because of the danger of intensifying impacts, for example, over the top discomfort and laziness.

Chamomile

Chamomile is a blooming plant that likewise happens to be one of the most well-known natural drugs on the planet.

The blossoms are regularly used to make tea; however, the leaves may likewise be dried and utilized for making tea, therapeutic concentrates, or effective packs.

For a huge number of years, chamomile has been utilized as a solution for sickness, looseness of the bowels, stoppage, stomach torment, urinary tract diseases, wounds, and upper respiratory contaminations.

This spice packs more than 100 dynamic mixes, a significant number of which are thought to add to its various advantages.

A few test-cylinder and creature considers have exhibited calming, antimicrobial, and cell reinforcement movement. However deficient human exploration is accessible.

However, a couple of little human investigations propose that chamomile treats looseness of the bowels, passionate unsettling influences just as squeezing related to the premenstrual condition (PMS), and torment and irritation connected to osteoarthritis.

Chamomile is ok for the vast majority yet may cause a hypersensitive response—particularly in case you're sensitive to comparable plants, for example, daisies, ragweed, or marigolds.

Chapter 12: Dr. Sebi's Natural Erectile Dysfunctions Cure

Definition of Disease

Before looking at how to treat erectile dysfunctions, there is a need to define what a disease is. According to Dr. Sebi, the term disease has been miss-interpreted by departmentalizing or sectionalizing it, which has made a lot of people to believe that the disease called; diabetes is different from sinusitis, erectile dysfunction is different from pneumonia, bronchitis is different from arthritis, sickle cell anemia is different from hypertension and a lot more because that was exactly what the western education want us to believe.

How to Cure the Root-Cause of Erectile Dysfunctions

According to Dr. Sebi, to cure the root cause of erectile dysfunction, there are two steps that cannot be avoided if you desire results. However, these steps are:

- Cleansing: Cleansing has to do with getting rid of mucus or detoxifying the body system using spring water, alkaline fruits smoothies, Irish sea moss, and the cleansing herbs.

- Revitalizing: Revitalizing has to do with nourishing and replenishing the body system and strengthening the immune system from the energy or damage that it has suffered as a result of a disease.

- Dieting: Although the steps are just the first two steps, Dr. Sebi stated that a lot of people were not able to be free from disease completely because, after the cleansing and revitalizing process, they now return to eating acidic food that is making them be vulnerable to the disease again. However, dieting is changing your eating habit. That is, eating foods from Dr. Sebi's nutritional guide. (I will talk about that soon).

Cleansing or Detoxification

Cleansing or detoxification is an alternative medication used in getting rid of all the acidic and toxins content (mucus) that have accumulated in the body which has made the body system to be vulnerable to disease. Until we stop eating, preserved/canned food, our body will be filled with toxins that have either short or long term effects on the human's health. However, the way to a healthy, happy, and sick-free lifestyle is to cleanse or detoxify the body system of all the toxins that make the body vulnerable to disease.

How to Undergo a Cleanse

When talking about cleansing, most doctors will only talk about the cleansing of the colon but Dr. Sebi, disagree with their opinion and state that, to do a cleanse, you will need to do an intra-cellular cleansing. That is the cleansing of each cell from the body system. However, to do an intra-cellular cleansing, you will need to cleanse the following:

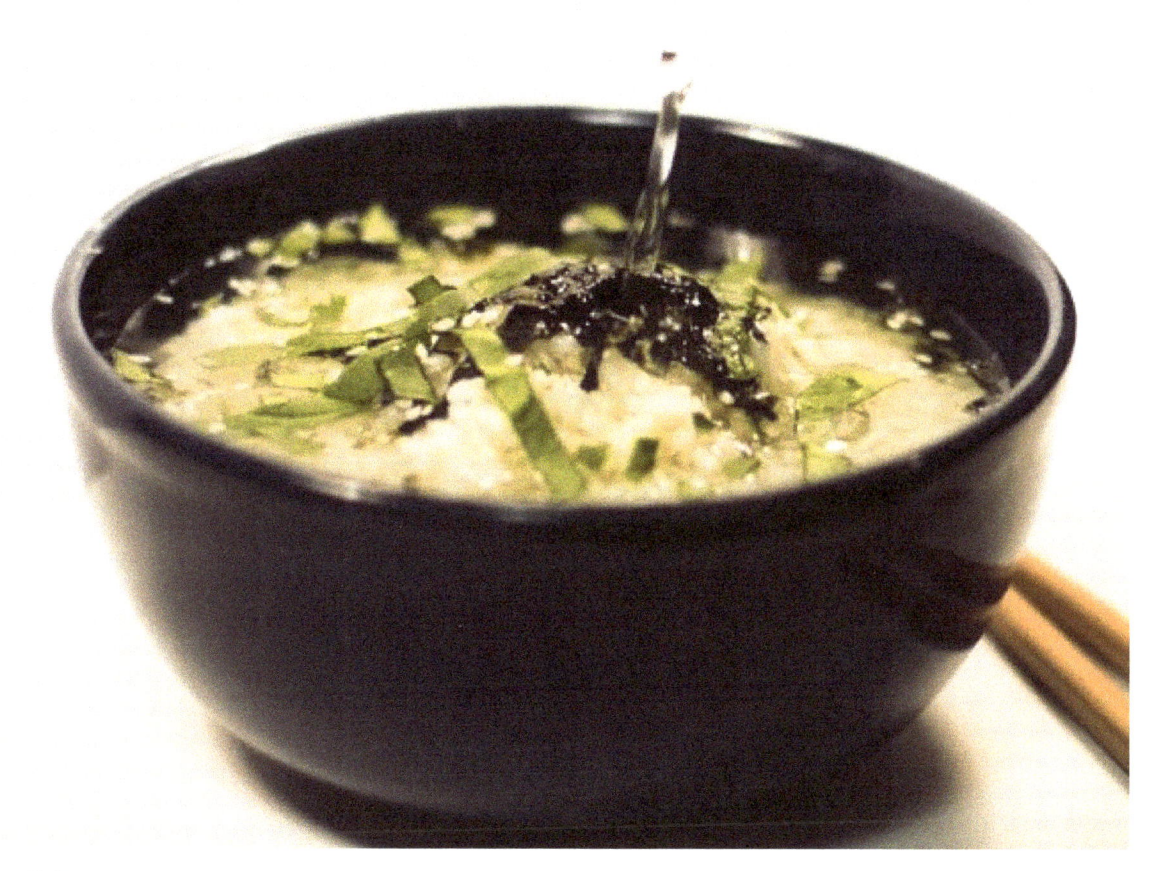

- Colon.
- Lymphatic gland
- Skin
- Kidney
- Liver
- Gallbladder.

The Various Types of Cleansing

Although there are various types of detoxification, I am going to center on fasting, which is the one approved by late Dr. Sebi.

Under the fasting method of detoxification, there are various types of fasting which include:

- **Dry fasting:** Under this type of fasting, you will abstain from food, water, juice, anything eatable or drinkable.

- **Liquid fasting:** under this type of fasting, you are to abstain from anything solid and consume only liquid-like; juice and any other liquid stuff without alcohol.
- **Water fasting:** under this type of fasting, you are to abstain from anything solid, juice, smoothies, etc. and consume only water.
- **Fruit fasting:** under this type of fasting, you are to avoid anything solid but survive mainly on fruit.
- **Raw food fasting:** under this type of fasting, you are to abstain completely from cooked food and survive mainly on veggies and fruit.
- **Smoothie fasting:** smoothie fasting is just like the fruit fasting; the only difference is the fact that under smoothie fasting, the fruit will be blended, and you will also consume blended veggies.

Bear in mind that Dr. Sebi approved 12 days fast with alkaline herbs, sea moss, spring water, and green smoothies which, must be made with fruit that is in Dr. Sebi's nutritional guide list.

The Step by Step Guide on How to Do an Intra-Cellular Cleansing

I will walk you through a step by step guide on how to do an intra-cellular cleansing with Dr. Sebi approved fast, alkaline herbs, diets, and green smoothies.

Let's get started. Irrespective of the type of fast (cleanse) that you want to undergo, you will still get results. Dr. Sebi recommends water fasting, but on the occasion that you won't be able to do the water fast, you can do the green smoothies or raw fruits and veggies fast.

There are symptoms that you will experience during the process of detoxifying or cleansing your body system, but you don't need to worry as the symptoms won't last more than a week. These symptoms include:

- The tongue might be discolored
- Insomnia or sleeplessness
- Experience cold or flu
- You might experience rashes or itching, pain, and ache
- Expel mucus
- Lack of energy (fatigue)
- You might experience breakouts
- Your bowel movement will change
- Blood pressure might be low (although this symptom is rare)

Chapter 13: The Major Risk Factors of Sexually Transmitted Diseases

Many factors can make you be at risk of having one or more sexually transmitted diseases. Some of these factors are:

- Underlining sexually transmitted infection.
- Tender or unhealthy age.
- Multiple sexual partners.
- Unsafe sex.
- Immune destroying drugs.
- Alcohol.
- Infectious homosexuality or bisexuality.
- The use of needle via injection/via sharp objects.

Underlining Sexually Transmitted Infection

Underlining infection means having a sexually transmitted infection before having another one. When you notice an unappealing discharge from your vaginal or blister in your penis, you do not have to engage in unprotected sex because this will make it very easy for you to contract another STDs.

The initial symptom you have, though not yet diagnosed, is a sign of an infection that you undermined. Since you already have exposure to std, it means that your sexual lifestyle might be putting you at risk.

Unhealthy Age

Sexually transmitted diseases, most times, do not affect elders. It occurs in the ages between 16 and 25. The vaginal of young is very susceptible to most of the causative agents of sexually transmitted diseases.

Ultimately, the young are more open to having multiple sexual partners and having sex that is not protected without paying attention to the fact that it might cause more harm than good.

Multiple Sexual Partners

Engaging in sexual intercourse with multiple individuals is one of the major factors that can put you at risk. You might think you are the only one that has multiple partners but, you also do not have it at the back of your mind that one or more of your sexual partners also have more sex partners. So, this is a long chain that you have to break to prevent yourself from these diseases.

Unsafe Sex

When you have intercourse without using any form of protection, you are putting yourself at serious risk. Vaginal or anal penetration by an infected individual who refuses to wear a latex condom will expressively increase your risk of having the infection.

Many sexually transmitted diseases, especially the ones caused by viruses, cannot be prevented with the use of latex condoms according to the report, but it can help you to some extent than having intercourse unsafely.

Immune Destroying Drugs

The use of drugs necessary for the treatment of erectile problems misused by individuals through having multiple sexes to confirm if the drug is effective brings about the exposure of sexually transmitted diseases.

Alcohol

Drinking can be awful for your sexual wellbeing from various perspectives. Individuals who normally use liquor, especially in social circumstances, are possibly less selective about whom they decide to engage in sexual relations with.

Dr. Sebi's History

Dr. Sebi was perceived as a well-known botanist who has rewarded a few people experiencing a few sicknesses, for example, herpes, HIV, cancer, diabetes, fibroid, hypertension, illicit drug use, body torment, explicitly transmitted maladies... and then some.

Specialist Sebi was a pathologist, botanist, characteristic advisor, conceived in Honduras in 1933. He was the top of the Usha research foundation in Honduras.

Dr. Sebi's basic eating regimens and spices are exceptionally successful against a few ailments. A portion of his antacid spices contains extraordinary detoxifying and purifying constituents.

His examinations and exploration of various types of soluble spices and plants have been in presence for a long time. During his examination and discoveries on plants and spices, he started to watch the plants that are viable against a few ailments and thus use them to fix victims that are experiencing various illnesses.

Specialist Sebi likewise gained data from his grandma, who with the assistance of a customary cultivator in Mexico, caused him to get mending from his burdensome sicknesses. These diseases are; corpulence, impotency, asthma, and diabetes.

Specialist Sebi likewise found that numerous normal soluble vegetables and organic products are stacked with materials that can empower, balance out, clean the body in the cell and intra-cell level.

He later centered on African plants and spices and proposed that most plants, for example, vegetables and organic products that are antacid, are fit for detoxifying the body and permit the body to be in a basic structure in this way forestalling the attack of illnesses.

These antacid plants play out their capacities by wiping out harmful parts that are amassed in the body and permitting significant minerals that are exhausted by the acidic degree of the body to get renewed.

Specialist Sebi contended that basic plants are equipped for battling infections. He said that maladies could possibly get by in the body when the acidic level is at its pinnacle. Along these lines, instilling a basic eating regimen can help evacuate abundance acids and restore the body back to its typical state/condition.

The Significance of Dr. Sebi's Diet

- Fights against sexually transmitted diseases.
- It contains very low fat, which prevents heart diseases and other heart malfunctions.
- Prevents and treats cancer.
- Prevents and treats stroke.
- It contains no cholesterol.
- It contains no alcohol.
- Prevents and cures diabetes.
- Cause most individuals who engage in the intake of the diet to experience loss of weight.
- Treats and prevents high blood pressure.
- It contains very low saturated fats, which also prevent major heart-related diseases.
- It contains no processed sugar.

Dr. Sebi's Forbidden Foods

Dr. Sebi's diets shun many foods that are not alkaline. Most of the foods you love eating are highly acidic, and this prevents the fast healing and cure in the body.

Examples of such foods include:

- Soy and soy products.
- Corn.
- Fish and seafood.
- Colors and flavors.
- Poultry products.
- Alcoholic products.
- The meat of all kinds.
- Eggs.
- Processed foods.
- Canned fruits.
- Foods fortified with vitamins and minerals
- Garlic.
- Genetically modified organism fruits.
- Seedless fruits.
- Foods with yeast or other components such as baking powder.
- Wheat.
- Fast foods.
- Genetically modified organism vegetables.
- Dairy products.
- Sugar

Chapter 14:   Dr. Sebi's Foods

All of the foods on Dr. Sebi's nutritional guide are healthy and will help to heal your body, but some foods are better than others. We will discuss the top ten foods that are on Dr. Sebi's nutritional guide. These foods will help your body in many different ways, and we will go over just how beneficial they are.

Peaches

The number of minerals and antioxidants that are present in peaches will help to slough off dead cells, and they are great at revitalizing and hydrating other cells. While peaches are most commonly associated with Georgia State, they were first cultivated in China. They are full of phosphorous, manganese, copper, potassium, niacin, Vitamin E, Vitamin A, Vitamin C, and dietary fiber.

Since peaches contain phosphorous, along with many other minerals, it helps to strengthen the teeth and bones. Phosphorous also helps to aid in the prevention of bone diseases, such as decalcification, which is what ends up causing osteoporosis. Consuming foods, like peaches, that are high in phosphorous as well as Vitamin C and calcium, play important parts in strengthening gums and jawbones, which keep teeth healthy.

Antioxidants, like zinc and Vitamin C, are needed for the normal functioning of the immune system. These antioxidants affect collagen healing, and, as such, wound healing. They also help to fight off infections. Zinc also contains anti-aging properties and also interferes with the aging process of the reproductive organs in men because it boosts the testosterone levels. Peaches, whether eaten or used on the skin, is a natural moisturizer. It has also been found that peaches also have a positive effect on the scalp to lower the chance of hair loss.

It has also been found that peaches decrease neurodegenerative disorders, like Alzheimer's. It can also decrease a person's risk of macular degeneration.

Plums

Plums will help to improve the immune defense of the body because it contains so many antioxidants. Plums contain more than 15 minerals and vitamins, as well as antioxidants and fiber. The dried version of plums is called prunes, and we all know that they are commonly used to help relieve constipation. Since the fiber content is insoluble, it helps to prevent constipation.

The antioxidants in plums help to reduce inflammation, and they can protect your cells from free radical damage. They have a high polyphenol antioxidant content, which positively affects bone health and can help to lower your risk for diabetes and heart disease. There are some studies that say that plums contain twice as much polyphenol antioxidants as peaches.

There are also properties in the plums that can help to regulate blood sugar. Even though they are high in carbs, plums don't cause a large increase in blood sugar levels once eaten. This is because of their adiponectin content, which is a hormone that helps to regulate blood sugar.

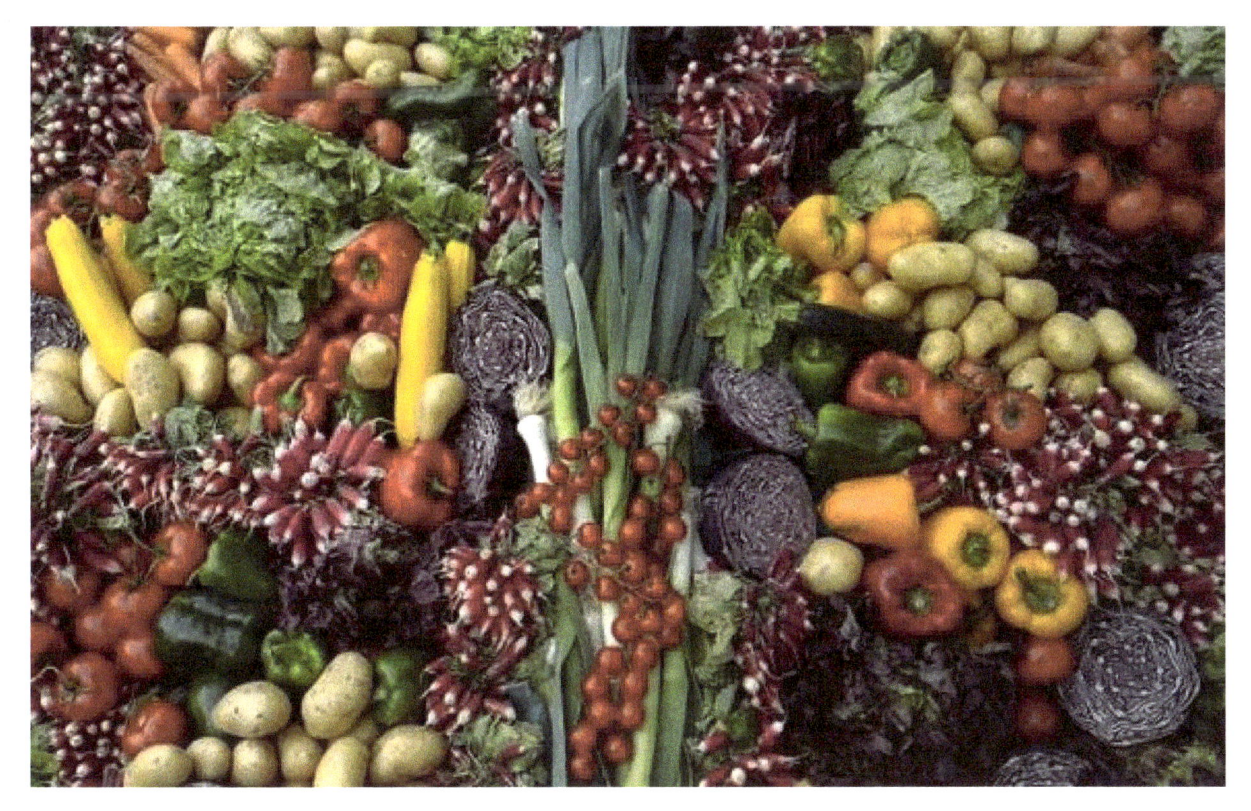

Watercress

It has been found that watercress is great at reversing the damage done to the DNA and white blood cells. Watercress is often overlooked but holds a lot of nutrients. It has a slightly peppery taste. Watercress was once considered a weed but was cultivated in the UK during the early 1800s. Its antioxidant content could help to lower a person's risk for chronic diseases.

Oxidative stress is connected to many chronic illnesses, which include cardiovascular disease, cancer, and diabetes. Fortunately, the antioxidants in watercress are able to protect your cells from oxidative stress, which will lower your odds of developing these illnesses. Watercress contains compounds that could help to protect you from cancer. It contains high amounts of phytochemicals, which lowers your cancer risk. It releases isothiocyanates when cut or chewed. Isothiocyanates include phenylmethyl sulforaphane and isothiocyanate, which are known to protect people against cancer.

Watercress also has dietary nitrates that help to improve the health of blood vessels by decreasing the thickness and stiffness of blood vessels and by reducing inflammation. It can also help to lower your cholesterol levels.

Watercress also contains phosphorous, potassium, magnesium, and calcium, which are all great for bone health. It can also boost the immune system because of its high vitamin C levels. Its vitamin C levels, along with its carotenoids, can help your eye health.

Cantaloupes

Cantaloupes contain phytochemicals and beta-carotene that help to fight off toxins. They also contain a healthy dose of antioxidants. According to the USDA, cantaloupes contain more beta-carotene than mangoes, nectarines, tangerines, peaches, oranges, grapefruit, and apricots. They contain the same amount of beta-carotene as carrots.

Beta-carotene is a carotenoid. Carotenoids are pigments that provide bright colors to fruits and vegetables. When you eat beta-carotene, your body converts it to vitamin A or works as an antioxidant to fight off free radicals that attack your body. Vitamin A is very nutrient for the immune system, red blood cells, and eye health.

A cup of balled cantaloupe has more than 100% of the recommended daily value in vitamin C. Vitamin C helps in the production of collagen, muscle, cartilage, and blood vessels. Cantaloupe also contains folate, which is vitamin B9. Folate is the term for vitamin B9 that is naturally present. Folic acid is what is used when vitamin B9 is added to foods or made into a supplement. Folate is great for women of childbearing age because it helps to prevent neural-tube birth defects.

Cantaloupe is also very high in water. In fact, it is 90% water. Besides water, it contains fiber. Both of these can help to prevent constipation and can help you to feel fuller longer.

Wakame

Researchers have found that wakame contains fucoxanthin that can inhibit the accumulation of fat in your cells and can also stimulate fat oxidation. Wakame has been cultivated in Korea and Japan for centuries. When added to salads and soups, it adds a unique texture and taste. It is very low in calories, only five per serving, but it is full of nutrients. A small amount of wakame can boost your intake of calcium, magnesium, folate, manganese, and iodine.

Chapter 15: Diagnosing and Acceptance

If you are struggling to come to terms with the fact that you have herpes, take a step back, and strive to think of it for what it is—a virus. A person who is ill with a cold doesn't blame himself for contracting sickness, and he is aware that his life isn't over due to the fact of it. Herpes is simply another infection, and while it would possibly affect your body in different ways, you can still treat and manage it just like any problem. It would take some time for you to get used to the way of life adjustments you'll have to implement to prevent passing the disease; however, having herpes doesn't have to change who you are essentially as a person. In fact, many people who have been diagnosed with herpes realize that their illness has made them a better person! When you carry a disease that can be passed to other people, you have to make some changes in your lifestyles to take accountability for yourself and for your actions. You can't go on living carelessly without any concern for others; you need to turn out to be a stronger as well as a more caring person in order to live through the period of your herpes.

Changes in the Lifestyle

While it is true that certain behaviors can increase your risk of contracting the disease, it is hard to come to terms with the idea that it might be your fault that you have herpes. Because herpes is a sexually transmitted infection (STI), your risk for contracting it increases with the number of sexual partners you have. People who only have a one-lifetime sexual partner have the lowest risk of contracting the disease, though it can still be spread through non-sexual contact. It is important to remember that the herpes virus can be transmitted through a number of different methods. You can contract oral herpes simply by sharing a glass of water with an infected person who has active sores or is currently shedding the virus. For oral contact, even a minimal amount of saliva can be enough to transmit the disease. Unlike some STIs, the host does not have to show open wounds in order to transmit the disease to an uninfected partner. If the person is unaware that they have herpes, or if they are aware but do not inform you of the risk, it cannot be your fault if you contract it even if it isn't technically your fault that you've contracted the herpes virus, you need to ask yourself some hard questions regarding whether or not it could have been prevented.

In summary:

- Having multiple sexual partners
- Contact with an open sore or crusted-over sore
- Unprotected sexual activity (oral, vaginal, anal, penetrative, etc.)
- Skin contact during asymptomatic shedding of the virus
- Close contact with an infected partner (touching, kissing, etc.)
- Contact with bodily fluids of an infected partner (saliva, blood, semen, vaginal

discharge)

Risk factors for outbreaks

During your life, you may undergo periods of remission. Periods at some stage in which your herpes flare-ups are called "outbreaks," and there are factors that may boom your hazard for an outbreak. A few of the factors that could result in outbreaks are:

Stress: Research has proven a hyperlink among durations of continual stress and recurrent herpes outbreaks, mainly in girls. Even brief-term stressors like an acute injury, flying in a plane, a stressful presentation at work can lead to an outbreak simply as easily as long-time period stressors like financial issues, ups and downs in a relationship, issues at the workplace, etc.

Menstruation: A study at the national institute of dental and craniofacial research discovered that oral herpes outbreaks could be brought about by way of menstruation in ladies. The hormonal modifications that occur during menstruation may perhaps be responsible for the extended chance for an outbreak because it may be a stressful time for both the mind and body. There are also a few research that advises that tampon use ought to worsen genital herpes outbreaks, as can the sporting of tight undies with sanitary pads. To help reduce the chances of a herpes outbreak for the duration of menstrual periods, try the use of non-chlorinated feminine hygiene products.

Exercise: A high-intensity workout is a form of stress for the body, and it can affect your immune activity, making way for a herpes outbreak. Exercise can additionally lead to immoderate perspiration and chafing, which can contribute to the development of herpes sores and lesions. Mild types of exercise, like taking walks or running, are the least probable to set off an outbreak.

Nutrition: Your dietary habits can play a vital role in increasing or decreasing your chance for a herpes outbreak. Some foods that are most likely to trigger an outbreak consist of coffee, alcohol, nuts, chocolate, dairy products, corn, soda, and unprocessed foods. Lysine is a dietary compound that can assist in preventing an outbreak; however, ingredients containing l-arginine (like chocolate and coffee) can actually suppress lysine.

Daylight/sunburn: Excessive exposure to daylight and sunburn can trigger the chances for an HSV-1 outbreak, especially when combined with emotional stress. Ultraviolet rays can simply block the activity of immune cells inside the pores and skin, which could lead to herpes outbreaks. Sunburn can cause skin inflammation, which also can result in outbreaks.

Dehydration: While your body is dehydrated, it exerts extra pressure, and the herpes virus may take benefit of one of these weak points and trigger an outbreak. This is common when your lips are cracked and dry due to dehydration.

Chapter 16: Benefits of Dr. Sebi's Diet

So, what is the usefulness of this diet? And why is Dr. Sebi's diet good for you?

Following this diet helps improve the health of people suffering from kidney disease. As would be explained below, some of the benefits of an alkaline diet include; helping to stop signs of aging, gradual loss of organs and cellular functions, slowing down the degeneration of bone mass and tissues which the availability of too much of acid in the body can rob us of important mineral nutrients which alkaline diet supplies.

Protects Muscle Mass and Bone Density

Researchers are of the view that when someone consumes more alkalizing fruits and vegetables, that individual is bound to be protected from Sarcopenia (decreased bone strength and muscle wasting due to aging), and as such, the intake of minerals which alkaline diet supplies plays a pivotal role in the development and maintenance of the structure of the bone.

By balancing the ratio of the important minerals like calcium, magnesium, and phosphate needed for maintaining lean muscle mass and building bones, an alkaline diet supports bone health. Also, there is improved production of growth hormones and vitamin D absorption through the alkaline diet, which helps protect bones and reduce other chronic health challenges.

Increased Muscle Mass

With having more muscle mass, one accomplishes many things even though that is far from your goal. A high level of muscle mass helps to increase your metabolic rate and burn away more fat. Dr. Sebi's diet has been known to preserve and increase your muscle mass.

There exists a study between two groups of men. One group followed a healthy eating pattern while the other operated on the 80/20 principle. Both groups operated on the same diet and the same workout. Our interest is the group that operated the 80/20 rule.

In the course of eight weeks, both groups gained an equal amount of muscle mass, only that the group that operated the alkaline diet lost more fat. It was evident that not only does one gain muscle mass operating on the alkaline diet, one tends to lose fat simultaneously also. The reason behind this is the increased growth hormone gained as a reason for alkalizing. With this hormone, there is a lot less muscle breakdown and more fat burnt, which is why this diet is vital for preserving and building muscle mass.

Increase Energy Levels

Feeling tired and lethargic because of a sugar crash causes the insulin level to spike up, which brings down your energy level and sends a signal to your brain, telling it to relax. With an Alkaline diet, you have more energy because there's no sign of insulin spikes throughout the day.

Since your body is in a normal starvation mode, you experience more energy because your body goes into a fight or flight response. This is when your body produces adrenaline throughout the day, giving you the needed energy to get along because your body feels it has to go on a hunting mission to get food. Note here that you will feel less energized at the beginning of your diet journey because it is still in the process of adjusting to these new changes. After the initial week or two, you will start noticing more energy to do more work, which in turn makes you feel a lot better.

Reduce Risk of Stroke and Hypertension

The increase in the production of growth hormone and the decrease of inflammation is one of the anti-aging effects derives from the consumption of Dr. Sebi's alkaline diet, which has led to protection against common health problems like hypertension, stroke, high cholesterol, kidney stones, and improved cardiovascular health. Research finds that growth hormone supports body composition and lowers the risk factors of a heart disease, which is the leading cause of death in the U.S.

An estimated 610,000 Americans die from it every year. Other contributing factors are an unhealthy lifestyle, which includes poor nutrition and low activity level. The risk of heart disease is being reduced when you abstain from red meat and consume a diet rich in low-fat dairy, seeds, fruits, and vegetables. A healthy body weight derives from the consumption of an alkaline diet produces fewer calories, which can also assist your heart.

Lowers Chronic Pain and Inflammation

Between the alkaline diet and reduced levels of chronic pain, we see a connection with the aid of studies carried out. It is found that chronic back pain, muscle spasms, headaches, inflammation, joint pain, and menstrual symptoms are the by-product of chronic acidosis. In Germany, a study conducted by the Society for Minerals and Trace Elements found out that 76 of our 82 patients with chronic back pain exposed to a daily dosage of alkaline supplement for four weeks reported a major decrease in pain as measured by the "Arhus rating scale for people with low back pain."

Body Detox and Cell Cleaning

When it comes to living a long and healthy life, detoxing the body is very important. Many methods exist out there through which people detox their bodies, and some of these methods don't usually work. It has been proven time and time again how the Alkaline diet helps detox the human body both on a cellular and digestive level, which makes it a superior cleaning agent when it comes to the body.

On a Cellular Level, an alkaline diet detoxifies the body by removing the bad cells and replacing them with healthier and stronger cells in a process called Autophagy. With this process comes benefits like; stronger immune system, prevention of diseases, insulin sensitivity, and reduction in the risk of cancer, which is great news.

Considering how the body can be detoxified with the help of the alkaline diet from a digestive level, one can see that there is a connection between the stomach and the brain. This is according to studies carried out, which implies that if the digestive system is not functioning at its best, the brain won't either, and is the reason people call the human gut a second brain.

Chapter 17: Dealing With the Herpes Stigma

If you've followed the recommendations in this book, herpes should no longer be a major issue for you. We've discovered how herpes outbreaks are primarily related to dietary and lifestyle conditions, and some proper nutrients, supplements, and habit changes can quickly rid yourself of the pesky virus.

The reason herpes is "the world's most annoying virus" is not so much because of the outbreaks, as it is the social stigma associated with having it.

Herpes is considered a social taboo. It's used as an insult against people (that **** probably has herpes), is used to defame people as "sluts" or "whores" (nonsense, you can catch HSV-2 from light contact) and it's used by people who probably have HSV-2 without realizing it to denigrate others.

Which is a shame considering it's one of the most benign illnesses. HSV-1 does have some dangerous health ramifications, but HSV-2 (genital herpes) does not—unless you have an autoimmune disorder like HIV.

So why would anybody make something seem worse than it really is? The answer is profit.

Because it's such a common illness, by scaring or shaming the people who catch it, it's possible to up the sales of Valtrex or whatever the latest pharmaceutical is. That's tens of millions of potential customers.

This is why many doctors indirectly exaggerate HSV in the media or on commercials. You'll never hear them say, "if you're one of the 2-4% who actually develops chronic HSV symptoms..." As far as they're concerned, everybody who is infected needs immediate pharmaceutical treatment.

So now you have to deal with the ramifications of this.

Telling Your Partner About HSV

So, now you're in the awkward position of having to explain to your significant other about being infected with genital herpes. Mainstream advice says: "tell your partner right away, always use condoms and take anti-viral medication to lessen your partner's chance of contracting the disease."

What this common advice does not mention is the fact most people are terrified of HSV, and it's not uncommon, at all, for boyfriends and girlfriends to leave their partners over such a matter. This is not an easy subject to bring up!

In addition, there's no mention of the severe side-effects of anti-viral, and some doctors suggest taking them for the rest of your life to keep your partner from becoming infected!

While yes, obviously you need to tell your partner right away, I suggest approaching the topic from a slightly different frame of mind:

Explain You Have Hsv-2 Not "Genital Herpes"

Hysteria and taboos sometimes surround words and concepts more than anything else. Call the virus what it really is. One of the reasons genital herpes is a bit of a misnomer is because sometimes HSV-2 isn't even located on the genitals, so if you're diagnosed with it, consult with your doctor to see if it's even latent on your nether region or not.

Explain the Virus Is Dormant and Prove It With a Medical Test

Prove your low viral count and dormant nature of the illness by having a urine test.

Give a Copy of This Book and Explain Hsv-2 Is Not a Threat

You can use the amazon lending option to give your partner a free copy of this book herpes is only a threat if it endangers the integrity of your relationship. Explain the truth that catching HSV-2 is not a big deal, unlike what media/society/commercials say. Furthermore, provide some of the pamphlets provided by the herpes virus association.

Explain That You Take Natural Anti-Virals and You Lead a Lifestyle to Minimize Chances of Spreading It

Don't take dangerous anti-viral pharmaceuticals if you're not having reoccurring outbreaks, and you don't need it. But, reassure your partner that you're taking all the necessary precautions to prevent infecting anybody else.

Ask Him/Her If They've Ever Had a Cold Sore Before

If so, they are infected with HSV-1, a far more dangerous form of herpes. Explain 30-40% of the adult population also has HSV-2, and the number is growing.

Tell My Partner

This is a moral question, for which the answer is obviously "yes", but I can perfectly understand why many people debate the idea. Given the severe social taboo of the virus, we've almost reached a point where people have no choice but to hide the fact they're infected, and I don't blame them. I don't condone it, but I perfectly understand why people feel this way.

It comes down to you, you can either be honest about your illness and risk having your partner leave you, or be a liar and hide it, and if it becomes apparent later that you're infected (or if he/she catches it from you), you'll risk having your partner leave you, and you'll be called a liar.

However, the big problem with revealing to a partner about herpes infection is that it's not realistic at the beginning of a relationship to wear the disease around your neck as a badge of dishonor. If you're single, and you meet the future love of your life, and you guys are tearing each other's clothes off in the heat of passion, do you really think this is a good time to say "wait, baby, I'm infected with genital herpes!"

Seriously, you'll never date again. Until the time the social taboo of HSV-2 is lifted, this is going to remain a big issue for everybody who's infected (which is currently 60+ million Americans).

For this reason, if you opt to not disclose herpes, make sure your viral count is as low as it can go, and obviously wear a condom for added protection. The odds of a new partner contracting herpes, in this case, is very small.

Obviously, if you're having any kind of outbreak whatsoever, you have to refrain from sex. And furthermore, if you're entering a relationship or a reoccurring series of physical encounters, reread the above steps for explaining your infection properly so as not to harm your relationship.

Chapter 18:   HIV

HIV harms the immune system by killing the white blood cells that you need to fight off infections. This places a person at risk for developing some serious infections and certain types of cancers. Once HIV reaches its final stages, it becomes AIDS, but not everybody who contracts HIV will develop AIDS. For a long time, people thought HIV and AIDS were one and the same, but they aren't.

The most common way for HIV to be spread is through unprotected sex with an HIV positive person. It can also be spread through shared drug needles or contact with the blood of an infected person. Women are also able to give it to their children during childbirth or pregnancy.

Some of the first signs of an HIV infection could be flu-like symptoms and swollen glands. These could also come and go within a couple of weeks to a month. You may not experience severe symptoms until several months or years later. You could experience a primary infection or acute HIV. Most of those who have been infected will develop flu-like symptoms within a couple of months after exposure. This is what is known as the primary infection. Some of the most common signs of the primary infection are:

- Swollen lymph glands, mostly in the neck
- Painful mouth sores and sore throat
- Rash
- Joint pain and muscle aches
- Headache
- Fever

It is possible that these symptoms could be so mild that they may go unnoticed. However, how much of the virus you have in your bloodstream is very high during this stage. This is why the infection will spread more easily during this time than once you reach the next stage.

The next stage is the latent clinical infection or chronic HIV. For some, they will still have swollen lymph nodes. Otherwise, there aren't any really specific symptoms and signs. HIV will say in the body and your white blood cells. If one does not get diagnosed and receive some sort of therapy, this stage can last for ten years. Some people will develop severe secondary diseases a lot sooner.

With better antiviral medicines, most HIV patients don't develop AIDS. If left untreated, HIV will normally turn into AIDS within ten years. Once AIDS develops, the immune system has already been severely damaged. It places a person at a higher risk of opportunistic cancers or infections, which are a disease that a person with a healthy immune system wouldn't have to worry about. The most common signs and symptoms of these secondary infections could include:

- Skin bumps or rashes
- Weight loss
- Persistent and unexplained fatigue
- Persistent white spots or odd lesions in your mouth or on the tongue
- Chronic diarrhea
- Recurring fever
- Soaking night sweats

HIV can only be spread through sex or contact with blood, or from mother to child during childbirth, pregnancy, or breastfeeding. When it comes to contact with blood, the blood has to entire a mucous membrane, such as the nose, mouth, anus, or vagina. Simply touching infected blood won't spread HIV, and once the blood is dried, it isn't dangerous.

The most common ways for HIV to be spread are:

- **Sex:** This is one of the most common ways for it to be spread. You can get infected by having unprotected oral, anal, or vaginal sex with an infected person whose vaginal secretions, semen, or blood enters your body. The virus is able to enter into the body through mouth sores or through small tears that can occur in the vagina or rectum during sex.
- **Blood Transfusions:** At one time, people could end up contracting HIV through a blood transfusion. Nowadays, American blood banks and hospitals screen the blood for HIV antibodies, so the odds of this happening now are small.
- **Sharing Needles:** The second most common way for HIV to be spread is by sharing contaminated intravenous drug paraphernalia. This also puts you at a higher risk of contracting other infectious diseases, like hepatitis.
- **Breastfeeding, Pregnancy, or Delivery:** HIV-positive Mothers can pass it onto their babies. Mothers who make sure that they are receiving treatment are able to lower the risk of passing it along.

Some rumors and lies were spread during the HIV epidemic in the '80s, and unfortunately, some of those have persisted. All of these beliefs can be dispelled through simple research and common sense. The most common misconception is how it is spread. Many people are afraid to touch an HIV-positive person because they think they can contract it that way, but you can't. HIV cannot be contracted through ordinary contact. This means that you are not able to get it by shaking hands, dancing, kissing or hugging somebody that is infected. It also cannot be spread through insect bites, water, or air. It is actually very hard to catch.

HIV also doesn't care about your color or sexual orientation. While the bulk of the infections in the US back in the '80s seemed to affect men who had sexual intercourse with other men, it is now clear that it can be spread through heterosexual sexual intercourse as well. People of any sexual orientation, sex, race, or age can become infected.

Chapter 19: Precautions Regarding pH Balance & the Alkaline Diet

As with beginning any diet or new way of eating, there are some important factors to consider when choosing the alkaline diet. First, determine if you have any health conditions that could be impacted by a change in your pH levels. For most, if not all, health conditions, an alkaline diet is one of the best plans to follow, though it's always a good idea to clear any potential issues with a medical professional. If you have any allergies or food sensitivities, this could be the result of a temporary sensitivity or effect of a condition that may be resolved through a change in diet. If the food(s) you have an allergic reaction to happen to be acidic in nature, then the solution is as simple as eliminating them from your diet. If the food item is more alkaline, it can be substituted for an alternative until the sensitivity disappears or changes altogether.

When adapting to an alkaline-based meal plan, always note your body's reaction to certain foods and combinations of foods. Even when you reduce the level of acidity in your diet, avoid adding too much sugar or salt to your foods. Fruits have their natural sugar, fructose, which is easily digested and used by the body, unlike processed or artificial sweeteners. Salt is good as long as we get the required amount through our diet, though adding too much can elevate blood pressure and contribute to hypertension.

Unless you have severe allergies or must avoid certain foods due to conflicts with medication or other medical conditions, the alkaline diet is a very nutritious way to eat. By planning your meals carefully, you can ensure that all nutrient requirements are met and to avoid deficiencies. General guidelines to take into consideration when beginning the alkaline diet are fairly easy to follow:

- **Drink plenty of water.** If eight glasses a day is too much to strive for, then drink natural teas and sparkling water.
- **Keep track of any adverse reactions during your diet.** If your body reacts in a negative way, such as indigestion or high blood pressure, it could be that some of the foods you are selecting may not be as alkaline as perceived.
- **Stay active.** This is a good idea regardless of the diet you follow, as exercise prevent many conditions, improve cardiovascular function, heart health, and increase oxygen levels in your body.
- **Make small changes at first to incorporate alkaline foods into your diet without making a drastic overhaul of your diet.** This will allow your body to become adjusted to the new types of foods you'll be getting used to over some time.

Achieve Permanent Results

The alkaline diet can produce very positive results on your health and well-being. If you suffer from chronic pain and conditions associated with a highly acidic environment, this way of eating will provide substantial relief. The success of your diet determines how well and consistent it is followed and incorporated into your lifestyle. Some people consider dieting as a temporary, and once they achieve a specific goal or level of weight loss or a similar result, they switch back to their previous food choices. To achieve permanent results, consistency in the way you eat, exercise, and live are essential in maintaining good health. Incorporating alkaline foods into your everyday meals and food options is the best way to meet your goals and maintain the benefit of a healthy lifestyle indefinitely.

Keeping a consistently healthy and budget-friendly shopping list that includes a roster of your favorite alkaline foods is a good way to stay on track. If you find yourself leaning towards more acidic food options, weigh the benefits of incorporating the food items into your current diet, or find a suitable substitute, if possible. Once your body grows accustomed to alkaline foods, you'll notice a shift in your cravings and what you enjoy. This is a positive change that indicates your body is adjusting to a new set of "rules" for eating, and over time, this will become routine and easy.

Chapter 20: Healthy Lifestyle

There is, of course, a healthy lifestyle question. Once you've made up your mind to change the way you think about this problem and then you have also determined the best physical treatment to apply in your case, it's time to ponder how you can perfect your lifestyle. This isn't geared towards boosting the ego, however. The goal is to make yourself feel happy, have peace, and prepare your mind for the best things that can happen to you. The storm has passed; your skies are clear.

You will have to make big, drastic changes but don't worry. Just remind yourself that the battle is all in your mind. It has to start there and end there. But how can you strengthen your resolve and your thinking for a better and healthier lifestyle?

Train your mind

Our mind is a trainable piece of machinery. First, you can train your brain in such a way that you can have a mind that has the ability to focus, and for our discussion, the object of focus is a "healthy lifestyle" appropriate for genital herpes sufferers.

Mind focus is very important

Here is the challenge when someone is trying to train the mind to be focused. Every day, so many things demand our attention. There are emails, people, calls, and in the business setting, clients that we need to attend to.

Understand that the brain is prone to get disturbed by distractions. How do you overcome distractions so that you can stay focused and true to the promise to change – for example, a promise that "that was the last stick that I will ever smoke" or a pledge "that I will exercise one hour a day to fill myself with fresh oxygen?"

- **Refrain from multitasking.** Multitasking reduces your intelligence. In fact, you tend to make more mistakes when multitasking. Plus, the emotional rewards are high, so you become emotionally high as well, which may lead to forgetting about the tasks which deserve more attention.

- **Do the most important things in the morning.** The brain gets tired as the day goes by. Every decision that we make drains the brain, but typically, what we do is work on simple things in the morning, leaving the difficult ones to be attended to towards the end of the day. Whatever lifestyle changes you are applying, do it while you can still call it "morning." Or if it works better for you, determine the time of the day when your mind can focus best, and then allocate that time to doing the toughest or most important tasks.

- **Train your mind like you are training your muscles.** This means focusing on only one task every time and sticking to finishing it no matter what. You may not be able to do this easily at the first attempt so, do it in time "chunks." At first, you can have five minutes for that task, 10 minutes the next time you tackle it, and so on. If you get distracted, just go back to the task at hand.

Health tasks at hand

You may be led to believe that you need a special set of life changes to implement because of the uniqueness of your condition. Don't ever believe that. You have a disease that's common to many, and the required life changes are just the common ones. There are variations, perhaps, but even if there really are variations, they need not be so outstanding for making things complicated. You can start out with the following healthy living strategies:

- **Strengthen your immune system**: Every part of the body functions better when shielded from external assaults and boosted by the things that improve overall health. Some of your most powerful enemies are smoking, bad eating habits, daily activities that promote the sedentary type of lifestyle, and things that cause people to put on more weight. Smoking is poisonous while bad food choices can cause gastrointestinal problems. You are required to exercise so that it will be easier for your body to release toxins and take in fresh oxygen. If your work environment requires you to sit down in front of a computer for hours, it's time to find another job. Your body is designed to do a lot of movements, so keep moving. Do gardening and a lot of climbing of stairs. Start getting involved in sports or fitness.

  Fruits and vegetables can help. These are foods that will keep you away from common diseases like the flu. If you experience fewer incidences of flu, it's probably because there's something good that's happening to your immune system. Yogurt is another powerful food as it has the ability to rid our intestines and stomach of harmful bacteria. If the gastrointestinal tract is clean, it will become easier for your system to absorb nutrients, which in turn can help in promoting blood circulation. Oats and barley are perfect sources of fiber. Some studies discovered these food items to have the power to protect animals from contracting influenza, anthrax, and herpes. Consume garlic, shellfish, and chicken soup as well.

- **Reduce stress:** Thank goodness we are now aware of the demons that stress can bring into our lives. It has been shown that there is a big link between stress and illness. Make sure you learn about stress and how it can affect your physical and mental well-being.

  For starters, do meditation activities which have been discovered to have the ability to change brain neural pathways. You can also use deep breathing, which can lower your blood pressure and heart rate.

  Another strategy is spending your time "at the moment." When you do that, you will be able to focus on your senses. That will help you relax and help you feel in control. You can also do relationship strengthening, water decompression, and laughing out loud for this purpose.

- **Strengthen your relationship:** You must strive to be happy, and one of the ways you can easily achieve that is by developing relationships. This is time to be social rather than reclusive. You have to be more aggressive and assertive because, just like everyone, you deserve to have space in the social sphere where you can build and strengthen relationships.

While there, be the one to first promote peace rather than trouble. While you strengthen yourself, try to strengthen others as well. It will feel so good you'd probably sense the demonic viruses hurriedly getting from away from you.

There are so many demons that we face every day, so be aware of these forces all the time. You can actually take everything that's happening to you as parts of one big spiritual battle. Strive to win and to be free.

Chapter 21: Alkaline Diet Recipes to Get Rid of Herpes

1. Tofu Frittata With Corn and Vegan Cheese Recipe

Simple and easy, this 15-minute frittata blends tofu, peppers, corn, and vegan cheese with creamy avocado for a one-pot meal that can be enjoyed any time of the day.

Preparation time: 15 minutes

Cooking time: 10 minutes

Servings: 4

Ingredients:

2 tablespoons extra-virgin olive oil

3 links tofu, cut into quarters

1 small onion, diced

Kosher salt and freshly ground black pepper

½ cup crumbled feta, preferably Bulgarian

1 jalapeño, diced

1 yellow bell pepper, diced

1 orange bell pepper, diced

1 ripe avocado, diced

½ cup cilantro leaves

1 ear of corn then kernels cut off the cob

Directions:

Adjust the broiler rack from the heat source to 10 inches, and preheat the broiler to high.

Heat oil over medium-high heat in a 12-inch skillet, until shimmering. Attach the onion and cook, stirring for about 2 minutes, until softened. Top with pepper and salt. Stir in jalapeño, bell peppers, corn, and tofu and cook for about 6 minutes until browned.

Switch to broiler and cook for around 3 minutes, until the top is set. Allow the frittata to cool a bit, then use a spatula to loosen the bottom and sides. Flip out the frittata carefully using a plate larger than the saucepan. Cut into wedges and serve with sliced cilantro and avocado.

Nutrition:

Calories: 240

Carbohydrates: 4g

Fat: 18g

Protein: 17g

2. Alkaline Cauliflower Fried Rice

Preparation time: 5 minutes

Cooking time: 5 minutes

Servings: 4

Ingredients:

1 zucchini (courgette)

1 inch fresh root ginger

1 inch fresh root turmeric

1 large cauliflower

1/2 bunch of kale (any variety)

1 tablespoon coconut oil

1 bunch of coriander

1/2 bunch parsley (any variety)

1 bunch mint

1 tablespoon tamari soy sauce or bragg liquid aminos

1 lime

4 spring onions

2 handfuls almonds

Optional

1 green chili

Instead of ginger and fresh turmeric, use 1 teaspoon of each powdered

Directions:

Begin by making the rice of cauliflower—it's very easy—just split the cauli into small florets and chop it into your blender or food processor and pulse until it's like rice. Unless you don't have the blender, you can only grate it and get an effect that is very close.

Now is veggie preparation time, so thinly slice your kale, quarter and then thinly slice the courgette (zucchini) and chop all your herbs roughly (discard the basil and parsley stems, but keep the coriander stems) next, prepare your ginger and turmeric—first by peeling them (for quick peeling, just scrape back of a spoon over the ginger/turmeric—sweet!) And then rub them in a big bowl.

Stir the coriander into the mix including the stems as this begins warming up.

Stir in the cauliflower after 30 seconds and then the kale after another 2 min-3 minutes, add the spring onions and then the rest of the herbs, the bragg/tamari and stir through—and then remove from the heat—the total cooking time will be less than 5 minutes—you don't want it to go too soft!

Now chop and mix the almonds roughly, season to taste, and add lime juice according to your favorite.

Nutrition:

Calories: 109.5

Fat: 7.5g

Cholesterol: 93.5g

Carbohydrates: 6.8g

Protein: 5.3g

3. Creamy Avocado Cilantro Lime Dressing Recipe

Preparation time: 20 minutes

Cooking time: 10 minutes

Servings: 6-8

Ingredients:

¼ cup olive oil

¼ teaspoon of sea salt

½ cup cilantro, chopped

¼ cup plain goat yogurt

Juice of ½ lime

1 teaspoon lime zest

1 avocado

1 clove garlic, peeled

½ jalapeno, chopped

¼ teaspoon pepper

½ teaspoon cumin

Directions:

Place/put all the ingredients in a food processor or mixer and mix it until well balanced.

Nutrition:

Calories: 123

Protein: 1g

Fat: 12g

Carbohydrate: 3.6g

Sugar: 0.8g

4. Creamy Avocado Dressing

Preparation time: 5 min

Cooking time: 5 min

Servings: 4

Ingredients:

1/4 teaspoon ground black pepper

Water, as needed

1 whole large avocado

1 clove garlic, peeled

1/2 tablespoon fresh lime or lemon juice

3 tablespoons olive oil or avocado oil

1/4 teaspoon kosher salt

Directions:

Put the peeled clove of garlic, lime or lemon juice, avocado, olive oil, salt, and pepper into a mini food processor.

Process till smooth, stopping a few times to scrape the sides down. Thin the salad dressing out with some water (1/4 cup to 1/2 cup) before a perfect consistency is achieved.

Maintain/keep at least a week in an airtight container, but 3 to 4 days is best.

Nutrition:

Calories: 38.2

Total fat: 2.6g

Saturated fat: 0.6g

Cholesterol: 1.2mg

Sodium: 8.8mg

Potassium: 76.9mg

Total carbohydrates: 3.6g

Dietary fiber: 1.0g

Sugars: 0.9g

5. Southwestern Avocado Salad Dressing

This avocado salad dressing salad packs a punch of cilantro and lime flavor. It is full of good avocado fat and adds a delicious twist to every salad in the southwest!

Preparation time: 5 minutes

Cooking time: 1 hour

Servings: 8

Ingredients:

1 ripe avocado

1 cup buttermilk

1/2 teaspoon garlic powder

1/2 teaspoon chipotle chili powder

1/2 teaspoon salt

1/4 cup cilantro

Juice of 1/2 lime

1 teaspoon ranch seasoning powder homemade or store-bought

Directions:

Break the avocado in half, extract the pit from the flesh and scoop the skin.

Attach all the other ingredients together to a mixer.

Blend in until creamy and smooth.

Prior to serving, refrigerate for one hour.

Keeps in the refrigerator for 3 days.

Nutrition:

Calories: 61 - Calories from fat: 36

Total fat: 4g - Saturated fat: 1g

Cholesterol: 3mg - Total carbohydrates: 4g

Dietary fiber: 1g - Sugars: 1g

Protein: 1g

6. Brain-Boosting Smoothie Recipe

Preparation time: 5 minutes

Cooking time: 5 minutes

Servings: 1

Ingredients:

½ avocado

½ banana

½ cup blueberries

6 walnuts

1 scoop vanilla whey protein powder

½ cup of water

Directions:

Add/put all ingredients to blender then blend until a smooth texture is reached.

Nutrition:

Calories: 400

Fat: 13g

Protein: 7g

Carbohydrates: 68g

Fiber: 10g

Sugar: 50g

Vitamin A: 70% RDA

Vitamin C: 201% RDA

Calcium: 9% RDA

Iron: 27% RDA

7. Lemon Avocado Salad Dressing

This creamy dressing, with its strong lemon taste, is a refreshing change of pace, not one that you can find on the shelves of the groceries. My uncle shared the recipe with me in California.

Preparation time: 5 minutes

Cooking time: 5 minutes

Servings: 2-3

Ingredients:

2 tablespoons olive oil

1 garlic clove, minced

1/2 teaspoon seasoned salt

1 medium ripe avocado, peeled and mashed

1/4 cup water

2 tablespoons sour cream

2 tablespoons lemon juice

1 tablespoon minced fresh dill or 1 teaspoon dill weed

1/2 teaspoon honey

Salad greens, cherry tomatoes, sliced cucumbers, and sweet red and yellow pepper strips

Directions:

In a blender, combine the first nine ingredients; cover and process until blended. Serve with salad greens, tomatoes, cucumbers, and peppers. Store in the refrigerator.

Nutrition:

Calories: 38.2 - Total fat: 2.6 g

Saturated fat: 0.6 g - Cholesterol: 1.2mg

Carbohydrate: 3.6g - Fiber: 1.0g

8. Avocado Salad With Bell Pepper and Tomatoes

Avocado shells make convenient vessels made with the scooped-out flesh for a vivid salad. The dressing is flavored with lime juice, garlic, and a pinch of cayenne. The salad may also be used as a quesadillas topping, or as a new filling for tacos.

Preparation time: 5 minutes

Cooking time: 5 minutes

Servings: 2-3

Ingredients:

Coarse salt

1 firm, ripe avocado, halved and pitted

6 cherry tomatoes, halved

1 teaspoon extra-virgin olive oil

Juice of 1/2 lime

1 scallion, trimmed and thinly sliced

1 tablespoon chopped fresh cilantro leaves, with whole leaves for garnish

1 small garlic clove, minced

Pinch of cayenne pepper

1/2 yellow bell pepper, ribs & seeds removed, diced

Directions:

Whisk the olive oil, lime juice, garlic, and cayenne together in a small bowl. Season with the salt.

From the avocado halves, scoop out the flesh, conserve shells, and chop. Switch to a bowl and add chopped cilantro, bell pepper, onions, scallion.

Drizzle with salt and season with dressing. Stir gently to mix. Mix spoon into allocated containers. Garnish with whole leaves of cilantro and serve right away.

Nutrition:

Calories: 424 - Fiber: 16.36g

Saturated fat: 5g - Carbohydrates: 31.25g

Fat: 34.63g Protein: 6.6g

9. Avocado Salad

Preparation time: 10 minutes

Cooking time: 5 minutes

Servings: 4

Ingredients:

1 avocado, finely chopped

3 tablespoons boiled corn

1 tomato, thinly chopped

1 tablespoon extra-virgin olive oil

Salt to taste

1 tablespoon lemon juice

3 green onions, chopped

Directions:

In a large bowl, whisk in chopped avocado and lemon juice.

In the same bowl, mix it with other ingredients, except for tomato.

Serve on slices of bread with sliced tomatoes.

Nutrition:

Calories: 119

Fat: 8.7g

Cholesterol: 125mg

Carbohydrates: 3.4g

Protein: 7.2g

10. Avocado Vegan Caprese Salad

Preparation time: 5 minutes

Cooking time: 5 minutes

Servings: 1

Ingredients:

1 1/2 teaspoons balsamic vinegar

Generous pinch of sugar

3 slices fresh vegan cheese

Fresh basil leaves

2 cups fresh arugula

2-3 campari or cocktail style tomatoes sliced

1/2 avocado pitted and sliced

1 tablespoon extra-virgin olive oil

Kosher salt and freshly ground black pepper

Directions:

In a serving bowl, add the arugula, onion, avocado slices, and vegan cheese.

Fill with leaves of broken or slivered basil.

With the balsamic vinegar, sugar, whisk the extra virgin olive oil in a small bowl and season with kosher salt and freshly ground black pepper to taste and pour over the salad.

Throw coat and serve.

Nutrition:

Calories: 164.2

Fat: 11.8g

Cholesterol: 10.0mg

Carbohydrates: 11.6g

Fiber: 4.7g

Sugar: 5g

Protein: 5.4g

11. Avocado Seitan Salad With Arugula

Preparation time: 10 minutes

Cooking time: 5 minutes

Servings: 1

Ingredients:

2 green onions, sliced thinly

8 cherry tomatoes, halved (or a mix of yellow and red)

¾ pound seitan fillet

1 avocado, pitted, peeled and chopped

1 small (raw) zucchini, thinly sliced in half-moons

4 radishes, thinly sliced

1 recipe avocado citrus dressing

Directions:

Preheat to 400 ° f on the oven. Line a small saucepan with parchment paper.

Arrange the seitan on the pan, skin down, and bake for 10 to 12 minutes until just cooked.

Warm slightly, cut fat, flake flesh, and set aside.

Divide arugula between serving plates. Top with seitan and avocado, courgettes, red onion, and tomatoes.

Serve in citrus dressing with creamy avocado

Nutrition:

Calories: 320 - Fat: 32g

Cholesterol: 5mg - Potassium: 210mg

Carbohydrates: 6g

Fiber: 3g - Protein: 6g

12. Dr. Sebi Alkaline Spaghetti Squash Recipe

Preparation time: 10 minutes

Cooking time: 30 minutes

Servings: 4

Ingredients:

1 spaghetti squash

Grapeseed oil

Sea salt

Cayenne powder (optional)

Onion powder (optional)

Directions:

Preheat your oven to 375°f

Carefully chop off the ends of the squash and cut it in half.

Scoop out the seeds into a bowl.

Coat the squash with oil.

Season the squash and flip it over for the other side to get baked. When properly baked, the outside of the squash will be tender.

Allow the squash to cool off, then, use a fork to scrape the inside into a bowl.

Add seasoning to taste.

Dish your alkaline spaghetti squash!

Nutrition:

Calories: 672

Carbohydrates: 65g

Fat: 47g

Protein: 12g

13. Dr. Sebi Alkaline Mushroom Chickpea Burgers Recipe

Preparation time: 20 minutes

Cooking time: 30 minutes

Servings: 8

Ingredients:

2 portobello mushrooms

2 cups cooked chickpeas

2 tablespoons Onion powder

2 tablespoons Himalayan sea salt

2 tablespoons Oregano

1/2 cup cilantro

1/4 cup garbanzo bean flour

1/2 tablespoon. Cayenne

1/2 cup green peppers

1/2 cup red and white onions

Food processor or blender

1/4 measurement cup

Directions:

Chop the mushrooms into chunks and dice the vegetables.

Place all the ingredients in a food processor and pulse for 3 seconds.

Check for consistency, if it's too wet, add more flour then scoop into a bowl.

Set your cooker to medium heat and sprinkle grapeseed oil into the skillet.

Scoop the blend into a cup and turn it over to your cooking surface.

Allow the blend to for 5 minutes on each side. Apply caution when flipping so that the blend can stay together.

Your alkaline mushroom/chickpea burgers are ready to be served.

Nutrition:

Calories: 225 - Carbohydrates: 22.5g

Fat: 14.2g - Protein: 11.4g

14. Dr. Sebi Alkaline Veggie Fajitas Recipe

Preparation time: 10 minutes

Cooking time: 20 minutes

Servings: 6-12

Ingredients:

Fixings:

1/2 cups cut green and red peppers

1/2 cups cut red and white onions

3 cups cut mushrooms

2 tablespoon Ocean salt

2 tablespoon Onion powder

2 tablespoon Sweet basil

2 tablespoon Oregano

1/2 tablespoon Cayenne powder

Juice from 1/2 of a lime

Grapeseed oil

Alkaline spelt tortillas

Alkaline guacamole (discretionary)

Alkaline mango salsa (discretionary)

If you would prefer not to utilize mushrooms in this formula, you can essentially preclude them and cut each preparing down the middle

Directions:

Make your mushrooms, bell peppers, and onions into long strips.

Set your cooker to medium heat then sprinkle a tablespoon of grapeseed oil on the skillet.

Sprinkle another tablespoon of grapeseed oil on a large skillet.

Mix your vegetables and seasoning, then, sauté for 5 minutes.

Serve them on spelt tortillas with the guacamole and salsa.

Your alkaline veggie fajitas are ready to be dished.

Nutrition:

Calories: 257 - Fat: 2g - Saturated fat: 0.4g

Protein: 12.9g - Carbohydrate: 50.3g

Sugar: 8g

15. Dr. Sebi Alkaline Roasted Tomato Sauce Recipe

Preparation time: 15 minutes

Cooking time: 40 minutes

Servings: 6

Ingredients:

18 Roma tomatoes

1/2 red bell pepper

1/2 sweet onion

1/2 red onion

1 medium shallot

1/8 cup grapeseed oil

1 tablespoon agave

3 teaspoons sea salt

3 teaspoons basil

2 teaspoons oregano

2 teaspoons onion powder

1/8 teaspoon cayenne powder

Equipment

Blender

Cookie sheet

Parchment paper

Pot—at least 4 quart

Directions:

Preheat your oven to 400° f.

Chop the vegetables in half and place them in a bowl.

Sprinkle grapeseed oil and a teaspoon of both basil and sea salt.

Sprinkle the chopped vegetables in the mixture until it is fully coated.

Place all the vegetables on a cookie sheet.

Bake in the oven for 30 minutes.

Toss the roasted vegetables into a blender and blend on high speed.

Pour the pasta and the remaining ingredients into a pot. Allow it to cook for 20 minutes.

Nutrition:

Calories: 25

Fat: 2g

Sodium: 80mg

Carbohydrate: 2g

16. Dr. Sebi Alkaline Vegan Hot Dogs Recipe

Preparation time: 20 minutes

Cooking time: 40 minutes

Servings: 10

Ingredients:

1 cup garbanzo beans

1 cup spelt flour

1/2 cup aquafaba

1/3 cup green pepper, diced

1/3 cup onion, diced

1/4 cup shallots, diced

1 tablespoon Onion powder

2 tablespoon Smoked sea salt

1 tablespoon Coriander

1/2 tablespoon Ginger

1/2 tablespoon Dill

1/2 tablespoon Fennel

1/2 tablespoon Crushed red pepper (optional)

Alkaline electric ketchup (optional)

Grapeseed oil for sautéing

Alkaline electric buns (optional)

When trying to make hotdog buns, all you have to do is follow the recipe to roll the dough then bake on a taco rack. In the absence of a rack, flatbread or tortillas can be used instead.

Tools:

Hotdog mold

Food processor

Parchment paper

Taco rack (optional)

Directions:

Sprinkle grapeseed oil in your skillet, add vegetables and garbanzo beans then sauté for 5 minutes.

Place the remaining vegetables and other ingredients in a food processor until it is well blended.

Scoop the mixture into your hand, then, make hotdog shapes with them and wrap with parchment paper afterward.

The molded hotdogs should be steamed for 40 minutes.

Once the steaming process is done, unwrap the hotdogs.

Sprinkle grapeseed oil in a skillet and cook the hotdogs for 10 minutes on medium heat.

Your alkaline electric hotdogs are ready to be dished.

Nutrition:

Calories: 159.2 - Carbohydrates: 6.3g

Fat: 3.3g - Protein: 25.5g

17. Dr. Sebi Alkaline Avocado Mayo Recipe

Preparation time: 10 minutes

Cooking time: 10 minutes

Servings: 1 cup

Ingredients:

Juice from half of a lime

1 avocado

1/4 cup cilantro

1/2 tablespoon Sea salt

1/2 tablespoon Onion powder

2-4 tablespoon Olive oil

Pinch of cayenne powder

Blender or hand mixer

Directions:

Remove the pit of the avocado and scoop the insides into a blender.

Add the rest of the ingredients and blend at a high speed.

For hand mixers, add all other ingredients except the oil which should be added slowly until the desired consistency is reached.

Dish your alkaline avocado mayo!

Nutrition:

Calories: 45

Fat: 4.5g

Sodium: 100mg

Carbohydrate: 0.5g

18. Dr. Sebi Alkaline Quinoa Milk Recipe

Preparation time: 10 minutes

Cooking time: 5 minutes

Servings: 4

Ingredients:

1 cup cooked white quinoa

3 cups spring water

6-8 dates

1 pinch sea salt (optional)

1 pinch cloves (optional)

Blender

Milk bag or cheesecloth

Directions:

Make a perfect blend of these ingredients in a blender.

Sieve with milk bag or cheesecloth.

Enjoy your well-deserved Dr. Sebi alkaline quinoa milk recipe.

Nutrition:

Calories: 111

Sugar: 3.2g

Sodium: 5mg

Fat: 1.6g

Saturated fat: 0.2g

Carbohydrates: 20.7g

Fiber: 2.3g

19. Dr. Sebi Alkaline Spicy Kale Recipe

Preparation time: 10 minutes

Cooking time: 15 minutes

Servings: 4

Ingredients:

1 bunch of kale

1/4 cup onion, diced

1/4 cup red pepper, diced

1 tablespoon Crushed red pepper

1/4 tablespoon Sea salt

Alkaline "garlic" oil or grapeseed oil

Salad spinner (optional)

Note: if you happen to not have a salad spinner, you can as well air dry the kale.

Directions:

Rinse the kale, fold its leaves into halves, and cut off the stem.

Chop kale into bits and remove the water using a salad spinner.

Set your cooker to high and add 2 tablespoons of oil.

Sauté salt, pepper, and onions for 3 minutes.

Reduce the heat to low, add the chopped kale and cover for 5 minutes.

Crushed pepper should be introduced to the mix, stir and cover for another 3 minutes.

Dish your alkaline spicy kale!

Nutrition:

Calories: 85.2 - Fat: 1.2g

Sodium: 61.2mg - Carbohydrates: 18g

Fiber: 5.9g - Protein: 5.3g

20. Dr. Sebi Alkaline Buns Recipe

Preparation time: 20 minutes

Cooking time: 1 hour

Servings: 6

Ingredients:

2 1/4 cups - 2 1/2 cups spelt flour

1/2 cup hemp milk or walnut milk

1/4 cup aquafaba

1/4 cup sparkling spring water

1 tablespoon Agave

1 tablespoon Onion powder

1 1/2 tablespoon Sea salt

1 tablespoon Basil or oregano

2 tablespoon Grapeseed oil

1 tablespoon Sea moss gel (optional)

Sesame seeds (optional)

Baking sheet

Plastic wrap

Parchment paper

Note: Mixer with a dough hook, if you do not have a mixer, you can knead by hand.

Directions:

Add all the dry ingredients into a mixing bowl and blend perfectly.

Add the remaining ingredients and blend on low speed for a minute. Then, knead dough at medium speed for 5 minutes.

Sprinkle grapeseed oil on a baking sheet already laced with parchment paper.

Separate dough into parts, roll with hand to make shapes then place on a baking sheet.

Brush the top with oil then add sesame seeds.

Use a plastic wrap to cover the buns and allow it to sit for 30 minutes.

Set your oven to 350°f and bake for half an hour.

Allow the buns to cook and carefully cut them in half to enjoy your alkaline electric buns!

Nutrition:

Carbohydrates: 47g

Fat: 7g - Protein: 9g

21. Dr. Sebi Alkaline Strawberry Jam Recipe

Preparation time: 10 minutes

Cooking time: 20 minutes

Servings: 16 oz

Ingredients:

4 cups sliced strawberries

2/3 cups of raw agave

3 tablespoons of key lime juice

1/2 cup Irish moss gel

Directions:

Slice enough strawberries to fill up 4 cups.

Mash or blend to your desired texture.

Agave, lime juice, and strawberries should be added to the saucepan on high heat.

Cook for 10 minutes then add Irish moss gel.

Cook for 5 more minutes to make certain that the gel has been thoroughly dissolved.

Remove from heat and allow the sauce to cool down before refrigerating.

Dish your alkaline electric strawberry jam!

Nutrition:

Calories: 56

Carbohydrates: 13g

22. Dr. Sebi Alkaline Date Syrup Recipe

Preparation time: 10 minutes

Cooking time: 15 minutes

Servings: 16-24 oz

Ingredients:

1 cup dates, preferably pitted

1 cup of spring water

This sweetener can be easily dissolved in water, unlike date sugar.

Directions:

Boil spring water then remove from heat when boiled.

Place dates in the boiled water for at least 5 minutes.

Pour the dates and some water into a blender then blend for until it's smooth.

If the texture is too thick, add more water and blend again.

Keep it a refrigerator and dish with alkaline date syrup!

Nutrition:

Calories: 270

Potassium: 848mg

Sodium: 5mg

Carbohydrates: 67g

Fiber: 3g

Sugar: 61g

Protein: 1g

23. Chickpea Mashed Potatoes

Preparation time: 5 minutes

Cooking time: 30 minutes

Servings: 4

Ingredients:

2 cups chickpeas, cooked

¼ cup green onions, diced

2 teaspoons sea salt

2 teaspoons onion powder

1 cup walnut milk; homemade, unsweetened

Directions:

Plug in a food processor, add chickpeas to it, pour in the milk, and then add salt and onion powder.

Cover the blending jar with its lid and then pulse for 1 to 2 minutes until smooth; blend in water if the mixture is too thick.

Take a medium saucepan, place it over medium heat, and then add blended chickpea mixture in it.

Stir green onions into the chickpeas mixture and then cook the mixture for 30 minutes, stirring constantly.

Serve straight away.

Nutrition:

Calories: 145.8

Carbohydrates: 19.1g

Fat: 7.3g

Protein: 3.3g

24. Mushroom and Onion Gravy

Preparation time: 5 minutes
Cooking time: 18 minutes
Servings: 4

Ingredients:

1 cup sliced onions, chopped

1 cup mushrooms, sliced

2 teaspoons onion powder

2 teaspoons sea salt

1 teaspoon dried thyme

6 tablespoons chickpea flour

½ teaspoon cayenne pepper

1 teaspoon dried oregano

4 tablespoons grapeseed oil

4 cups spring water

Directions:

Take a medium pot, place it over medium-high heat, add oil and when hot, add onions, mushrooms, and then cook for 1 minute.

Season the vegetables with onion powder, salt, thyme, and oregano. Stir until mixed, and cook for 5 minutes.

Pour in water, stir in cayenne pepper, stir well, and then bring the mixture to a boil.

Slowly stir in chickpea flour, and bring the mixture to a boil again.

Remove pan from heat and then serve gravy with a favorite dish.

Nutrition:

Calories: 120 - Carbohydrates: 8.4g

Fat: 7.6g - Protein: 2.2g

25. Vegetable Chili

Preparation time: 5 minutes
Cooking time: 30 minutes
Servings: 6

Ingredients:

2 cups black beans, cooked

1 medium red bell pepper; deseeded, chopped

1 poblano chili; deseeded, chopped

2 jalapeño chilies; deseeded, chopped

4 tablespoons cilantro, chopped

1 large white onion; peeled, chopped

1 ½ tablespoon minced garlic

1 ½ teaspoon sea salt

1 ½ teaspoon cumin powder

1 ½ teaspoon red chili powder

3 teaspoons lime juice

2 tablespoons grapeseed oil

2 ½ cups vegetable stock

Directions:

Take a large pot, place it over medium-high heat, add oil and when hot, add onion and cook for 4–5 minutes until translucent.

Add bell pepper, jalapeno pepper, poblano chili, and garlic and then cook for 3–4 minutes until veggies turn tender.

Season the vegetables with salt, stir in cumin powder and red chili powder, then add chickpeas and pour in vegetable stock.

Bring the mixture to a boil, then switch heat to medium-low and simmer the chili for 15–20 minutes until thickened slightly.

Then remove the pot from heat, ladle chili stew among six bowls, drizzle with lime juice, garnish with cilantro, and serve.

Nutrition:

Calories: 224.2

Carbs: 42.6g

Fat: 1.2g

Protein: 12.5g

26. Wild Rice and Black Lentils Bowl

Preparation time: 10 minutes

Cooking time: 50 minutes

Servings: 4

Ingredients:

Wild rice

2 cups wild rice, uncooked

4 cups spring water

½ teaspoon salt

2 bay leaves

Black lentils

2 cups black lentils, cooked

1 ¾ cups coconut milk, unsweetened

2 cups vegetable stock

1 teaspoon dried thyme

1 teaspoon dried paprika

½ of medium purple onion; peeled, sliced

1 tablespoon minced garlic

2 teaspoons creole seasoning

1 tablespoon coconut oil

Plantains

3 large plantains, chopped into ¼-inch-thick pieces

3 tablespoons coconut oil

Brussels sprouts

10 large brussels sprouts, quartered

2 tablespoons spring water

1 teaspoon sea salt

½ teaspoon ground black pepper

Directions:

Prepare the rice: take a medium pot, place it over medium-high heat, pour in water, and add bay leaves and salt.

Bring the water to a boil, then switch heat to medium, add rice, and then cook for 30–45 minutes or more until tender.

When done, discard the bay leaves from rice, drain if any water remains in the pot, remove it from heat, and fluff by using a fork. Set aside until needed.

While the rice boils, prepare lentils: take a large pot, place it over medium-high heat and when hot, add onion and cook for 5 minutes or until translucent.

Stir garlic into the onion, cook for 2 minutes until fragrant and golden, then add remaining ingredients for the lentils and stir until mixed.

Bring the lentils to a boil, then switch heat to medium and simmer the lentils for 20 minutes until tender, covering the pot with a lid.

When done, remove the pot from heat and set aside until needed.

While rice and lentils simmer, prepare the plantains: chop them into ¼-inch-thick pieces.

Take a large skillet pan, place it over medium heat, add coconut oil and when it melts, add half of the plantain pieces and cook for 7–10 minutes per side or more until golden-brown.

When done, transfer browned plantains to a plate lined with paper towels and repeat with the remaining plantain pieces; set aside until needed.

Prepare the sprouts: return the skillet pan over medium heat, add more oil if needed, and then add brussels sprouts.

Toss the sprouts until coated with oil, and then let them cook for 3–4 minutes per side until brown.

Drizzle water over sprouts, cover the pan with the lid, and then cook for 3–5 minutes until steamed.

Season the sprouts with salt and black pepper, toss until mixed, and transfer sprouts to a plate.

Assemble the bowl: divide rice evenly among four bowls and then top with lentils, plantain pieces, and sprouts.

Serve immediately.

Nutrition:

Calories: 333 - Carbohydrates: 49.2g

Fat: 10.7g - Protein: 6.2g

27. Spaghetti Squash With Peanut Sauce

Preparation time: 15 minutes

Cooking time: 15 minutes

Servings: 4

Ingredients:

1 cup cooked shelled edamame; frozen, thawed

3-pound spaghetti squash

½ cup red bell pepper, sliced

¼ cup scallions, sliced

1 medium carrot, shredded

1 teaspoon minced garlic

½ teaspoon crushed red pepper

1 tablespoon rice vinegar

¼ cup coconut aminos

1 tablespoon maple syrup

½ cup peanut butter

¼ cup unsalted roasted peanuts, chopped

¼ cup and 2 tablespoons spring water, divided

¼ cup fresh cilantro, chopped

4 lime wedges

Directions:

Prepare the squash: cut each squash in half lengthwise and then remove seeds.

Take a microwave-proof dish, place squash halves in it cut-side-up, drizzle with 2 tablespoons water, and then microwave at high heat setting for 10–15 minutes until tender.

Let squash cool for 15 minutes until able to handle. Use a fork to scrape its flesh lengthwise to make noodles, and then let noodles cool for 10 minutes.

While squash microwaves, prepare the sauce: take a medium bowl, add butter in it along with red pepper and garlic, pour in vinegar, coconut aminos, maple syrup, and water, and then whisk until smooth.

When the squash noodles have cooled, distribute them evenly among four bowls, top with scallions, carrots, bell pepper, and edamame beans, and then drizzle with prepared sauce.

Sprinkle cilantro and peanuts and serve each bowl with a lime wedge.

Nutrition:

Calories: 419 - Carbohydrates: 32.8g

Fat: 24g - Protein: 17.6g

28. Cauliflower Alfredo Pasta

Preparation time: 10 minutes

Cooking time: 30 minutes

Servings: 4

Ingredients:

Alfredo sauce

4 cups cauliflower florets, fresh

1 tablespoon minced garlic

¼ cup nutritional yeast

½ teaspoon garlic powder

¾ teaspoon sea salt

½ teaspoon onion powder

½ teaspoon ground black pepper

½ tablespoon olive oil

1 tablespoon lemon juice, and more as needed for serving

½ cup almond milk, unsweetened

Pasta

1 tablespoon minced parsley

1 lemon, juiced

½ teaspoon sea salt

¼ teaspoon ground black pepper

12 ounces spelt pasta; cooked, warmed

Directions:

Take a large pot half full with water, place it over medium-high heat, and then bring it to a boil.

Add cauliflower florets, cook for 10–15 minutes until tender, drain them well, and then return florets to the pot.

Take a medium skillet pan, place it over low heat, add oil and when hot, add garlic and cook for 4–5 minutes until fragrant and golden-brown.

Spoon garlic into a food processor, add remaining ingredients for the sauce in it, along with cauliflower florets, and then pulse for 2–3 minutes until smooth.

Tip the sauce into the pot, stir it well, place it over medium-low heat, and then cook for 5 minutes until hot.

Add pasta into the pot, toss well until coated, taste to adjust seasoning, and then cook for 2 minutes until pasta gets hot.

Divide pasta and sauce among four plates, season with salt and black pepper, drizzle with lemon juice, and then top with minced parsley.

Serve straight away.

Nutrition:

Calories: 360 - Carbohydrates: 59g

Fat: 9g - Protein: 13g

29. Sloppy Joe

Preparation time: 8 minutes

Cooking time: 12 minutes

Servings: 4

Ingredients:

2 cups Kamut or spelt wheat, cooked

½ cup white onion, diced

1 Roma tomato, diced

1 cup chickpeas, cooked

½ cup green bell peppers, diced

1 teaspoon sea salt

1/8 teaspoon cayenne pepper

1 teaspoon onion powder

1 tablespoon grapeseed oil

1 ½ cups barbecue sauce, alkaline

Directions:

Plug in a high-power food processor, add chickpeas and spelt, cover with the lid, and then pulse for 15 seconds.

Take a large skillet pan, place it over medium-high heat, add oil and when hot, add onion and bell pepper, season with salt, cayenne pepper, and onion powder, and then stir until well combined.

Cook the vegetables for 3–5 minutes until tender. Add tomatoes, add the pulsed mixture, pour in barbecue sauce, and then stir until well mixed.

Simmer for 5 minutes, then remove the pan from heat and serve sloppy joe with alkaline flatbread.

Nutrition:

Calories: 333 - Carbohydrates: 65g

Fat: 5g - Protein: 14g

30. Kale Chickpea Mash

Kale and chickpea produce a healthy and yummy lunch dish that has a wide range of health benefits. It's perfect for people on the Dr. Sebi diet.

Preparation time: 15 minutes

Cooking time: 12 minutes

Servings: 1

Ingredients:

1 shallot

3 tablespoons garlic

A bunch of kale

1/2 cup boiled chickpea

2 tablespoons coconut oil

Sea salt

Directions:

Add some garlic in olive oil

Chop shallot and fry it with oil in a nonstick skillet.

Cook until the shallot turns golden brown.

Add kale and garlic in the skillet and stir well.

Add chickpeas and cook for 6 minutes. Add the rest of the ingredients and give a good stir.

Serve and enjoy

Nutrition:

Calories: 149 - Total fat: 8g

Saturated fat: 1g - Net carbohydrates: 13g

Protein: 4g - Sugars 6g

Fiber 3g

Sodium 226mg

Potassium 205mg

31. Quinoa and Apple

The combination of quinoa and apple yields a delicious and filling lunch dish that can be carried to work in your lunch box.

Preparation time: 15 minutes

Cooking time: 12 minutes

Servings: 1

Ingredients:

1/2 cup quinoa

1 apple

1/2 lemon

Cinnamon to taste

Directions:

Cook quinoa according to the packet directions.

Grate the apple and add to the cooked quinoa. Cook for 30 seconds.

Serve in a bowl then sprinkle lime and cinnamon. Enjoy.

Nutrition:

Calories: 229

Total fat: 3.2g

Net carbs: 32.3g

Protein: 6.1g

Sugars: 4.2g

Fiber: 3.3g

Sodium: 35.5mg

Potassium: 211.8mg

32. Warm Avo and Quinoa Salad

This is an amazing alkaline quinoa dish that will blow your mind away. It's an easy dish that will be ready in less than 20 minutes.

Preparation time: 5 minutes

Cooking time: 12 minutes

Servings: 4

Ingredients:

4 ripe avocados, quartered

1 cup quinoa

0.9 lb. Chickpeas, drained

1 oz flat-leaf parsley

Directions:

Add quinoa in a pot with 2 cups of water. Bring to boil then simmer for 12 minutes or until all the water has evaporated. The grains should be glassy and swollen.

Toss the quinoa with all other ingredients and season with salt and pepper to taste.

Serve with olive oil and lemon wedges. Enjoy.

Nutrition:

Calories: 354

Total fat: 16g

Saturated fat: 2g

Net carbs: 31g

Protein: 15g

Sugars: 6g

Fiber: 15g

Sodium: 226mg

Potassium: 205mg

33. Kale Pesto Pasta

There is no better way to eat your green than by making this cool kale pesto pasta. Make sure to try at your home for lunch.

Preparation time: 15 minutes

Cooking time: 12 minutes

Servings: 1

Ingredients:

1/2 cup walnuts

1 bunch kale

2 cups basil, fresh

1/4 cup oil

2 limes, freshly squeezed

Salt and pepper

1 zucchini, spiralized

Asparagus, cherry tomatoes, and spinach leaves for garnish

Directions:

Soak the walnuts overnight.

Add the walnuts with all other ingredients except the zucchini in a food processor and pulse until well blended.

Add the zucchini mix and serve garnished with asparagus, cherry tomatoes and spinach. Enjoy.

Nutrition:

Calories: 176

Total fat: 17g

Saturated fat: 3g

Net carbohydrates: 5g

Protein: 4g

Fiber: 1g

Sodium: 314mg

34. Spinach With Chickpeas and Lemon

If looking for an alkaline lunch to carry in your lunch box as part of a busy lifestyle, this flavorful easy recipe is the one for you.

Preparation time: 5 minute

Cooking time: 10 minutes

Servings: 2

Ingredients:

3 tablespoons oil

1 onion, thinly sliced

4 garlic cloves, minced

1 tablespoons ginger, grated

1/2 container cherry tomatoes

1 lemon, freshly zested and juiced

1 tablespoon red pepper flakes, crushed

1 can chickpeas

Salt to taste

Directions:

Add oil in a skillet and cook onions until browned. Add garlic cloves, ginger, tomatoes, zest, and pepper flakes. Cook for 4 minutes.

Add chickpeas and cook for 3 more minutes. Add spinach and cook until they start to wilt.

Add lemon juice and season with salt to taste. Cook for 2 more minutes.

Serve and enjoy.

Nutrition:

Calories: 209 - Total fat: 8.1g

Saturated fat: 1g - Total carbohydrates: 28.5g

Protein: 22.5g - Fiber: 6g

Sodium: 372mg

Potassium: 286mg

35. Raw Green Veggie Soup

A delightful and welcoming flavorsome soup that is completely energizing and uplifting especially during Dr. Sebi's diet.

Preparation time: 5 minutes

Cooking time: 5 minutes

Servings: 1

Ingredients:

1 avocado

1 zucchini, chopped

2 celery stalks, chopped

2 cups spinach

1/4 cup parsley, fresh

2 sliced green peppers

1/8 onion, chopped

1 garlic clove

1/4 cup almonds, soak overnight, and rinse

Salt to taste

1-1/2 cup water

1 lemon juice

Diced watermelon radish for garnish

Directions:

Add all the ingredients in a food processor except salt.

Pulse until smooth or until the desired consistency is desired.

Pour the soup in a saucepan to warm a little bit before seasoning with salt and squeezed lemon.

Garnish with watermelon radish and enjoy.

Nutrition:

Calories: 48.9 - Fat: 0.4g - Carbs: 10.6g - Protein: 3.1g - Sugars: 1.9g - Fiber: 3.9g

36. Kale Caesar Salad

An easy and classic way to enjoy your kale during lunchtime. The dish is filling and complements Dr. Sebi's diet.

Preparation time: 5 minutes

Cooking time: 12 minutes

Servings: 1

Ingredients:

1 bunch of curly kale, washed

1 cup sunflower seeds

1/3 cup almond nuts

1/8 tablespoon chipotle powder

2 garlic cloves

1-1/4 water

1-1/2 tablespoon agave syrup

1/2 tablespoon sea salt

Directions:

Wash and pat dry the curly kale and remove the center membrane .tear the kale leaves into small sizes.

Add all other ingredients in a blender and blend until smooth and creamy.

Pour half of the mixture over the kale and toss until well coated.

Pour the remaining mixture and mix until the kales are well coated on the curls and folds.

Let rest for 10 minutes then serve on plates. Sprinkle sunflower seeds and enjoy.

Nutrition:

Calories: 157 - Total fat: 6g - Saturated fat: 2g - Carbs: 18g - Protein: 9g - Sugars: 1g

Fiber: 2g - Sodium: 356mg

37. Red and White Salad

The macadamia nuts and avocado oil add a beautiful buttery flavor to this salad. You can also use your favorite nuts and oil.

Preparation time: 5 minutes

Cooking time: 10 minutes

Servings: 2

Ingredients:

3 radishes

1 fennel bulb, greens removed

1/2 jicama, peeled and halved

2 celery stalks

Juice from 1 lime

1/4 cup avocado oil

Salt to taste

Macadamia nuts

Directions:

Slice radish, fennel, jicama, and celery using a mandolin slicer on the thinnest setting.

Toss them in a mixing bowl with lime and oil. Season with salt then top with nuts.

Enjoy.

Nutrition:

Calories: 197

Total fat: 9g

Saturated fat: 4g

Total carbs: 20g

Protein: 7g

Sugars: 1g

Fiber: 2g

Sodium: 366mg

38. Almond Milk

This is an awesome alternative to cow milk that is healthy, cheap, and very easy to make. Serve the milk with your favorite alkaline side for a filling lunch.

Preparation time: 5 minutes

Cooking time: 10 minutes

Servings: 2

Ingredients:

1.7oz almonds, sliced

133.8 oz filtered water

1 tablespoon sunflower granules

2 dates, stones removed

Directions:

Soak the almonds for a few hours ahead of time.

Add all the ingredients in a blender and blend for 2 minutes.

Pour the milk in a container through a straining cloth. Carry in your lunch box or store in a fridge for up to 3 days.

You can use almond pulp in cakes or almond mixes.

Nutrition:

Calories 90

Total fat: 2.5g

Total carbohydrates: 16g

Protein: 1g

Sugars: 4g

Sodium: 140mg

Potassium: 140mg

39. Creamy Kale Salad With Avocado and Tomato

This alkaline bowl is healthy, delicious, and filling. It's also very easy to assemble and can be carried to work in your lunchbox.

Preparation time: 5 minutes

Cooking time: 10 minutes

Servings: 2

Ingredients:

2 handful of kale

2 cherry tomatoes

1 ripe avocado

Juice from 1 lime

1 garlic clove, crushed

1 tablespoon agave

1/2 tablespoon paprika

1/2 tablespoon black pepper

Directions:

Wash kale and tomatoes and roughly chop them. Place them in a mixing bowl.

Peel the avocado and add it to the mixing bowl.

Add lemon juice and the rest of the ingredients to the bowl and mix them thoroughly.

Serve and enjoy.

Nutrition:

Calories: 179.2 - Total fat: 14.1g

Saturated fat: 1.9g - Carbohydrates: 13.5g

Protein: 3.7g - Sugars: 6g

Fiber: 6.1g

Sodium: 77mg

Potassium: 624mg

40. Creamy Broccoli Soup

This is a thick and flavorful soup recipe. It is simple quick and the most delicious soup to serve for lunch.

Preparation time: 5 minutes

Cooking time: 10 minutes

Servings: 5

Ingredients:

2 cups vegetable stock

4 cups broccoli, chopped

1 red pepper, chopped

1 avocado

2 onions, chopped

2 celery stalks, sliced

Ginger to taste

1 tablespoon salt

Directions:

Warm vegetable stock in a small pot. Add broccoli and season with salt to taste. Simmer for 5 minutes.

Add the broccoli in a blender with pepper, avocado, onions, and celery stalks. Add some water for thinning then blend until smooth.

Serve when warm with ginger to your liking. Garnish with a lemon slice. Enjoy.

Nutrition:

Calories: 270 - Total fat: 18g

Saturated fat: 11g - Total carbohydrates: 17g

Protein: 12g

Sugars: 5g

Fiber: 3.5g

Sodium: 470g

41. Caprese Stuffed Avocado

The sweet juicy cherry tomatoes are tossed in basil pesto together with boccoccini balls then stuffed in avocado halves for a delightful light lunch.

Preparation time: 5 minutes

Cooking time: 10 minutes

Servings: 4

Ingredients:

1/2 cup cherry tomatoes

4 oz baby bocconcini balls

2 tablespoons basil pesto

1 tablespoon minced garlic

1/4 oil

Salt and pepper to taste

2 ripe avocados

2 tablespoons balsamic glaze

Basil for serving

Directions:

In a mixing bowl, add cherry tomatoes, bocconcini balls, basil pesto, garlic, salt and pepper to taste. Toss until well combined and all flavors have blended.

Half the avocados and arrange them on a platter.

Spoon the mixture in the avocado halves and drizzle with balsamic glaze.

Top with basil and serve. Enjoy.

Nutrition:

Calories: 341

Total fat: 29g

Saturated fat: 7g

Total carbohydrates: 15g

Protein: 8g

Sugars: 4g

Fiber: 6g

Sodium: 220mg

Potassium: 550mg

Conclusion

Herpes ailment is a drawn-out corrupting that is acknowledged by herpes simplex virus (HSV). The genital locale, the oral area, the skin, and the butt-driven district are the areas of the body that is influenced by this sullying. This ailment is known for an incredibly drawn out stretch, and it commonly assaults people causing several tribulations; some are smooth, and some are perilous.

The genital herpes is one of the most by and large saw kinds of herpes simplex sickness. The genital herpes pollution is an explicitly transmitted affliction that results in genital and butt-driven disturbs. There might be wounds that likewise sway the mouth and face. Dr. Sebi was a notable cultivator that restored many individuals experiencing herpes, and different maladies, for example, disease, aids, hypertension, fibroid, diabetes, body torment, illicit drug use, and so forth.

All Dr. Sebi's spices and diet are profoundly powerful in rewarding infections. Dr. Sebi's spices and plant-based eating regimens help to purge and detoxify the body, making them the ideal solution for the herpes simplex infection. Dr. Sebi utilizes homegrown treatment, diet changes, and other powerful common recuperating strategies to fix herpes. In the event that you are experiencing the herpes infection, and you have attempted present day medication and different types of treatment and nothing worked, at that point, Dr. Sebi's spices and plant-based weight control plans are what you need.

You evidently know now what really is Dr. Sebi herpes fix. Really, Dr. Sebi's answer for herpes is constantly appearing at each side of the world. The purpose behind the so fiery widespread is genuinely not a colossal number of dollars spent on pills or worldwide eminence considering how some huge name is getting a handle on it. It is to reach the hearts of herpes patients in such a case that its adequacy.

All in all, Dr. Sebi's herpes fix is a compelling one with zero symptoms. At the point when you eat well nourishments, your insusceptible framework will have the quality it needs to fend off intruders. This treatment is expensive, yet it additionally vows to assuage you of your condition, why not spend the additional sum. Dr. Sebi had once been prosecuted for demonstrating this fix works, think about what, he won since he wasn't feigning when he said his item works.

Dr. Sebi's herpes cure is a perpetual solution for herpes, which keeps you away from herpes episodes as well as encourages you from the different reactions that antivirals may give you. Dr. Sebi's herpes cure can possibly work when done appropriately and with the correct spices and the best quality items so ensure you read the book and even investigate different assets to ensure you are prepared to begin the procedure. In any case, there's as yet an opportunity that this treatment won't work for you and could conceivably work for your companion, relative, neighbor, or who else in light of the fact that your body is not quite the same as their body. Your body may respond an alternate way, so if things don't beat that, it's smarter to make an arrangement and counsel your doctor.

I hope you will be able to implement in your life what you have learned in this book!

Dr. Sebi Cookbook

Table of Contents

INTRODUCTION **189**

DOCTOR SEBI'S FOOD LIST **190**
    VEGETABLES 192
    FRUITS 192
    ALKALINE GRAINS 192
    ALKALINE SUGARS 192
    DIETS DESIGNED BY DR. SEBI 193
    LIST OF FOODS TO AVOID IN DR. SEBI'S DIET 193
    APPROVED PRODUCTS 193
    IRON PLUS 193
    GREEN FOOD 194
    BROMIDE PLUS POWDER/BROMIDE PLUS CAPSULES 194
    BIO FERRO TONIC/BIO FERRO CAPSULES 194
    BANJU 195
    BODY CARE 195
    HERBAL TEAS 196
    FOODS TO AVOID 197

HOW TO FOLLOW THE DIET **198**
    RULES TO FOLLOW 198
    HOW TO PREPARE THE BODY 198
    MEAL PLAN 198
    WHAT YOU SHOULD NOT EAT 201
    A 7-DAY ALKALINE MEAL PLAN 201
    INSTRUCTIONS TO DETOX YOUR BODY WITH ALTERNATIVE THERAPIES 202

SOUPS **203**

SALADS **223**

MAIN DISHES **231**

SAUCES **248**

SPECIAL INGREDIENTS **256**

SNACKS & BREAD **260**

DESSERTS **274**

SMOOTHIES **291**

CONCLUSION **307**

Introduction

Dr. Sebi felt the Western solution to illness was unsuccessful. He held that acidity and mucus — for starters, bacteria, and viruses — induced sickness.

A big dietary hypothesis is that illness can exist only in acidic conditions. To avoid or eliminate the disease, the purpose of the diet is to maintain alkaline conditions in the body. The official website of the food offers botanical medicines helping to detoxify the body.

Methodology

Often, stretching for the additional mile, you get to the areas you had only dreamed about. They were going well on Dr. Sebi's alkaline diet, which will be the battle that ultimately contributes to a balanced lifestyle. Dr. Sebi's alkaline diet is an assumption that certain products, such as berries, vegetables, roots, and legumes, leave a chemical residue or ash behind in the body. The body is strengthened by the critical ingredients of rock, such as calcium, magnesium, titanium, zinc, and copper. The avoidance of asthma, malnutrition, exhaustion, and even cancer is an alkaline diet. Here are ten strategies to adopt this diet effectively, following these strategies to see results immediately:

1. **Drink water.** Water is probably our body's most famous (after oxygen) resource. Drink between 8-10 glasses of water to keep the body well hydrated (filtered to cleaned).
2. **Avoid acidic drinks like tea, coffee, or soda.** Our body also attempts to regulate acid and alkaline content. There is no need to blink in carbonated beverages as the body refuses carbon dioxide as waste!
3. **Breathe.** Oxygen is the explanation that our body works, and if you provide the body with adequate oxygen, it should perform better. Sit back and enjoy two to five minutes of slow breaths. Nothing is easier than performing Yoga.
4. **Avoid food with preservatives and food colours.** Our body has not been programmed to absorb such substances, and the body then absorbs them or retains them as fat, so they do not damage the liver. Chemicals create acids, such that the body neutralizes them either by generating cholesterols or blanching iron from the RBCs (leading to anaemia) or by extracting calcium from bones (osteoporosis).
5. **Avoid artificial sweeteners.** These sweeteners, which tend to be high in low fat, are potentially detrimental to the body. In addition, Saccharin, a primary ingredient in sweeteners, triggers cancer. Keep away from these things, therefore. Go for less healthy food, still a decent one.
6. **Exercise.** Alkaline and the acidic clement will also be matched. A little acid (because of muscles) often regulates natural bodywork.
7. **Satiate your urges for a snack by eating vegetables or soaked nuts.** Whenever we are thirsty, we still consume a little fast food. Establish a tradition of consuming fresh vegetables or almonds, even walnuts.

Doctor Sebi's Food List

Many individuals in the U.S. suffer from different diseases ranging from cancer, hypertension, diabetes, mental disabilities, and many more. Many of these junks and fast foods are disease-causing substances (contains too much acid) not because they contain pathogens but because they contain elements such as an increasing amount of acid that increase weight and clogged up in the body.

The accumulation of all these substances in the body brings about an increased amount of fatty acids and cholesterol, which later blocks up the blood vessels and hinders the free flow of blood.

Many of these substances cause genetic materials in the body to make a mistake and bring about the growth of abnormal cells, which subsequently result in cancer.

Nowadays, dieters have embraced the intake of alkaline food not only because they know the importance of clean and prolong life.

Acidic foods are majorly the foods we eat. Such foods are meat, grains, eggs, fish, alcohol, etc. These foods increase the body's acidic level. The intake of alkaline foods will cause your blood to become soluble and therefore inhibit you from having diseases.

When you take a plant diet that has a reduced acid diet, it replaces the animal protein with excess acid. This will promote your kidney because it makes it reduce its work of removing the excess acids present in animal diets.

Besides, bone diseases and many bones associated problems are at times are related to the consumption of some foods that are high in acid. Then, to avoid any bone infections in the body, you must endeavour to eat alkaline diets.

The foods designed by Dr. Sebi are straightforward to acquire around you, and they are cheap and do expensive activities in your body. These foods make you remain lean, clean, and healthy.

Dr. Sebi classified the foods into different categories. These categories are:

- Fruits
- Vegetables
- Alkaline Grains
- Alkaline Sugars

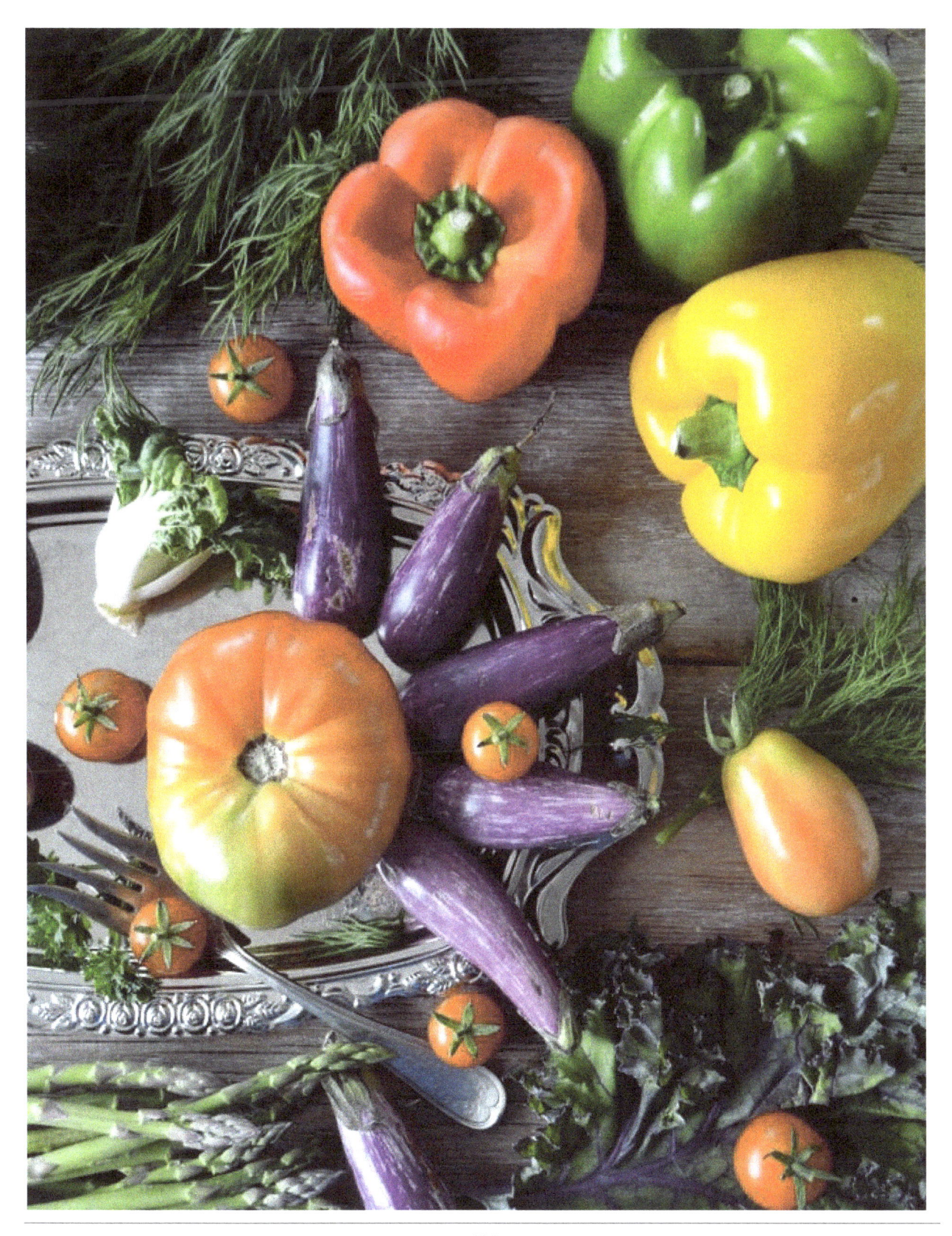

Vegetables

- Cucumber
- Tomatillo
- Turnip greens.
- Wakame
- Onions
- Dandelion greens
- Cherry and plum tomato
- Dulse
- Garbanzo beans
- Izote flower and leaf
- Kale
- Mushrooms except for Shitake
- Arame
- Wild Arugula
- Avocado
- Amaranth
- Bell Pepper
- Chayote
- Hijiki
- Nopales
- Nori
- Zucchini
- Watercress
- Lettuce except for iceberg
- Olives
- Purslane verdolaga
- Squash
- Okra

Fruits

- Apples
- Pears
- Limes
- Mango
- Berries
- Melons
- Prickly pear
- Cherries
- Soursops
- Dates
- Figs
- Grapes
- Prunes
- Raisins
- Papayas
- Bananas
- Cantaloupe
- Currants
- Orange
- Soft jelly coconuts
- Peaches
- Plums

Alkaline Grains

- Spelt
- Fonio
- Quinoa
- Rye
- Kamut
- Tef
- Wild rice
- Amaranth

Alkaline Sugars

- 100% Pure agave syrup extracted from cactus
- Dried date sugar

Diets Designed by Dr. Sebi

The diets designed by Dr. Sebi are essential for the prevention and cure of cancer disease and many other conditions. All sufferers of cancer disease are expected to consume only foods approved by Dr. Sebi, although the diets might be severe for those who are addicted to acidic foods such as rice, soy, beans, alcohol, junks, and many more.

List of Foods to Avoid in Dr. Sebi's Diet

Some foods are disregarded in Dr. Sebi's food list because you must do away with them. Most of these foods could be dangerous for your health, especially for cancer patients.

These foods contain an increasing amount of acidic contents and are not advised to be taken by a cancer patient. Although these foods are suitable for the mouth, they are not good for the body. Dr. Sebi tagged them as forbidden foods. These foods are listed below:

- Alcoholic beverages
- Fish and seafood
- Meat of all kind
- Poultry products
- Colorants and flavours
- Processed foods
- Canned foods and fruits
- Soy and soy products
- Corn
- Genetically modified organism fruits
- Eggs
- Wheat
- Seedless fruits
- Foods with yeast or other components such as baking powder
- Fast foods
- Sugar
- Foods fortified with vitamins and minerals
- Garlic
- Genetically modified organism vegetables
- Dairy foods

Approved Products

While food plays the most significant part in the Dr. Sebi diet, there are products that he recommends you take. Various sites sell Dr. Sebi supplements. Some are more luxurious and expensive than others, but they are all the same things. The goal of the supplements is to provide your body with nutrients that it needs to function correctly. Some supplements are specific to men and women as well, so make sure that you pay attention. Most websites will also provide you with grouped products that offer you everything you need for general health or to heal a specific ailment.

Iron Plus

Iron plus is meant to help purify the entire body. It contains chaparral, which, as we have talked about, is a powerful antioxidant. Iron plus also contains:

- Bugleweed
- Palo guaco
- Hombre grande

- Blue vervain
- Chaparral
- Elderberry

Green Food

This is a multi-mineral supplement that is made up of herbs from Africa and offers chlorophyll-rich food that nourished the body. It contains ortiga, which is well known as an anti-inflammatory. It can also help with gout, rheumatism, influenza, hemorrhage, cardiovascular system, locomotor system disorders, gastrointestinal tract disorders, urinary tract infections, and kidney disorders. It is also great at helping poor circulation and purifying the blood. Ortiga has also been used to improve the symptoms of hay fever. Green food contains:

- Bladderwrack
- Nopal
- Tila
- Nettle

Bromide Plus Powder/Bromide Plus Capsules

This is meant to help your thyroid gland and bones. It is excellent for people who suffer from dysentery, respiratory issues, pulmonary illnesses, and bad breath. It is a natural diuretic, improves the digestive system, regulates the bowels, and suppresses the appetite. It contains bladderwrack, which is a seaweed that lives in the Baltic Sea, Atlantic Ocean, and the Pacific Ocean. It is one of the sources of iodine. It is full of mannitol, alginic, potassium, bromine, and beta-carotene. It contains bladderwrack and Irish sea moss.

Bio Ferro Tonic/Bio Ferro Capsules

Bio Ferro contains the right ingredients to purify and nourish the blood. It includes a yellow dock root, which is an herb that acts as a digestive bitter to help improve digestion. It is a detoxifier and blood purifier and especially helps the liver. Yellow dock root also helps the metabolism of fats and stimulates bile production. It can also help with bowel movements and get rid of waste lingering in the intestinal tract. It will also increase urination. Bio Ferro contains:

- Cocolmeca
- Yellow dock root
- Burdock root
- Chaparral
- Elderberry

Bio ferro capsules work the same way as the tonic. They have slightly different ingredients even though they do the same thing. The capsules contain:

- Yellow dock root
- Nopal
- Nettle
- Burdock root
- Chaparral

Banju

The banju tonic is made from potent ingredients to make a tonic that helps to stimulate the central nervous system and brain. It contains:

- Bugleweed
- Valerian root
- Burdock root
- Blue vervain
- Elderberry

Body Care

Uterine Oil and Wash

As you can presumption by the name, this is meant for women. This helps to cleanse and restore the flora and fauna of the vagina. The red clover in the wash acts as a blood purifier, improves circulation, and acts as an expectorant. It also contains isoflavones and flavonoids, which help to produce estrogen. Red clover is excellent at treating conditions that are associated with menopause. The ingredients in the wash include:

- Red clover
- Sage
- Arnica
- Lupulo

Tooth Powder

This is a natural powder that you can use as a toothpaste that will help stop gum disease and tooth decay. It contains Encino and myrrh gum powder.

Hair Food Oil

This is meant to nourish the scalp and hair. It is gentle on the skin so that it can be used every day. It helps stimulate hair growth. It contains:

- French vanilla
- Coconut oil
- Batana oil
- Olive oil

Eyewash

This product naturally cleanses and nourishes the eye. It contains the only eyebright, which is commonly used to help treat many different eye diseases. It can also aid to reduce the inflammation in the eye caused by conjunctivitis and blepharitis.

Eva Salve

This salve is meant to tone and nourish the skin. The unique combination of ingredients in eva salve provides natural minerals the skin needs like potassium phosphate, fluorine, and calcium, which your skin needs to maintain elasticity. It also contains sage which is a powerful antioxidant that helps to fight off free radical damage. Eva salve contains:

- Manzo
- Eucalyptus
- Sage
- Arnica
- Olive oil
- Lily of the valley
- Nopal
- Shea butter
- Estro

Herbal Teas

- Stomach relief tea
- Stress relief tea
- Immune support tea
- Energy booster tea
- Cold and cough tea
- Blood pressure balance tea

Foods to Avoid

Any foods that are not covered in the Dr. Sebi vitamins manual aren't accredited, which includes:

- Canned fruit or vegetables
- Seedless fruit
- Eggs
- Dairy
- Fish
- Red meat
- Rooster
- Soy products
- Processed meals, including take-out or eating place meals
- Fortified ingredients
- Wheat
- Sugar (except date sugar and agave syrup)
- Alcohol
- Yeast or foods rose with yeast
- Meals made with baking powder

Furthermore, many greens, grains, nuts, and seeds are banned on the diet. Only foods indexed inside the guide can be eaten. The food regimen limits any food this is processed, animal-primarily based, or made with leavening.

How to Follow the Diet

Rules to Follow

To follow Dr. Sebi's diet, you need to strictly adhere to his rules, which are present on his website. Here is a list of his guidelines below:

1. Do not eat or drink any product or ingredient not mentioned in the approved list for the diet. It is not recommended and should never be consumed when following the diet.
2. You have to drink almost one gallon (or more than three liters) of water every day. It is recommended to drink spring water.
3. You have to take Dr. Sebi's mixtures or products one hour before consuming your medications.
4. You can take any of Dr. Sebi's mixtures/products together without any worry.
5. You need to follow the nutritional guidelines stringently and punctually take Dr. Sebi's mixtures/products daily.
6. You are not allowed to consume any animal-based food or hybrid products.
7. You are not allowed to consume alcohol or any kind of dairy product.
8. You are not allowed to consume wheat, only natural growing grains as listed in the nutritional guide
9. The grains mentioned in the nutritional guide can be available in different forms, like pasta and bread, in different health food stores. You can consume them.
10. Do not use fruits from cans; also, seedless fruits are not recommended for consumption.
11. You are not allowed to use a microwave to reheat your meals.

How to Prepare the Body

It should be clear that it is a restrictive diet low in calories. Many people believe that because of this reason, it cannot be used as a standard way to lose weight as it puts too much stress on the body of a new dieter. Because it is low in calories and an intensive diet, weight loss can be seen, but the person needs to assess whether they are capable of handling a low caloric diet. Being too ambitious with this diet might turn fatal, so if you want to try the diet, be careful!

This diet has been suggested to be followed throughout one's entire life, which might not be possible for a new dieter. With any diet, if you start cutting foods strongly and then revert to your old routine of eating unhealthy meals, the chances are that the weight loss and benefits you see will get reversed. This is a risk in this diet as well. When starting, set reasonable goals and don't go too strongly. Let your body first get used to it and then start setting up more ambitious goals.

Meal Plan

Starting the diet can be daunting, so here is a list of meal ideas that you can copy from. For the first few days, follow it so that you get used to the diet.

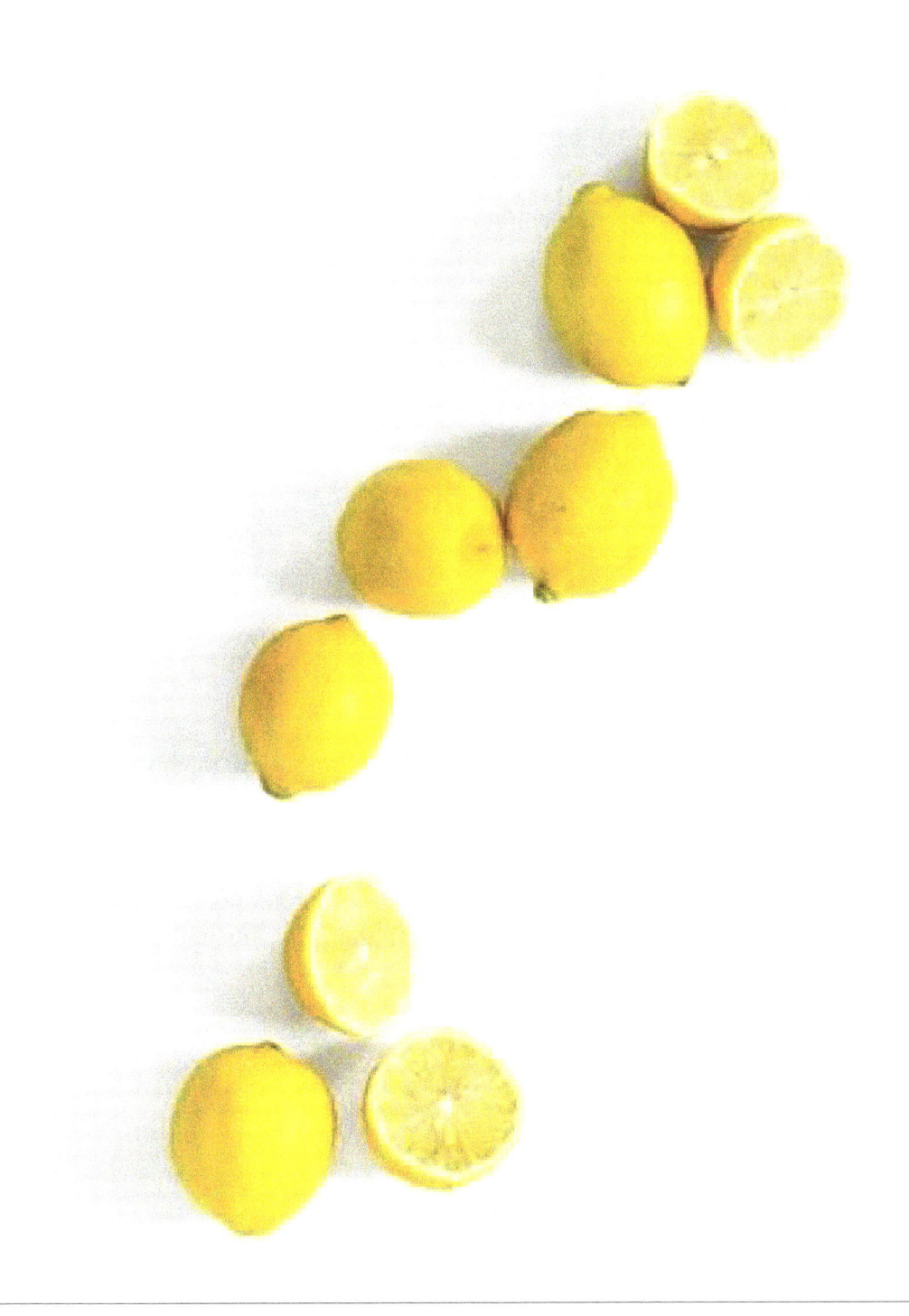

Breakfast

1. Banana pancakes with agave syrup (more than one is recommended).

2. A strawberry and banana smoothie with added hemp seeds and water.

3. Cooked quinoa with coconut milk (pure) and agave syrup for sweetness (add a fruit of your choice as well).

Lunch

1. A salad made up of kale, tomatoes, onions, avocados, and chickpeas with olive oil and dressing of herbs.

2. A pizza made with spelt flour, Brazil nut cheese topped with different vegetables like tomatoes, etc.

3. A pasta made of spelt with different vegetables, and lime and olive oil dressings.

Evening Snack

1. A smoothie made by cucumbers, kale, a few pieces of ginger, and one or two apples.

2. Herbal tea accompanied by the fruit of your choice.

3. Blueberry muffins made by spelt and teff flour, coconut milk (pure), agave syrup, and blueberries.

Dinner

1. A wild rice stir-fry with vegetables of your choice.

2. A burger made up of spelt flour bread; tomatoes, onions, and kale as vegetables; and a chickpea patty.

3. Thick vegetable soup made up of zucchini, mushrooms, peppers, spices, sea salt, onions, and seaweed powder.

Drink Water

Smoothies are a drink, and by drinking them, you are ultimately fulfilling your water intake for the day. Dr. Sebi's diet requires you to drink one gallon of water daily, but that can be difficult. Dehydration is a serious problem that can lead to anxiety. To prevent that, you need to drink lots of water, which the smoothie diet helps you with.

What You Should Not Eat

Foods that are not listed in the nutritional guide are not allowed to be consumed. Some examples of such foods are given below:

1. Any canned product, be it fruits or vegetables, listed in the nutritional guide
2. Seedless fruits like grapes
3. Eggs
4. Any type of dairy product
5. Fish
6. Any type of poultry
7. Red meat
8. Soy products
9. Processed foods
10. Restaurant foods and delivered foods
11. Hybrid and fortified foods
12. Wheat
13. White sugar
14. Alcohol
15. Yeast and its products
16. Baking powder

Some other foods and ingredients have been cut off. You only need to follow the nutritional guide to know what you have to eat.

A 7-Day Alkaline Meal Plan

Among the diverse body parts, the liver is among one of the significant organs, for it has considerable capacity in body detoxification. Through this body detoxification, synthetics and other outside substances like poisons and even defecation, pee, and sweat are expelled from the body. These substances originate from the unsafe nourishments that we eat like handled and non-regular rich nourishments, liquor drinks that we devour, cigarettes that we smoke, and even drugs that we expend for anti-infection treatment and hormone elective drugs. These substances are the ones that our bodies attempt to take out every day.

When there are many harming materials inside the body, the liver needs to keep keeping up until its ability runs out. When this is dismissed, vast amounts of poisons can be gathered in the body and will cause many body issues and diseases. To anticipate this and keep up excellent health, we should experience a detoxification diet and take significant consideration of our liver.

A liver detoxification plan can be completed either on a three-day, seven-day, or twenty-one-day program. This depends on a firm focus on a diet with unprocessed and natural foods grown from the ground, entire grains, and water cure with enough measure of water or liquid other option. Nourishments that are wealthy in fat or sugar, caffeine, liquor drinks, unnatural and human-made nourishment, drugs, and low-quality nourishments would all be able to must be put to a stop, at any rate, seven days before the diet plan.

One to Three Days. This is the period to start your fluid diet plan where you need to drink around ten to twelve glasses of water ordinarily alongside frequently crushed lime juice. Even though it can indeed be challenging to execute this diet because of the weariness and slightness, light exercise can be included as a request to affix the method of flushing the poisons out of the body. Additionally, you should shun taking in any sort of milk or dairy item.

Four to Six Days. Fresh organic products, vegetables, and entire grains can be expended like celery, apples, carrots, oranges, which would all be able to be blended into one juice. The juice can incorporate your selection of leafy foods. Even though healthy nourishments are devoured, there are as yet liquid choices, for example, natural teas for around a few cups every day. Concerning suppers, they can incorporate cut and bubbled vegetables like celery, carrots, broccoli, and spinach. Besides, you can likewise utilize soups that can be taken in at regular intervals.

Seven Days. Along with the leafy foods, the liquids are expended together. They would all be able to be arranged by having them crude or steamed. Additionally, you can consume rosemary tea and dandelion options, which can be useful for this period.

You can generally change the sorts of foods grown from the ground that you will use as long as you oblige the strategy. When the seventh day is a doe, you can participate in the typical diet; finally, however, there is still a restriction on liquor consumption for around one entire week after the detoxification diet. You have to end the food once you feel torment, disorder, and squeamishness. Most likely, this detoxification diet can have an enormous impact on the advancement and support of a healthy lifestyle.

Instructions to Detox Your Body With Alternative Therapies

Conventional Chinese Medicine (TCM) is a fantastic asset when figuring out how to detox your body, and is mainly prescribed for treating stomach related issue, for example, bad-tempered inside syndrome; ceaseless skin conditions like dermatitis; weariness and despair; hormonal awkward nature, for example, PMS; endometriosis and poor sperm tally, and barrenness (both male and female). It can create results with interminable conditions that Western methods neglect to help. At the point when joined with a detox diet, it can make perceptible upgrades to a people's health and prosperity.

Self-finding and treatment of ailments are not suggested; however, at some TCM focuses, you can portray your side effects to the specialist behind the counter and get a suitable cure on the spot. TCM can be useful for treating individuals experiencing withdrawal from drug and liquor addictions. Liquor makes liver and nerve bladder uneven characters, which realizes a mix of unnecessary moistness and warmth.

Numerous drugs are prepared through the liver, making it warmed and blocked, so the liver's blood gets frail and insufficient. TCM equations center on clearing and supporting the liver and nerve bladder, while simultaneously treating the heart, to help quiet the brain and sensory system. Consolidating TCM with figuring out how to detox your body yourself is probably the best thing you can accomplish for your health.

Soups

42. Creamy Avocado-Broccoli Soup

Preparation Time: 10 minutes

Cooking Time: 15 minutes

Servings: 1-2

Ingredients:

2-3 flowers broccoli
1 small avocado
1 yellow onion
1 green or red pepper
1 celery stalk
2 cups of vegetable broth (yeast-free)
Celtic sea salt to taste

Directions:

Warm vegetable stock (don't bubble). Include hacked onion and broccoli, and warm for a few minutes. At that point, put the avocado, pepper, and celery in the blender and blend until the soup is smooth (include some more water whenever wanted). Season and serve warm. Delicious!!

Nutrition:

Calories: 60g - Carbohydrates: 11g
Fat: 2 g - Protein: 2g

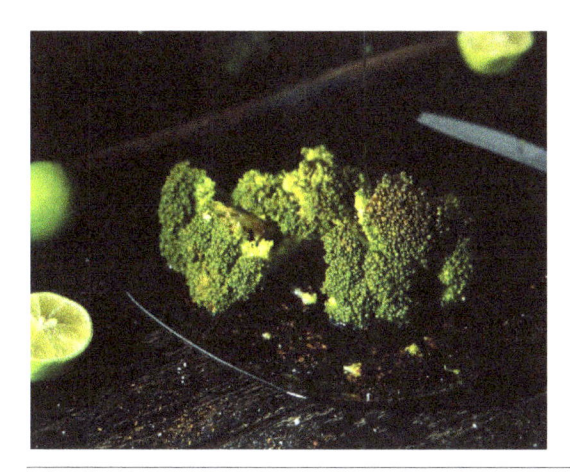

43. Fresh Garden Vegetable Soup

Preparation Time: 7 minutes

Cooking Time: 20 minutes

Servings: 1-2

Ingredients:

2 huge carrots
1 little zucchini
1 celery stem
1 cup of broccoli
3 stalks of asparagus
1 yellow onion
1 quart of (antacid) water
4-5 tsps. of sans yeast vegetable stock
1 tsp. new basil
2 tsps. Ocean salt to taste

Directions:

Put water in a pot, include the vegetable stock just as the onion and boil it.
In the meantime, cleave the zucchini, the broccoli, and the asparagus, and shred the carrots and the celery stem in a food processor.
When the water is bubbling, it would be ideal if you turn off the oven as we would prefer not to heat up the vegetables. Simply put them all in the high temp water and hold up until the vegetables arrive at wanted delicacy. Permit to cool somewhat, at that point put all fixings into a blender and blend until you get a thick, smooth consistency.

Nutrition:

Calories: 43
Carbohydrates: 7g
Fat: 1 g

44. Rawsome Gazpacho Soup

Preparation Time: 7 minutes

Cooking Time: 3 hours

Servings: 3-4

Ingredients:

500g tomatoes
1 small cucumber
1 red pepper
1 onion
2 cloves of garlic
1 small chili
1 quart of water (preferably alkaline water)
4 tbsp. cold-pressed olive oil
Juice of one fresh lemon
1 dash of cayenne pepper
Sea salt to taste

Directions:

Remove the skin of the cucumber and cut all vegetables in large pieces.
Put all ingredients except the olive oil in a blender and mix until smooth.
Add the olive oil and mix again until oil is emulsified.
Put the soup in the fridge and chill for at least 2 hours (soup should be served ice cold).
Add some salt and pepper to taste, mix, place the soup in bowls, garnish with chopped scallions, cucumbers, tomatoes, and peppers and enjoy!

Nutrition:

Calories: 39
Carbohydrates: 8g
Fat: 0.5 g
Protein: 0.2g

45. Alkaline Carrot Soup with Fresh Mushrooms

Preparation Time: 10 minutes

Cooking Time: 20 minutes

Servings: 1-2

Ingredients:

4 mid-sized carrots
4 mid-sized potatoes
10 enormous new mushrooms (champignons or chanterelles)
1/2 white onion
2 tbsp. olive oil (cold squeezed, additional virgin)
3 cups vegetable stock
2 tbsp. parsley, new and cleaved
Salt and new white pepper

Directions:

Wash and strip carrots and potatoes and dice them.
Warm up vegetable stock in a pot on medium heat. Cook carrots and potatoes for around 15 minutes. Meanwhile finely shape onion and braise them in a container with olive oil for around 3 minutes.
Wash mushrooms, slice them to wanted size, and add to the container, cooking for an additional of approximately 5 minutes, blending at times. Blend carrots, vegetable stock and potatoes, and put the substance of the skillet into the pot.
When nearly done, season with parsley, salt, and pepper and serve hot. Appreciate this alkalizing soup!

Nutrition:

Calories: 75
Carbohydrates: 13g
Fat: 1.8g
Protein: 1 g

46. Swiss Cauliflower-Soup

Preparation Time: 10 minutes

Cooking Time: 15 minutes

Servings: 3-4

Ingredients:

2 cups cauliflower pieces
1 cup potatoes, cubed
2 cups vegetable stock (without yeast)
2 tbsp. new chives
1 tbsp. pumpkin seeds
1 touch of nutmeg and cayenne pepper

Directions:

Cook cauliflower and potato in vegetable stock until delicate and blend it.
Season the soup with nutmeg and cayenne, and possibly somewhat salt and pepper. Optionally, include some creamy vegan cheese and mix a couple of moments until the soup is smooth and prepared to serve. Enhance it with pumpkin seeds.

Nutrition:

Calories: 65
Carbohydrates: 13g
Fat: 2g
Protein: 1g

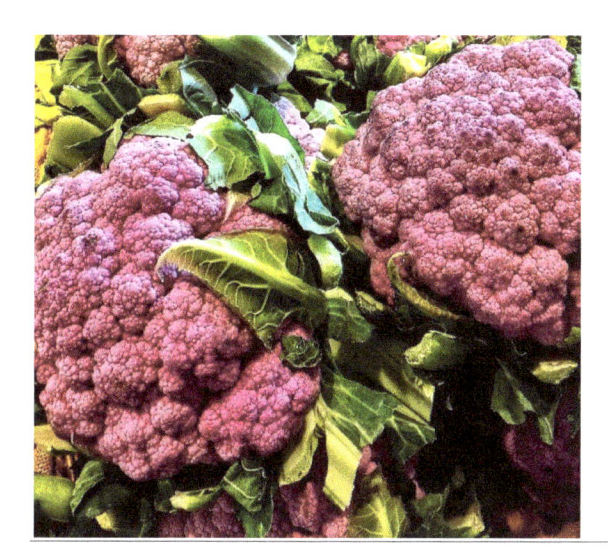

47. Chilled Parsley-Gazpacho with Lime & Cucumber

Preparation Time: 10 minutes

Cooking Time: 2 hours

Servings: 1

Ingredients:

4-5 middle-sized tomatoes
2 tbsp. olive oil, extra virgin, and cold-pressed
2 large cups fresh parsley
2 ripe avocados
2 cloves garlic, diced
2 limes, juiced
4 cups vegetable broth
1 middle-sized cucumber
2 small red onions, diced
1 tsp. dried oregano
1½ tsp. paprika powder
½ tsp. cayenne pepper
Sea salt and freshly ground pepper to taste

Directions:

In a pan, heat up olive oil and sauté onions and garlic until translucent. Set aside to cool down.
Use a large blender and blend parsley, avocado, tomatoes, cucumber, vegetable broth, lime juice, and onion-garlic mix until smooth. Add some water if desired, and season with cayenne pepper, paprika powder, oregano, salt, and pepper. Blend again and put in the fridge for at least 1, 5 hours.
Tip: Add chives or dill to the gazpacho. Enjoy this great alkaline (cold) soup!

Nutrition:

Calories: 48
Carbohydrates: 12 g
Fat: 0.8g

48. Chilled Avocado Tomato Soup

Preparation Time: 7 minutes

Cooking Time: 20 minutes

Servings: 1-2

Ingredients:

2 small avocados
2 large tomatoes
1 stalk of celery
1 small onion
1 clove of garlic
Juice of 1 fresh lemon
1 cup of water (best: alkaline water)
A handful of fresh lavage
Parsley and sea salt to taste

Directions:

Scoop the avocados and cut all veggies in little pieces.
Spot all fixings in a blender and blend until smooth.
Serve chilled and appreciate this nutritious and sound soluble soup formula!

Nutrition:

Calories: 68
Carbohydrates: 15g
Fat: 2g
Protein: .8g

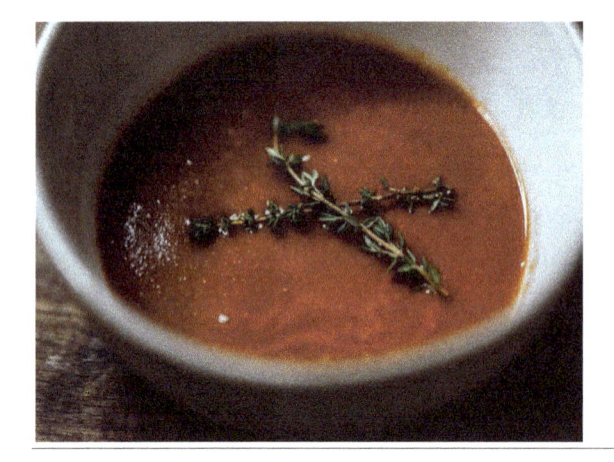

49. Pumpkin and White Bean Soup with Sage

Preparation Time: 10 minutes

Cooking Time: 40 minutes

Servings: 3-4

Ingredients:

1 ½ pound pumpkin
½ pound yams
½ pound white beans
1 onion
2 cloves of garlic
1 tbsp. of cold squeezed additional virgin olive oil
1 tbsp. of spices (your top picks)
1 tbsp. of sage
1 ½ quart water (best: antacid water)
A spot of ocean salt and pepper

Directions:

Cut the pumpkin and potatoes in shapes, cut the onion and cut the garlic, the spices, and the sage in fine pieces.
Sauté the onion and also the garlic in olive oil for around two or three minutes.
Include the potatoes, pumpkin, spices, and sage and fry for an additional 5 minutes.
At that point include the water and cook for around 30 minutes (spread the pot with a top) until vegetables are delicate.
At long last include the beans and some salt and pepper. Cook for an additional 5 minutes and serve right away. Prepared!! Appreciate this antacid soup. Alkalizing tasty!

Nutrition:

Calories: 78
Carbohydrates: 12g

50. Alkaline Carrot Soup With Millet

Preparation Time: 7 minutes

Cooking Time: 40 minutes

Servings: 3-4

Ingredients:

2 cups cauliflower pieces
1 cup potatoes, cubed
2 cups vegetable stock (without yeast)
Vegan cheese
2 tbsp. new chives
1 tbsp. pumpkin seeds
1 touch of nutmeg and cayenne pepper

Directions:

Cook cauliflower and potato in vegetable stock until delicate and blend it.
Season the soup with nutmeg and cayenne, and possibly somewhat salt and pepper. Include the vegan cheese and chives and mix a couple of moments until the soup is smooth and prepared to serve. It can be enhanced with pumpkin seeds.

Nutrition:

Calories: 65
Carbohydrates: 15g
Fat: 1g
Protein: 2g

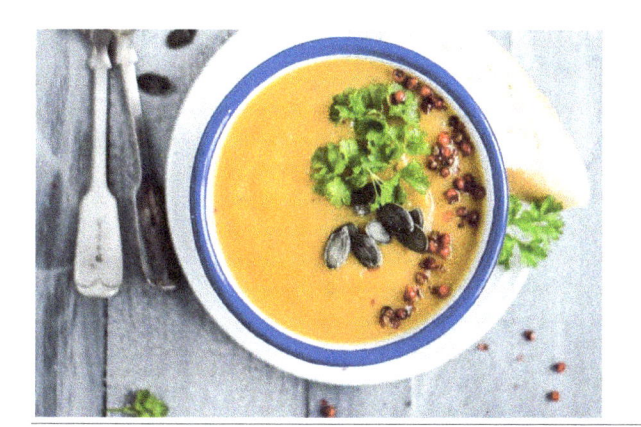

51. Alkaline Pumpkin Tomato Soup

Preparation Time: 15 minutes

Cooking Time: 30 minutes

Servings: 3-4

Ingredients:

1 quart of water (if accessible: soluble water)
400g new tomatoes, stripped and diced
1 medium-sized sweet pumpkin
5 yellow onions
1 tbsp. cold squeezed additional virgin olive oil
2 tsp. ocean salt or natural salt
Touch of cayenne pepper
Your preferred spices (discretionary)
Bunch of new parsley

Directions:

Cut onions in little pieces and sauté with some oil in a significant pot.
Cut the pumpkin down the middle, at that point remove the stem and scoop out the seeds.
At long last scoop out the fragile living creature and put it in the pot.
Include likewise the tomatoes and the water and cook for around 20 minutes.
At that point empty the soup into a food processor and blend well for a couple of moments. Sprinkle with salt pepper and other spices.
Fill bowls and trimming with new parsley. Make the most of your alkalizing soup!

Nutrition:

Calories: 78
Carbohydrates: 20
Fat: 0.5g
Protein: 1.5g

52. Alkaline Pumpkin Coconut Soup

Preparation Time: 10 minutes

Cooking Time: 15 minutes

Servings: 3-4

Ingredients:

2lb pumpkin
6 cups of water (best: soluble water delivered with a water ionizer)
1 cup low-fat coconut milk
5 ounces of potatoes
2 major onions
3 ounces leek
1 bunch of new parsley
1 touch of nutmeg
1 touch of cayenne pepper
1 tsp. ocean salt or natural salt
4 tbsp. cold squeezed additional virgin olive oil

Directions:

As a matter of first significance: cut the onions, the pumpkin, and the potatoes just as the hole into little pieces.
At that point, heat the olive oil in a significant pot and sauté the onions for a couple of moments.
At that point, include the water and heat up the pumpkin, potatoes, and the leek until delicate.
Include coconut milk.
Presently utilize a hand blender and puree for around 1 moment. The soup should turn out to be extremely velvety.
Season with salt, pepper, and nutmeg. Lastly, include the parsley and appreciate this alkalizing pumpkin soup hot or cold!

Nutrition:

Calories: 88 - Carbohydrates: 23g
Fat: 2.5 g - Protein: 1.8g

53. Cold Cauliflower-Coconut Soup

Preparation Time: 7 minutes

Cooking Time: 20 minutes

Servings: 3-4

Ingredients:

1 pound (450g) new cauliflower
1 ¼ cup (300ml) unsweetened coconut milk
1 cup of water (best: antacid water)
2 tbsp. new lime juice
1/3 cup cold squeezed additional virgin olive oil
1 cup new coriander leaves, slashed
Spot of salt and cayenne pepper
1 bunch of unsweetened coconut chips

Directions:

Steam cauliflower for around 10 minutes. At that point, set up the cauliflower with coconut milk and water in a food processor and get it started until extremely smooth. Include new lime squeeze, salt and pepper, a large portion of the cleaved coriander, and the oil and blend for an additional couple of moments.
Pour in soup bowls and embellishment with coriander and coconut chips. Appreciate!

Nutrition:

Calories: 65
Carbohydrates: 11g
Fat: 0.3g
Protein: 1.5g

54. Raw Avocado-Broccoli Soup With Cashew Nuts

Preparation Time: 10 minutes

Cooking Time: 30 minutes

Servings: 1-2

Ingredients:

½ cup of water (if available: alkaline water)
½ avocado
1 cup chopped broccoli
½ cup cashew nuts
½ cup alfalfa sprouts
1 clove of garlic
1 tbsp. cold-pressed extra virgin olive oil
1 pinch of sea salt and pepper
Some parsley to garnish

Directions:

Put the cashew nuts in a blender or food processor, include some water and puree for a couple of moments.
Include the various fixings (except for the avocado) individually and puree each an ideal opportunity for a couple of moments. Dispense the soup in a container and warm it up to the normal room temperature.
Enhance with salt and pepper. In the interim dice the avocado and slash the parsley.
Dispense the soup in a container or plate; include the avocado dices and embellishment with parsley.
That's it! Enjoy this excellent healthy soup!

Nutrition:

Calories: 48
Carbohydrates: 18g
Fat: 3g
Protein: 1.4g

55. Lemon-Tarragon Soup

Preparation Time: 10 minutes

Cooking Time: 10 minutes

Servings: 1-2

Cashews and coconut milk replace heavy cream in this healthy version of the lemon-tarragon soup, balanced by tart freshly squeezed lemon juice and fragrant tarragon. It's a light, airy soup that you won't want to miss.

Ingredients:

1 tablespoon avocado oil
½ cup diced onion
3 garlic cloves, crushed
¼ plus ⅛ teaspoon sea salt
¼ plus ⅛ teaspoon freshly ground black pepper
1 (13.5-ounce) can full-fat coconut milk
1 tablespoon freshly squeezed lemon juice
½ cup raw cashews
1 celery stalk
2 tablespoons chopped fresh tarragon

Directions:

In a medium skillet over medium-high warmth, heat the avocado oil. Add the onion, garlic, salt, and pepper, and sauté for 3 to 5 minutes or until the onion is soft.
In a high-speed blender, blend the coconut milk, lemon juice, cashews, celery, and tarragon with the onion mixture until smooth. Adjust seasonings, if necessary.
Fill 1 huge or 2 little dishes and enjoy immediately, or transfer to a medium saucepan and warm on low heat for 3 to 5 minutes before serving.

Nutrition:

Calories: 60 - Carbohydrates: 13 g
Protein: 0.8 g

56. Chilled Cucumber and Lime Soup

Preparation Time: 5 minutes

Cooking Time: 20 minutes

Servings: 1-2

Chilled soups are perfect for the hot summer months, and this easy soup is made with garden fresh vegetables with no cooking involved. Simply prepare the veggies, add them to a blender, and lunch is served!

Ingredients:

1 cucumber, peeled
½ zucchini, peeled
1 tablespoon freshly squeezed lime juice
1 tablespoon fresh cilantro leaves
1 garlic clove, crushed
¼ teaspoon of sea salt

Directions:

In a blender, blend the cucumber, zucchini, lime juice, cilantro, garlic, and salt until well combined. Add more salt, if necessary. Fill 1 huge or 2 little dishes and enjoy immediately, or refrigerate for 15 to 20 minutes to chill before serving.

Nutrition:

Calories: 48 - Carbohydrates: 8 g
Fat: 1g - Protein: .5g

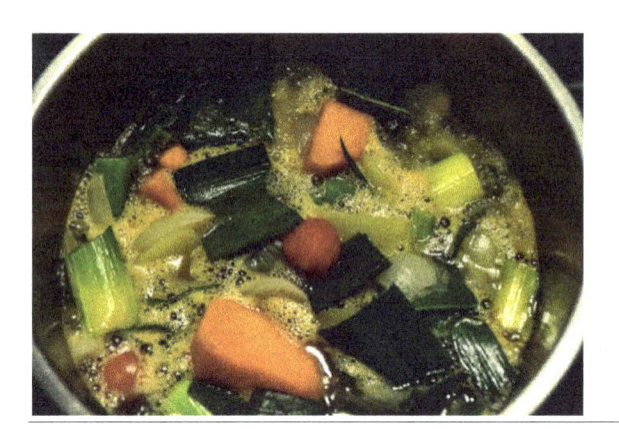

57. Coconut, Cilantro, and Jalapeño Soup

Preparation Time: 5 minutes

Cooking Time: 5 minutes

Servings: 1-2

This soup is a nutrient dream. Cilantro is a natural anti-inflammatory and is also excellent for detoxification. And one single jalapeño has an entire day's worth of vitamin C!

Ingredients:

2 tablespoons avocado oil
½ cup diced onions
3 garlic cloves, crushed
¼ teaspoon of sea salt
1 (13.5-ounce) can full-fat coconut milk
1 tablespoon freshly squeezed lime juice
½ to 1 jalapeño
2 tablespoons fresh cilantro leaves

Directions:

In a medium skillet over medium-high warmth, heat the avocado oil. Include the garlic, onion salt, and pepper, and sauté for 3 to 5 minutes, or until the onions are soft. In a blender, blend the coconut milk, lime juice, jalapeño, and cilantro with the onion mixture until creamy.
Fill 1 huge or 2 little dishes and enjoy it.

Nutrition:

Calories: 75
Carbohydrates: 13 g
Fat: 2 g
Protein: 4 g

210

58. Spicy Watermelon Gazpacho

Preparation Time: 5 minutes

Cooking Time: 5 minutes

Servings: 1-2

At first taste, this soup may have you wondering if you're lunching on a hot and spicy salsa. It has the heat and seasonings of a traditional tomato-based salsa, but it also has a faint sweetness from the cool watermelon. The soup is really hot with a whole jalapeño, so if you don't like food too hot, just use half a jalapeño.

Ingredients:

2 cups cubed watermelon
¼ cup diced onion
¼ cup packed cilantro leaves
½ to 1 jalapeño
2 tablespoons freshly squeezed lime juice

Directions:

In a blender or food processor, pulse to combine the watermelon, onion, cilantro, jalapeño, and lime juice only long enough to break down the ingredients, leaving them very finely diced and taking care to not over process.

Pour into 1 large or 2 small bowls and enjoy.

Nutrition:

Calories: 35
Carbohydrates: 12
Fat: .4 g

59. Roasted Carrot and Leek Soup

Preparation Time: 4 minutes

Cooking Time: 30 minutes

Servings: 3-4

The carrot, a root vegetable, is an excellent source of antioxidants (1 cup has 113 percent of your daily value of vitamin A), and fibre (1 cup has 14 percent of your daily value). This bright and colourful soup freezes well to enjoy later when you're short on time.

Ingredients:

6 carrots
1 cup chopped onion
1 fennel bulb, cubed
2 garlic cloves, crushed
2 tablespoons avocado oil
1 teaspoon of sea salt
1 teaspoon freshly ground black pepper
2 cups almond milk, plus more if desired

Directions:

Preheat the oven to 400°F. Line a baking sheet with parchment paper.
Cut the carrots into thirds, and then cut each third in half. Transfer to a medium bowl. Add the onion, fennel, garlic, and avocado oil, and toss to coat. Season with the salt and pepper, and toss again.
Transfer the vegetables to the prepared baking sheet, and roast for 30 minutes. Remove from the oven and allow the vegetables to cool.
In a high-speed blender, blend the almond milk and roasted vegetables until creamy and smooth. Adjust the seasonings, if necessary, and add additional milk if you prefer a thinner consistency.
Pour into 2 large or 4 small bowls and enjoy.

Nutrition:

Calories: 55 - Carbohydrates: 12g
Fat: 1.5 g - Protein: 1.8 g

60. Creamy Lentil and Potato Stew

Preparation Time: 10 minutes

Cooking Time: 30 minutes

Servings: 4

This is a hearty stew that is sure to be a favourite. It's a one-pot meal that is the perfect comfort food. With fresh vegetables and herbs along with protein-rich lentils, it's both healthy and filling. Any lentil variety would work, even a mixed, sprouted lentil blend. Another bonus of this recipe: It's freezer-friendly.

Ingredients:

2 tablespoons avocado oil
½ cup diced onion
2 garlic cloves, crushed
1 to 1½ teaspoons of sea salt
1 teaspoon freshly ground black pepper
1 cup dry lentils
2 carrots, sliced
1 cup peeled and cubed potato
1 celery stalk, diced
2 fresh oregano sprigs, chopped
2 fresh tarragon sprigs, chopped
5 cups vegetable broth, divided
1 (13.5-ounce) can full-fat coconut milk

Directions:

In a great soup pot over average-high hotness, heat the avocado oil. Include the garlic, onion, salt, and pepper, and sauté for 3 to 5 minutes, or until the onion is soft. Add the lentils, carrots, potato, celery, oregano, tarragon, and 2½ cups of vegetable broth, and stir.

Get to a boil, decrease the heat to medium-low, and cook, stirring frequently and adding additional vegetable broth a half cup at a time to make sure there is enough liquid for the lentils and potatoes to cook, for 20 to 25 minutes, or until the potatoes and lentils are soft.

Take away from the heat, and stir in the coconut milk. Pour into 4 soup bowls and enjoy.

Nutrition:

Calories: 85
Carbohydrates: 20g
Fat: 3g
Protein: 3g

61. Roasted Garlic and Cauliflower Soup

Preparation Time: 10 minutes

Cooking Time: 35 minutes

Servings: 1-2

Roasted garlic is always a treat, and paired with cauliflower in this wonderful soup, what you get is a deeply satisfying soup with savoury, rustic flavors. Blended, the result is a smooth, thick, and creamy soup, but if you prefer a thinner consistency, just add a little more vegetable broth to thin it out. Cauliflower is anti-inflammatory, high in antioxidants, and a good source of vitamin C (1 cup has 86 percent of your daily value).

Ingredients:

4 cups bite-size cauliflower florets
5 garlic cloves
1½ tablespoons avocado oil¾ teaspoon of sea salt
½ teaspoon freshly ground black pepper
1 cup almond milk
1 cup vegetable broth, plus more if desired

Directions:

Preheat the oven to 450°F. Line a baking sheet with parchment paper.

In a medium bowl, toss the cauliflower and garlic with the avocado oil to coat. Season with the salt and pepper, and toss again. Transfer to the prepared baking sheet and roast for 30 minutes. Cool before adding to the blender.

In a high-speed blender, blend the cooled vegetables, almond milk, and vegetable broth until creamy and smooth. Adjust the salt and pepper, if necessary, and add additional vegetable broth if you prefer a thinner consistency.

Transfer to a medium saucepan, and lightly warm on medium-low heat for 3 to 5 minutes.

Ladle into 1 large or 2 small bowls and enjoy.

Nutrition:

Calories: 48 - Carbohydrates: 11g
Protein: 1.5g

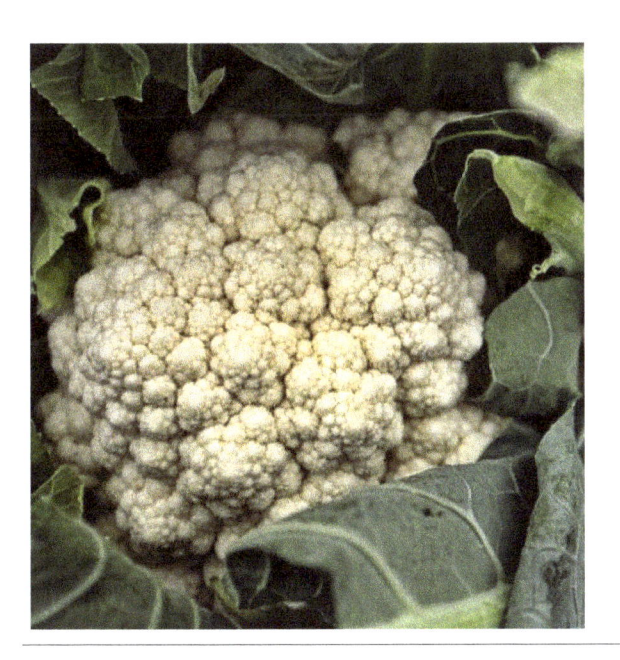

62. Beefless "Beef" Stew

Preparation Time: 10 minutes

Cooking Time: 0 minutes

Servings: 4

The potatoes, carrots, aromatics, and herbs in this soup meld so well together, you'll forget there's typically beef in this stew. Hearty and flavourful, this one-pot comfort food is perfect for a fall or winter dinner.

Ingredients:

1 tablespoon avocado oil
1 cup onion, diced
2 garlic cloves, crushed
1 teaspoon of sea salt
1 teaspoon freshly ground black pepper
3 cups vegetable broth, plus more if desired
2 cups water, plus more if desired
3 cups sliced carrot
1 large potato, cubed
2 celery stalks, diced
1 teaspoon dried oregano
1 dried bay leaf

Directions:

In a medium soup pot over medium heat, heat the avocado oil. Include the onion, garlic, salt, and pepper, and sauté for 2 to 3 minutes, or until the onion is soft.

Add the vegetable broth, water, carrot, potato, celery, oregano, and bay leaf, and stir. Get to a boil, decrease the heat to medium-low, and cook for 30 to 45 minutes, or until the potatoes and carrots are soft.

Adjust the seasonings, if necessary, and add additional water or vegetable broth, if a soupier consistency is preferred, in half-cup increments.

Ladle into 4 soup bowls and enjoy.

63. Creamy Mushroom Soup

Preparation Time: 5 minutes

Cooking Time: 20 minutes

Servings: 4

This savoury, earthy soup is a must-try if you love mushrooms. Shiitake and baby Portobello (cremini) mushrooms are used here, but you can substitute them with your favourite mushroom varieties. Full-fat coconut milk gives it that close-your-eyes-and-savor-it creaminess that pushes the soup into the comfort food realm—perfect for those cold evenings when you need a warm soup to heat up your insides.

Ingredients:

1 tablespoon avocado oil
1 cup sliced shiitake mushrooms
1 cup sliced cremini mushrooms
1 cup diced onion
1 garlic clove, crushed
¾ teaspoon of sea salt
½ teaspoon freshly ground black pepper
1 cup vegetable broth
1 (13.5-ounce) can full-fat coconut milk
½ teaspoon dried thyme
1 tablespoon coconut aminos

Directions:

In a great soup pot over average-high hotness, heat the avocado oil. Add the mushrooms, onion, garlic, salt, and pepper, and sauté for 2 to 3 minutes, or until the onion is soft.
Add the vegetable broth, coconut milk, thyme, and coconut aminos. Reduce the heat to medium-low, and simmer for about 15 minutes, stirring occasionally.
Adjust seasonings, if necessary, ladle into 2 large or 4 small bowls, and enjoy.

Nutrition:

Calories: 65 - Carbohydrates: 12g
Fat: 2g - Protein: 2g

64. Chilled Berry and Mint Soup

Preparation Time: 5 minutes

Cooking Time: 20 minutes

Servings: 1-2

There's no better way to cool down when it's hot outside than with this chilled, sweet mixed berry soup. It's light and showcases summer's berry bounty: raspberries, blackberries, and blueberries. The fresh mint brightens the soup and keeps the sweetness in check. This soup isn't just for lunch or dinner—you can try it as a quick breakfast, too! If you like a thinner consistency for this, just add a little extra water.

Ingredients:

FOR THE SWEETENER

¼ cup unrefined whole cane sugar, such as Sucanat
¼ cup water, plus more if desired

FOR THE SOUP

1 cup of mixed berries (raspberries, blackberries, blueberries)
½ cup of water
1 teaspoon freshly squeezed lemon juice
8 fresh mint leaves

Directions:

To prepare the sweetener

In a small saucepan over medium-low, heat the sugar and water, stirring continuously for 1 to 2 minutes, until the sugar is dissolved. Cool.

To prepare the soup

In a blender, blend the cooled sugar water

with the berries, water, lemon juice, and mint leaves until well combined.
Transfer the mixture to the refrigerator and allow chilling completely, about 20 minutes. Ladle into 1 large or 2 small bowls and enjoy.

Nutrition:

Calories: 89 - Carbohydrates: 12g
Fat: 6g - Protein: 2.2 g

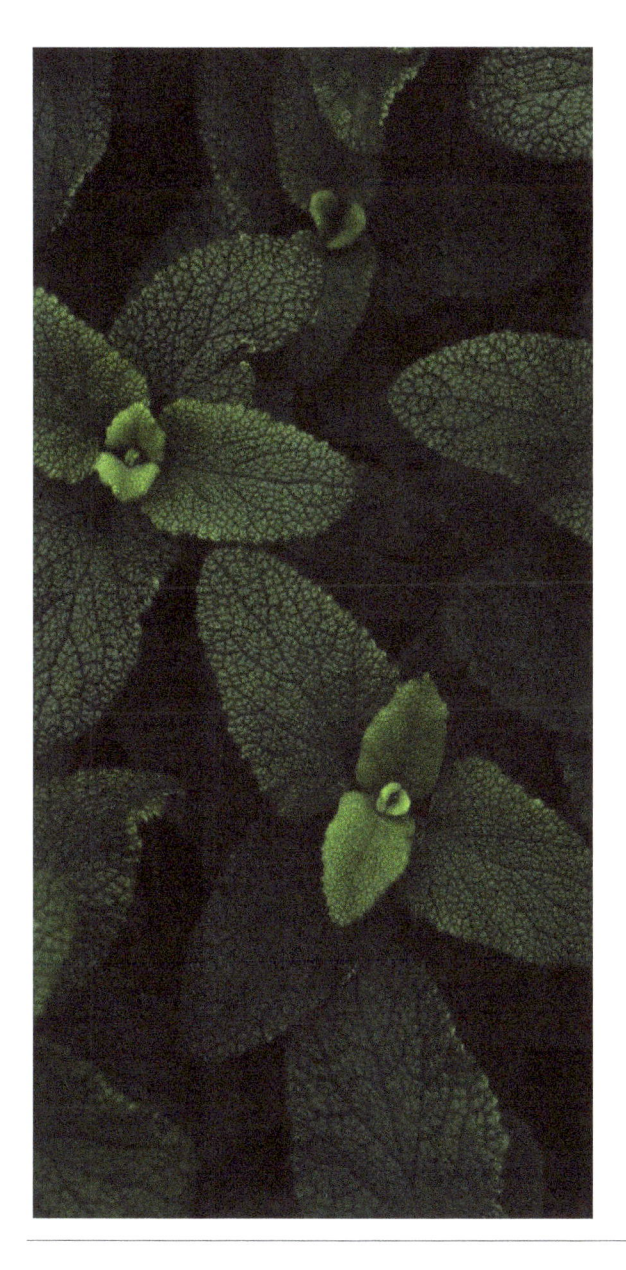

65. White Bean Soup

Preparation Time: 10 minutes

Cooking Time: 40 minutes

Servings: 6

Ingredients:

2 cups white beans, rinsed
¼ tsp. cayenne pepper
1 tsp. dried oregano
½ tsp. fresh rosemary, chopped
3 cups filtered alkaline water
3 cups unsweetened almond milk
3 garlic cloves, minced
2 celery stalks, diced
1 onion, chopped
1 tbsp. olive oil
½ tsp. sea salt

Directions:

Add oil into the instant pot and set the pot on sauté mode.
Add carrots, celery, and onion in oil and sauté until softened, about 5 minutes.
Add garlic and sauté for a minute.
Add beans, seasonings, water, and almond milk and stir to combine.
Cover pot with lid and cook on high pressure for 35 minutes.
When finished, release pressure naturally, then open the lid.
Stir well and serve.

Nutrition:

Calories 276
Fat 4.8 g
Carbohydrates 44.2 g
Sugar 2.3 g
Protein 16.6 g
Cholesterol 0 mg

66. Kale Cauliflower Soup

Preparation Time: 10 minutes

Cooking Time: 25 minutes

Servings: 4

Ingredients:

2 cups baby kale
½ cup unsweetened coconut milk
4 cups of water
1 large cauliflower head, chopped
3 garlic cloves, peeled
2 carrots, peeled and chopped
2 onion, chopped
3 tbsp. olive oil
Pepper
Salt

Directions:

Add oil into the instant pot and set the pot on sauté mode.
Add carrot, garlic, and onion to the pot and sauté for 5-7 minutes.
Add water and cauliflower and stir well.
Cover pot with lid and cook on high pressure for 20 minutes.
When finished, release pressure using the quick release, then open the lid.
Add kale and coconut milk and stir well.
Blend the soup utilizing a submersion blender until smooth.
Season with pepper and salt.

Nutrition:

Calories 261
Fat 18.1 g
Carbohydrates 23.9 g
Sugar 9.9 g
Protein 6.6 g
Cholesterol 0 mg

67. Healthy Broccoli Asparagus Soup

Preparation Time: 10 minutes

Cooking Time: 20 minutes

Servings: 6

Ingredients:

2 cups broccoli florets, chopped
15 asparagus spears, ends trimmed and chopped
1 tsp. dried oregano
1 tbsp. fresh thyme leaves
½ cup unsweetened almond milk
3 ½ cups filtered alkaline water
2 cups cauliflower florets, chopped
2 tsp. garlic, chopped
1 cup onion, chopped
2 tbsp. olive oil
Pepper
Salt

Directions:

Add oil in the instant pot and set the pot on sauté mode.
Add onion to the olive oil and sauté until onion is softened.
Add garlic and sauté for 30 seconds.
Add all vegetables and water and stir well.
Cover pot with lid and cook on manual mode for 3 minutes.
When finished, release pressure naturally, then open the lid.
Blend the soup utilizing a submersion blender until smooth.
Stir in almond milk, herbs, pepper, and salt.
Serve and enjoy.

Nutrition:

Calories 85
Fat 5.2 g
Carbohydrates 8.8 g
Sugar 3.3 g

Protein 3.3 g
Cholesterol 0 mg

68. Creamy Asparagus Soup

Preparation Time: 10 minutes

Cooking Time: 30 minutes

Servings: 6

Ingredients:

2 lbs. fresh asparagus cut off woody stems
¼ tsp. lime zest
2 tbsp. lime juice
14 oz. coconut milk
1 tsp. dried thyme
½ tsp. oregano
½ tsp. sage
1 ½ cups filtered alkaline water
1 cauliflower head, cut into florets
1 tbsp. garlic, minced
1 leek, sliced
3 tbsp. coconut oil
Pinch of Himalayan salt

Directions:

Preheat the oven to 400 F/ 200 C.
Line baking tray with parchment paper and set aside.
Arrange asparagus spears on a baking tray. Drizzle with 2 tablespoons of coconut oil and sprinkle with salt, thyme, oregano, and sage.
Bake in preheated oven for 20-25 minutes.
Add remaining oil in the instant pot and set the pot on sauté mode.
Put some garlic and leek to the pot and sauté for 2-3 minutes.
Add cauliflower florets and water in the pot and stir well.
Cover pot with a lid and select steam mode and set timer for 4 minutes.
When finished, release pressure using the quick release.
Add roasted asparagus, lime zest, lime juice, and coconut milk and stir well.
Blend the soup utilizing a submersion blender until smooth.
Serve and enjoy.

Nutrition:

Calories 265 - Fat 22.9 g
Carbohydrates 14.7 g
Sugar 6.7 g - Protein 6.1 g
Cholesterol 0 mg

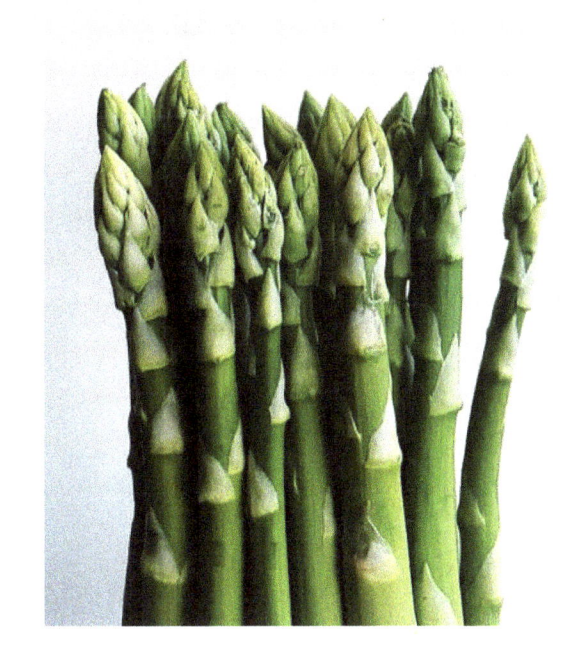

69. Quick Broccoli Soup

Preparation Time: 5 minutes

Cooking Time: 10 minutes

Servings: 6

Ingredients:

1 lb. broccoli, chopped
6 cups filtered alkaline water
1 onion, diced
2 tbsp. olive oil
Pepper
Salt

Directions:

Add oil into the instant pot and set the pot on sauté mode.
Add the onion in olive oil and sauté until softened.
Add broccoli and water and stir well.
Cover pot with top and cook on manual high pressure for 3 minutes.
When finished, release pressure using the quick release, and then open the lid.
Blend the soup utilizing a submersion blender until smooth.
Season soup with pepper and salt.
Serve and enjoy.

Nutrition:

Calories 73
Fat 4.9 g
Carbohydrates 6.7 g
Protein 2.3 g
Sugar 2.1 g
Cholesterol 0 mg

70. Green Lentil Soup

Preparation Time: 10 minutes

Cooking Time: 30 minutes

Servings: 4

Ingredients:

1 ½ cups green lentils, rinsed
4 cups baby spinach
4 cups filtered alkaline water
1 tsp. Italian seasoning
2 tsp. fresh thyme
14 oz. tomatoes, diced
3 garlic cloves, minced
2 celery stalks, chopped
1 carrot, chopped
1 onion, chopped
Pepper
Sea salt

Directions:

Add all ingredients except spinach into the direct pot and mix fine.
Cover pot with top and cook on manual high pressure for 18 minutes.
When finished, release pressure using the quick release, and then open the lid.
Add spinach and stir well.
Serve and enjoy.

Nutrition:

Calories 306
Fat 1.5 g
Carbohydrates 53.7 g
Sugar 6.4 g
Protein 21 g
Cholesterol 1 mg

71. Squash Soup

Preparation Time: 10 minutes

Cooking Time: 40 minutes

Servings: 4

Ingredients:

3 lbs. butternut squash, peeled and cubed
1 tbsp. curry powder
1/2 cup unsweetened coconut milk
3 cups filtered alkaline water
2 garlic cloves, minced
1 large onion, minced
1 tsp. olive oil

Directions:

Add olive oil in the instant pot and set the pot on sauté mode.
Add onion and cook until tender, about 8 minutes.
Add curry powder and garlic and sauté for a minute.
Add butternut squash, water, and salt and stir well.
Cover pot with lid and cook on soup mode for 30 minutes.
When finished, release pressure naturally for 10 minutes, then release using the quick release, and then open the lid.
Blend the soup utilizing a submersion blender until smooth.
Add coconut milk and stir well.
Serve warm and enjoy.

Nutrition:

Calories 254
Fat 8.9 g
Carbohydrates 46.4 g
Sugar 10.1 g
Protein 4.8 g
Cholesterol 0 mg

72. Tomato Soup

Preparation Time: 5 minutes

Cooking Time: 20 minutes

Servings: 4

Ingredients:

6 tomatoes, chopped
1 onion, diced
14 oz. coconut milk
1 tsp. turmeric
1 tsp. garlic, minced
1/4 cup cilantro, chopped
1/2 tsp. cayenne pepper
1 tsp. ginger, minced
1/2 tsp. sea salt

Directions:

Add all ingredients to the direct pot and mix fine.
Cover the instant pot with a lid and cook on manual high pressure for 5 minutes.
When finished, release pressure naturally for 10 minutes then release using the quick release.
Blend the soup utilizing a submersion blender until smooth.
Stir well and serve.

Nutrition:

Calories 81
Fat 3.5 g
Carbohydrates 11.6 g
Sugar 6.1 g
Protein 2.5 g
Cholesterol 0 mg

73. Basil Zucchini Soup

Preparation Time: 10 minutes

Cooking Time: 20 minutes

Servings: 4

Ingredients:

3 medium zucchinis, peeled and chopped
1/4 cup basil, chopped
1 large leek, chopped
3 cups filtered alkaline water
1 tbsp. lemon juice
3 tbsp. olive oil
2 tsp. sea salt

Directions:

Add 2 tbsp. oil into the pot and set the pot on sauté mode.
Add zucchini and sauté for 5 minutes.
Add basil and leeks and sauté for 2-3 minutes.
Add lemon juice, water, and salt. Stir well.
Cover pot with lid and cook on high pressure for 8 minutes.
When finished, release pressure naturally, then open the lid.
Blend the soup utilizing a submersion blender until smooth.
Top with remaining olive oil and serve.

Nutrition:

Calories 157
Fat 11.9 g
Carbohydrates 8.9 g
Protein 5.8 g
Sugar 4 g
Cholesterol 0 mg

74. Summer Vegetable Soup

Preparation Time: 5 minutes

Cooking Time: 20 minutes

Servings: 10

Ingredients:

1/2 cup basil, chopped
2 bell peppers, seeded and sliced
1/ cup green beans, trimmed and cut into pieces
8 cups filtered alkaline water
1 medium summer squash, sliced
1 medium zucchini, sliced
2 large tomatoes, sliced
1 small eggplant, sliced
6 garlic cloves, smashed
1 medium onion, diced
Pepper
Salt

Directions:

Combine all elements into the direct pot and mix fine.
Cover pot with lid and cook on soup mode for 10 minutes.
Release pressure using the quick release, then open the lid.
Blend the soup utilizing a submersion blender until smooth.
Serve and enjoy.

Nutrition:

Calories 84
Fat 1.6 g
Carbohydrates 12.8 g
Protein 6.1 g
Sugar 6.1 g
Cholesterol 0 mg

75. Spicy Carrot Soup

Preparation Time: 10 minutes

Cooking Time: 20 minutes

Servings: 6

Ingredients:

8 large carrots, peeled and chopped
1 1/2 cups filtered alkaline water
14 oz. coconut milk
3 garlic cloves, peeled
1 tbsp. red curry paste
1/4 cup olive oil
1 onion, chopped
Salt

Directions:

Combine all elements into the direct pot and mix fine.
Cover the pot with a lid, select the manual, and set the timer for 15 minutes.
Release pressure naturally, then open the lid.
Blend the soup utilizing a submersion blender until smooth.
Serve and enjoy.

Nutrition:

Calories 267
Fat 22 g
Carbohydrates 13 g
Protein 4 g
Sugar 5 g
Cholesterol 20 mg

76. Zucchini Soup

Preparation Time: 10 minutes

Cooking Time: 30 minutes

Servings: 10

Ingredients:

10 cups zucchini, chopped
32 oz. filtered alkaline water
13.5 oz. coconut milk
1 tbsp. Thai curry paste

Directions:

Combine all elements into the direct pot and mix fine.
Cover pot with lid and cook on manual high pressure for 10 minutes.
Release pressure using the quick release, then open the lid.
Use a blender to blend the soup until smooth.
Serve and enjoy.

Nutrition:

Calories 122
Fat 9.8 g
Carbohydrates 6.6 g
Protein 4.1 g
Sugar 3.6 g
Cholesterol 0 mg

77. Dill Celery Soup

Preparation Time: 10 minutes

Cooking Time: 30 minutes

Servings: 4

Ingredients:

6 cups celery stalk, chopped
2 cups filtered alkaline water
1 medium onion, chopped
1/2 tsp. dill
1 cup of coconut milk
1/4 tsp. sea salt

Directions:

Combine all elements into the direct pot and mix fine.

Cover pot with a lid and select soup mode; it takes 30 minutes.

Release pressure using the quick release, then open the lid carefully.

Blend the soup utilizing a submersion blender until smooth.

Stir well and serve.

Nutrition:

Calories 193 - Fat 15.3 g
Carbohydrates 10.9 g
Protein 5.2 g - Sugar 5.6 g - Cholesterol 0 mg

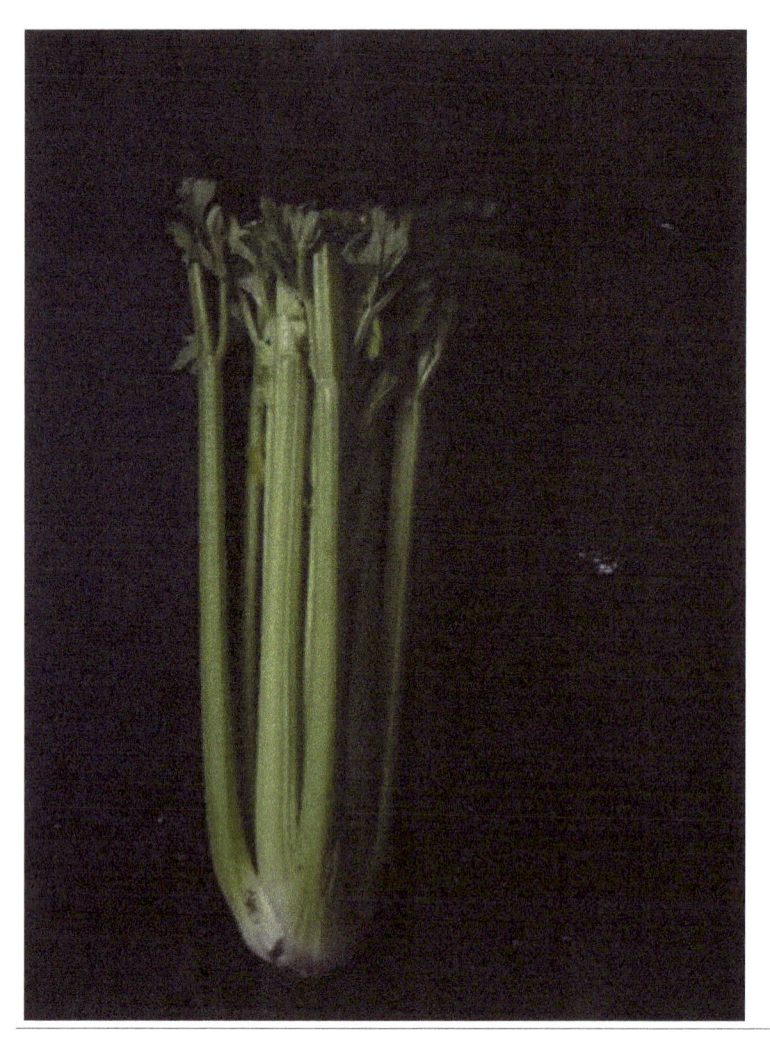

Salads

1. Thai Quinoa Salad

Preparation Time: 10 minutes

Cooking Time: 0 minutes

Servings: 1-2

Ingredients:

Ingredients used for dressing:

1 tbsp. sesame seed
1 tsp. chopped garlic
1 tsp. lemon, fresh juice
3 tsp. apple cider vinegar
2 tsp. tamari, gluten-free.
1/4 cup of tahini (sesame butter)
1 pitted date
1/2 tsp. salt
1/2 tsp. toasted sesame oil

Salad ingredients:

1 cup of quinoa, steamed
1 big handful of arugula
1 tomato cut in pieces
1/4 of the red onion, diced

Directions:

Add the following to a small blender: 1/4 cup + 2 tbsp. Filtered water, the rest of the ingredients, and blend. Steam 1 cup of quinoa in a steamer or a rice pan, then set aside. Combine the quinoa, the arugula, the tomatoes sliced, the red onion diced on a serving plate or bowl, add the Thai dressing and serve with a spoon.

Nutrition:

Calories: 100
Carbohydrates: 12 g

2. Green Goddess Bowl and Avocado Cumin Dressing

Preparation Time: 10 minutes

Cooking Time: 0 minutes

Servings: 1-2

Ingredients:

Ingredients for the dressing of avocado cumin:

1 avocado
1 tbsp. cumin powder
2 limes, freshly squeezed
1 cup of filtered water
1/4 seconds. sea salt
1 tbsp. olive extra virgin olive oil
Cayenne pepper dash
Optional: 1/4 tsp. smoked pepper

Tahini lemon dressing ingredients:

1/4 cup of tahini (sesame butter)
1/2 cup of filtered water (more if you want thinner, less thick)
1/2 lemon, freshly squeezed
1 clove of minced garlic
3/4 tsp. sea salt (Celtic Gray, Himalayan, Redmond Real Salt)
1 tbsp. olive extra virgin olive oil
Black pepper to taste

Salad ingredients:

3 cups of kale, chopped
1/2 cup of broccoli flowers, chopped
1/2 zucchini (make spiral noodles)
1/2 cup of kelp noodles, soaked and drained
1/3 cup of cherry tomatoes, halved.
2 tsp. hemp seeds

Directions:

Gently steam the kale and the broccoli (flash the steam for 4 minutes), set aside. Mix the zucchini noodles and kelp noodles and toss them with a generous portion of the smoked avocado cumin dressing. Add the cherry tomatoes and stir again. Place the steamed kale and broccoli and drizzle with the lemon tahini dressing. Top the kale and the broccoli with the noodles and tomatoes and sprinkle the whole dish with the hemp seeds.

Nutrition:

Calories: 89
Carbohydrates: 11g
Fat: 1.2g
Protein: 4g

3. Sweet and Savory Salad

Preparation Time: 10 minutes

Cooking Time: 0 minutes

Servings: 1-2

Ingredients:

1 big head of butter lettuce
1/2 of cucumber, sliced
1 pomegranate, seed or 1/3 cup of seed
1 avocado, 1 cubed
1/4 cup of shelled pistachio, chopped

Ingredients for dressing:

1/4 cup of apple cider vinegar
1/2 cup of olive oil
1 clove of garlic, minced

Directions:

Put the butter lettuce in a salad bowl. Add the remaining ingredients and toss with the salad dressing.

Nutrition:

Calories: 68 - Carbohydrates: 8g
Fat: 1.2g - Protein: 2g

4. Kale Pesto's Pasta

Preparation Time: 10 minutes

Cooking Time: 0 minutes

Servings: 1-2

Ingredients:

1 bunch of kale
2 cups of fresh basil
1/4 cup of extra virgin olive oil
1/2 cup of walnuts
2 limes, freshly squeezed
Sea salt and chili pepper
1 zucchini, noodle (spiralizer)
Optional: garnish with chopped asparagus, spinach leaves, and tomato.

Directions:

The night before, soak the walnuts to improve absorption. Put all the recipe ingredients in a blender and blend until the consistency of the cream is reached. Add the zucchini noodles and enjoy.

Nutrition:

Calories: 55 - Carbohydrates: 9 g
Fat: 1.2g

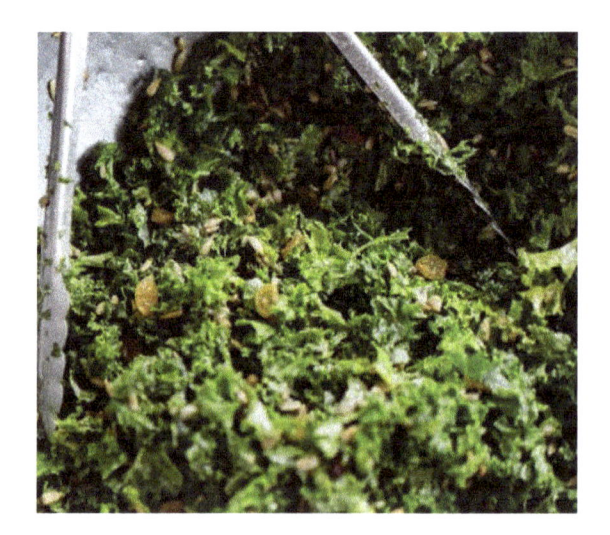

5. Beet Salad with Basil Dressing

Preparation Time: 10 minutes

Cooking Time: 0 minutes

Servings: 4

Ingredients:

Ingredients for the dressing:

¼ cup blackberries
¼ cup extra-virgin olive oil
Juice of 1 lemon
2 tablespoons minced fresh basil
1 teaspoon poppy seeds
A pinch of sea salt

For the salad:

2 celery stalks, chopped
4 cooked beets, peeled and chopped
1 cup blackberries
4 cups spring mix

Directions:

To make the dressing, mash the blackberries in a bowl. Whisk in the oil, lemon juice, basil, poppy seeds, and sea salt.
To make the salad: Add the celery, beets, blackberries, and spring mix to the bowl with the dressing.
Combine and serve.

Nutrition:

Calories: 192
Fat: 15g
Carbohydrates: 15g
Protein: 2g

6. Basic Salad with Olive Oil Dressing

Preparation Time: 10 minutes

Cooking Time: 0 minute

Servings: 4

Ingredients:

1 cup coarsely chopped iceberg lettuce
1 cup coarsely chopped romaine lettuce
1 cup fresh baby spinach
1 large tomato, hulled and coarsely chopped
1 cup diced cucumber
2 tablespoons extra-virgin olive oil
¼ teaspoon of sea salt

Directions:

In a bowl, combine the spinach and lettuces.
Add the tomato and cucumber.
Drizzle with oil and sprinkle with sea salt.
Mix and serve.

Nutrition:

Calories: 77
Fat: 4g
Carbohydrates: 3g
Protein: 1g

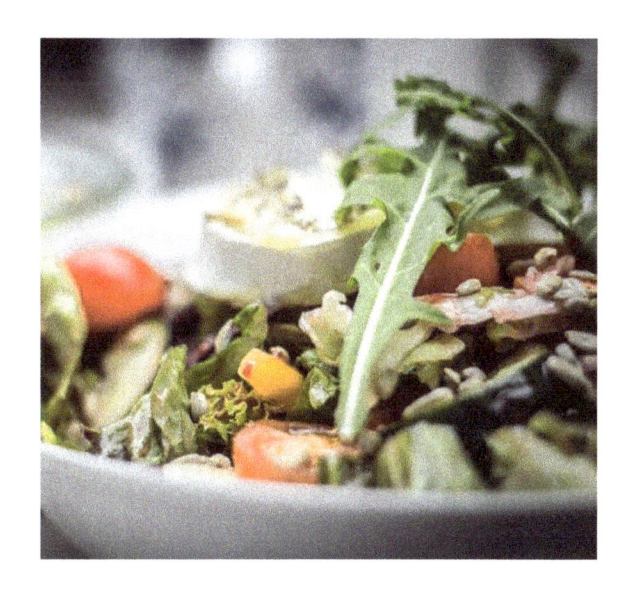

7. Spinach & Orange Salad with Oil Drizzle

Preparation Time: 10 minutes

Cooking Time: 0 minute

Servings: 4

Ingredients:

4 cups fresh baby spinach
1 blood orange, coarsely chopped
½ red onion, thinly sliced
½ shallot, finely chopped
2 tbsp. minced fennel fronds
Juice of 1 lemon
1 tbsp. extra-virgin olive oil
A pinch of sea salt

Directions:

In a bowl, toss together the spinach, orange, red onion, shallot, and fennel fronds. Add the lemon juice, oil, and sea salt. Mix and serve.

Nutrition:

Calories: 79
Fat: 2g
Carbohydrates: 8g
Protein: 1g

8. Fruit Salad with Coconut-Lime Dressing

Preparation Time: 5 minutes

Cooking Time: 0 minutes

Servings: 4

Ingredients:

Ingredients for the dressing:

¼ cup full-fat canned coconut milk
1 tbsp. raw honey
Juice of ½ lime
A pinch of sea salt

For the salad

2 bananas, thinly sliced
2 mandarin oranges, segmented
½ cup strawberries, thinly sliced
½ cup raspberries
½ cup blueberries

Directions:

To make the dressing: whisk all the dressing ingredients in a bowl.
To make the salad: Add the salad ingredients in a bowl and mix.
Drizzle with the dressing and serve.

Nutrition:

Calories: 141 - Fat: 3g
Carbohydrates: 30g - Protein: 2g

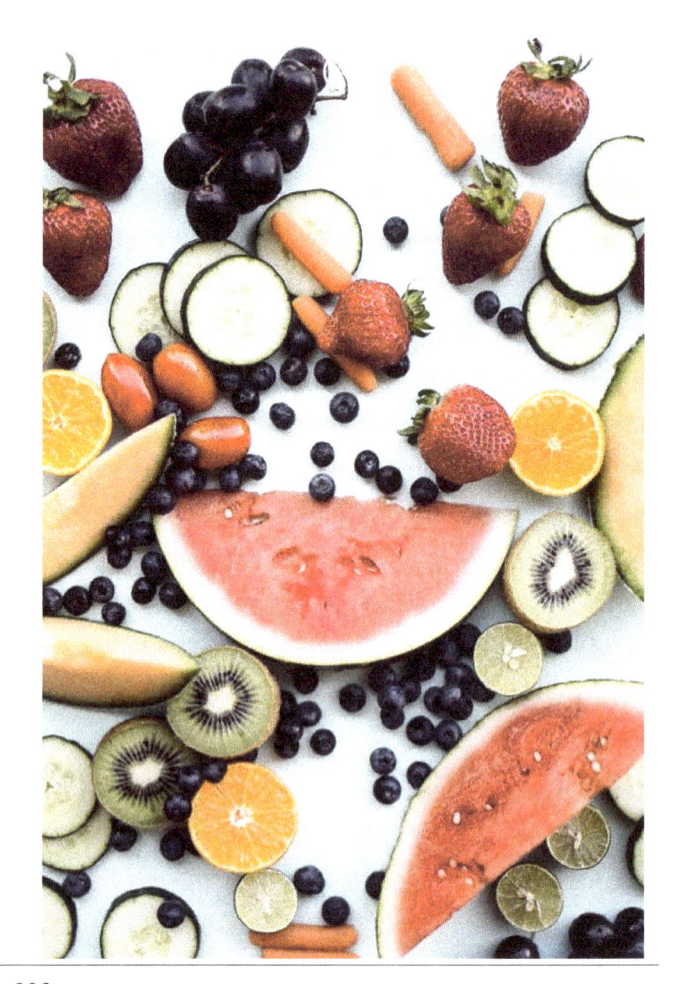

9. Cranberry and Brussels Sprouts with Dressing

Preparation Time: 10 minutes

Cooking Time: 0 minute

Servings: 4

Ingredients:

Ingredients for the dressing:

⅓ cup extra-virgin olive oil
2 tbsp. apple cider vinegar
1 tbsp. pure maple syrup
Juice of 1 orange
½ tbsp. dried rosemary
1 tbsp. scallion, whites only
A pinch of sea salt

For the salad

1 bunch scallions, greens only, finely chopped
1 cup Brussels sprouts, stemmed, halved, and thinly sliced
½ cup fresh cranberries
4 cups fresh baby spinach

Directions:

To make the dressing: In a bowl, whisk the dressing ingredients.
To make the salad: Add the scallions, Brussels sprouts, cranberries, and spinach to the bowl with the dressing.
Combine and serve.

Nutrition:

Calories: 267
Fat: 18g
Carbohydrates: 26g
Protein: 2g

10. Parsnip, Carrot, and Kale Salad with Dressing

Preparation Time: 10 minutes

Cooking Time: 0 minutes

Servings: 4

Ingredients:

Ingredients for the dressing:

⅓ cup extra-virgin olive oil
Juice of 1 lime
2 tbsp. minced fresh mint leaves
1 tsp. pure maple syrup
A pinch of sea salt

For the salad:

1 bunch kale, chopped
½ parsnip, grated
½ carrot, grated
2 tbsp. sesame seeds

Directions:

To make the dressing, mix all the dressing ingredients in a bowl.
To make the salad, add the kale to the dressing and massage the dressing into the kale for 1 minute.
Add the parsnip, carrot, and sesame seeds. Combine and serve.

Nutrition:

Calories: 214
Fat: 2g
Carbohydrates: 12g
Protein: 2g

11. Tomato Toasts

Preparation Time: 5 minutes

Cooking Time: 5 minutes

Servings: 4

Ingredients:

4 slices of sprouted bread toasts
2 tomatoes, sliced
1 avocado, mashed
1 teaspoon olive oil
1 pinch of salt
¾ teaspoon ground black pepper

Directions:

Blend the olive oil, mashed avocado, salt, and ground black pepper.
When the mixture is homogenous – spread it over the sprouted bread.
Then place the sliced tomatoes over the toasts.
Enjoy!

Nutrition:

Calories: 125 - Fat: 11.1g
Carbohydrates: 7.0g - Protein: 1.5g

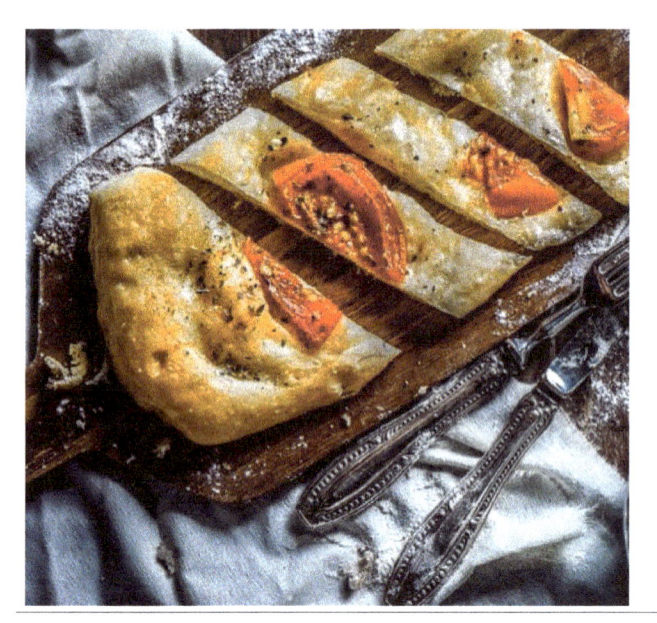

12. Every day Salad

Preparation Time: 10 minutes

Cooking Time: 40 minutes

Servings: 6

Ingredients:

5 halved mushrooms
6 halved cherry (plum) tomatoes
6 rinsed lettuce leaves
10 olives
½ chopped cucumber
Juice from ½ key lime
1 teaspoon olive oil
Pure sea salt

Directions:

Tear rinsed lettuce leaves into medium pieces and put them in a medium salad bowl. Add mushrooms halves, chopped cucumber, olives, and cherry tomato halves into the bowl. Mix well. Pour olive and key lime juice over the salad. Add pure sea salt to taste. Mix it all till it is well combined.

Nutrition:

Calories: 88 - Carbohydrates: 11g
Fat: .5g - Protein: .8g

13. Super-Seedy Salad with Tahini Dressing

Preparation Time: 10 minutes

Cooking Time: 0 minutes

Servings: 1-2

Ingredients:

1 slice stale sourdough, torn into chunks
50g mixed seeds
1 tsp. cumin seeds
1 tsp. coriander seeds
50g baby kale
75g long-stemmed broccoli, blanched for a few minutes then roughly chopped
½ red onion, thinly sliced
100g cherry tomatoes, halved
½ a small bunch flat-leaf parsley, torn

DRESSING

100ml natural yogurt
1 tbsp. tahini
1 lemon, juiced

Directions:

Heat the oven to 200°C/fan 180°C/gas 6. Put the bread into a food processor and pulse into very rough breadcrumbs. Put into a bowl with the mixed seeds and spices, season, and spray well with oil. Tip onto a non-stick baking tray and roast for 15-20 minutes, stirring and tossing regularly, until deep golden brown.

Whisk together the dressing ingredients, some seasoning, and a splash of water in a large bowl. Tip the baby kale, broccoli, red onion, cherry tomatoes, and flat-leaf parsley into the dressing, and mix well. Divide between 2 plates and top with the crispy breadcrumbs and seeds.

Nutrition:

Calories: 78
Carbohydrates: 6 g
Fat: 2g
Protein: 1.5g

14. Sebi's Vegetable Salad

Preparation Time: 10 minutes

Cooking Time: 0 minutes

Servings: 1-2

Ingredients:

4 cups each of raw spinach and romaine lettuce
2 cups each of cherry tomatoes, sliced cucumber, chopped baby carrots and chopped red, orange and yellow bell pepper
1 cup each of chopped broccoli, sliced yellow squash, zucchini and cauliflower.

Directions:

Just wash all these vegetables. Mix in a large mixing bowl and top off with a non-fat or low-fat dressing of your choice.

Nutrition:

Calories: 48
Carbohydrates: 11g
Protein: 3g

15. Greek Salad

Preparation Time: 10 minutes

Cooking Time: 0 minutes

Servings: 1-2

Ingredients:

1 Romaine head, torn in bits
1 cucumber sliced
1-pint cherry tomatoes, halved
1 green pepper, thinly sliced
1 onion sliced into rings
1 cup kalamata olives
1 ½ cups feta cheese, crumbled

For dressing combine:

1 cup olive oil
1/4 cup lemon juice
2 tsp. oregano
Salt and pepper

Directions:

Layer ingredients on a plate. Drizzle dressing over salad.

Nutrition:

Calories: 107
Carbohydrates: 18g
Fat: 1.2 g
Protein: 1g

16. Sebi's Alkaline Spring Salad

Preparation Time: 10 minutes

Cooking Time: 0 minutes

Servings: 1-2

Eating seasonal fruits and vegetables is a fabulous way of taking care of yourself and the environment at the same time. This alkaline-electric salad is delicious and nutritious.

Ingredients:

4 cups seasonal approved greens of your choice
1 cup cherry tomatoes
1/4 cup walnuts
1/4 cup approved herbs of your choice

For the dressing:

3-4 key limes
1 tbsp. of homemade raw sesame
Sea salt and cayenne pepper

Directions:

First, get the juice of the key limes. In a small bowl, whisk together the key lime juice with the homemade raw sesame "tahini" butter. Add sea salt and cayenne pepper, to taste. Cut the cherry tomatoes in half.
In a large bowl, combine the greens, cherry tomatoes, and herbs. Pour the dressing on top and "massage" with your hands.
Let the greens soak up the dressing. Add more sea salt, cayenne pepper, and herbs on top if you wish. Enjoy!

Nutrition:

Calories: 77
Carbohydrates: 11g

Main Dishes

17. Ginger-Maple Yam Casserole

Preparation Time: 10 minutes

Cooking Time: 40 minutes

Servings: 4

Ingredients:

2 yams, peeled and cut into ½-inch chunks
¼ cup fresh ginger, peeled and grated
2 tbsp. avocado oil
2 tbsp. pure maple syrup
4 tsp. cardamom
A pinch of sea salt

Directions:

Preheat the oven to 375F.
In a casserole dish, combine the yams, ginger, oil, maple syrup, cardamom, and salt. Mix well.
Cover and bake for 40 minutes.
Serve.

Nutrition:

Calories: 144 - Fat: 7g - Carbohydrates: 20g
Protein: 1g

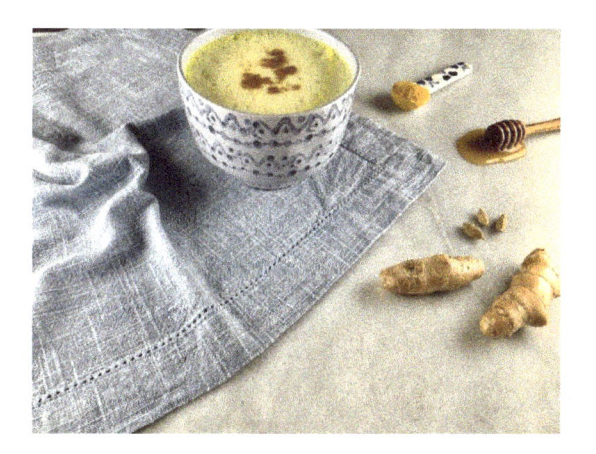

18. Layered Cabbage Roll Casserole

Preparation Time: 10 minutes

Cooking Time: 40 minutes

Servings: 4

Ingredients:

1 cup quinoa
½ red onion, finely chopped
4 garlic cloves, minced
4 white mushrooms, finely chopped
1 (28-ounce) can diced tomatoes, drained
2 cups low-sodium vegetable stock
¼ cup minced fresh basil
8 green cabbage leaves, whole

Directions:

Preheat the oven to 350F.
In a casserole dish, combine 2 tbsp. red onion, ¼ cup quinoa, 1 minced garlic clove, and 1 chopped mushroom. Add ¼ can of tomatoes, ½ cup stock, and 1 tbsp. basil. Stir to mix.
Top with 2 cabbage leaves. Repeat steps 2 and 3 until all of the ingredients are used up.
Cover and bake for 40 minutes.
Rest for 10 minutes and serve.

Nutrition:

Calories: 261
Fat: 2g
Carbohydrates: 51g
Protein: 12g

19. Vegetarian Pie

Preparation Time: 20 minutes

Cooking Time: 1 hour 20 minutes

Servings: 8

Ingredients:

Ingredients for topping:

5 cups of water
1¼ cups yellow cornmeal

For filing:

1 tbsp. extra-virgin olive oil
1 large onion, chopped
1 medium red bell pepper, seeded and chopped
2 garlic cloves, minced
1 tsp. dried oregano, crushed
2 tsp. chili powder
2 cups fresh tomatoes, chopped
2½ cups cooked pinto beans
2 cups boiled corn kernels

Directions:

Preheat the oven to 375 F. Lightly grease a shallow baking dish.
In a pan, add the water over medium-high heat and bring to a boil.
Slowly, add the cornmeal, stirring continuously.
Reduce the heat to low and cook covered for about 20 minutes, stirring occasionally.
Meanwhile, prepare the filling. In a large skillet, heat the oil over medium heat and sauté the onion and bell pepper for about 3-4 minutes.
Add the garlic, oregano, and spices and sauté for about 1 minute
Add the remaining ingredients and stir to combine.
Reduce the heat to low and simmer for about 10-15 minutes, stirring occasionally.
Remove from the heat.
Place half of the Cooked cornmeal into the Prepared baking dish evenly.
Place the filling mixture over the cornmeal evenly.
Place the remaining cornmeal over the filling mixture evenly.
Bake for 45-50 minutes or until the top becomes golden brown.
Remove the pie from the oven and set it aside for about 5 minutes before serving.

Nutrition:

Calories: 350
Fat: 3.9g
Carbohydrates: 58.2g
Protein: 16.8g

20. Ginger-Sesame Quinoa with Vegetables

Preparation Time: 10 minutes

Cooking Time: 30 minutes

Servings: 4

Ingredients:

1 cup quinoa
2 cups low-sodium vegetable stock
1 tbsp. tahini
4 tsp. fresh ginger, peeled and minced
A pinch of sea salt, plus more for seasoning
2 carrots, finely chopped
1 red bell pepper, finely chopped
1 cup snow peas, stringed and halved
2 tsp. sesame seeds
Sesame oil, for garnish

Directions:

Preheat the oven to 325F.
In a casserole dish, combine the stock, quinoa, tahini, ginger, and salt. Mix.
Add in the pepper, carrots, and snow peas. Mix well.

Cover and bake for 30 minutes.
Top with sesame seeds and a drizzle of sesame oil.
Adjust seasoning with salt and serve.

Nutrition:

Calories: 261
Fat: 3g
Carbohydrates: 46g
Protein: 10g

21. Butternut Squash, Apple Casserole with Drizzle

Preparation Time: 10 minutes

Cooking Time: 30 minutes

Servings: 4

Ingredients:

1 butternut squash, peeled, seeded, and cut into ½-inch chunks
2 Granny Smith apples, cored and cut into ½-inch chunks
1 white onion, cut into ½-inch chunks
4 garlic cloves, coarsely chopped
½ tbsp. avocado oil
½ tbsp. pure maple syrup
2 tsp. ground cinnamon
½ tsp. chili powder
A pinch of sea salt
A pinch of freshly ground black pepper

Directions:

Preheat the oven to 375F.
In a large casserole dish, combine the apples, squash, onion, garlic, oil, syrup, cinnamon, chili powder, salt, and pepper. Mix well.
Cover and bake for 30 minutes.
Serve.

Nutrition:

Calories: 123 - Fat: 2g
Carbohydrates: 28g - Protein: 2g

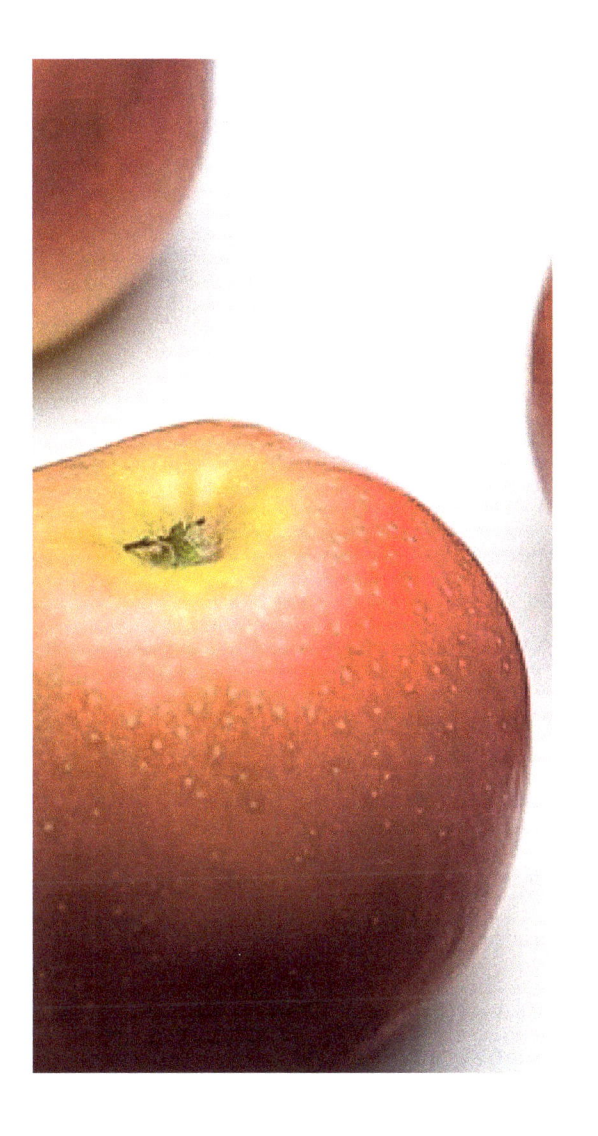

22. Mango, Quinoa, and Black Bean Casserole with Sauce

Preparation Time: 10 minutes

Cooking Time: 25 minutes

Servings: 4

Ingredients:

2 cups full-fat canned coconut milk
1 cup low-sodium vegetable stock
1 cup quinoa
2 cups black beans, drained and rinsed
1 mango, finely chopped
¼ cup minced fresh mint
A pinch of sea salt, for seasoning

Directions:

Preheat the oven to 425F.
In a casserole dish, combine the stock, milk, and quinoa.
Cover and bake for 25 minutes.
Remove the dish from the oven. Mix in the beans, mango, and fresh mint.
Season with salt and serve.

Nutrition:

Calories: 573
Fat: 23g
Carbohydrates: 75g
Protein: 15g

23. Pepper and Onion Masala

Preparation Time: 10 minutes

Cooking Time: 30 minutes

Servings: 2

Ingredients:

1 cup of brown rice
Boiling filtered water, for rinsing
2 tablespoons coconut oil
1 teaspoon cumin seeds
¼ teaspoon asafoetida
½ teaspoon ground turmeric
1 onion, rinsed and chopped
2 green chiles, rinsed and chopped
2 garlic cloves, chopped
1 (1-inch) piece fresh ginger, peeled and grated
3 tablespoons tomato paste
1 teaspoon chili powder
Himalayan pink salt
1 bell pepper, any color, rinsed and chopped
2 tablespoons of filtered water

Directions:

In a minor saucepan over average-low heat, associate the brown rice with enough boiling water to cover, and simmer for 25 to 30 minutes, until cooked. Drain and rinse with boiling filtered water.
Meanwhile, in a small non-stick skillet over medium heat, heat the coconut oil. Add the cumin seeds, asafoetida, and turmeric. Fry for 3 minutes, until golden.
Add the onion, green chiles, garlic, and ginger. Sauté for 5 minutes, until the onion is soft.
Stir in the tomato paste and chili powder, and season with salt. Mix well.
Add the bell pepper and water, and cook for 5 minutes.

Serve the rice with the hot masala.

Nutrition:

Calories: 520 - Total fat: 8g
Total carbohydrates: 81g
Fiber: 6g - Sugar: 4g - Protein: 4g

Nutrition:

Calories: 300 - Total fat: 19g
Total carbohydrates: 23g
Fiber: 9g - Sugar: 11g
Protein: 7g

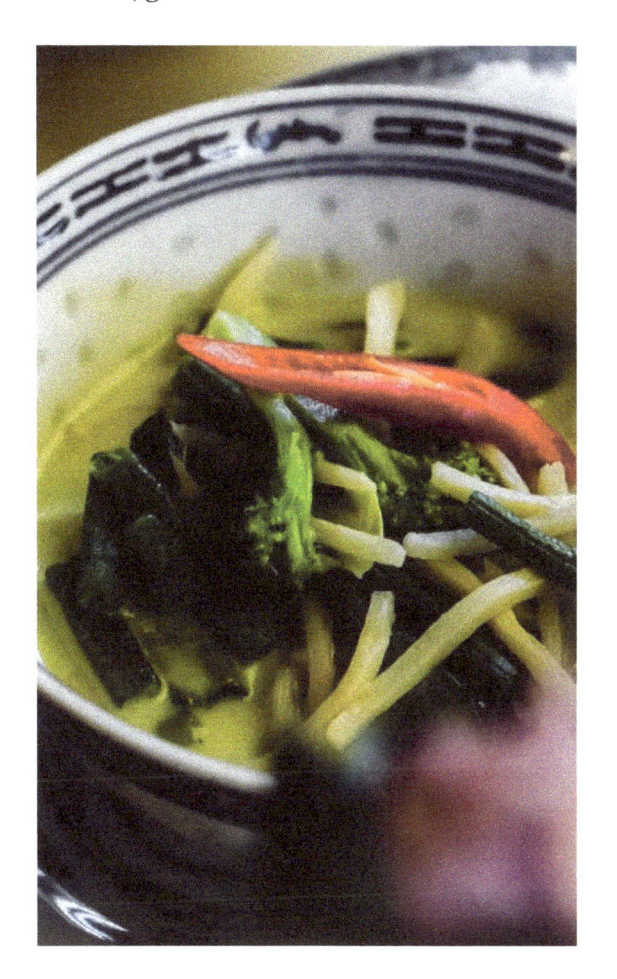

24. Red Thai Vegetable Curry

Preparation Time: 10 minutes

Cooking Time: 15 minutes

Servings: 4

Ingredients:

2 cups vegetable stock
1 sweet potato, rinsed and chopped
1 head broccoli, rinsed and chopped
1 eggplant, rinsed and chopped
1 zucchini, rinsed and chopped
1 red bell pepper, rinsed and chopped
1½ cups canned, full-fat coconut milk
1 tablespoon red Thai curry paste
2 kaffir lime leaves
1 (1-inch) piece fresh ginger, peeled and grated
Himalayan pink salt
Freshly ground black pepper
2 tablespoons coconut aminos
Juice of 1 lime

Directions:

In a large pot over high heat, bring the vegetable stock to a boil. Add the sweet potato, broccoli, eggplant, zucchini, red bell pepper, coconut milk, curry paste, lime leaves, and ginger. Reduce the heat to low and cook for 10 minutes, stirring frequently. Taste and season with salt and pepper. Simmer for 5 minutes more.
Remove the pot from the heat, stir in the coconut aminos and lime juice, and serve.

25. Thick Alkaline Minestrone

Preparation Time: 10 minutes

Cooking Time: 15 minutes

Servings: 2

Ingredients:

1 tablespoon coconut oil
¼ onion, rinsed and diced
2 garlic cloves, minced
½ cup sweet potato, scrubbed and cubed
½ cup zucchini, rinsed and cubed
½ cup eggplant, rinsed and cubed
½ cup carrot, rinsed and diced
½ cup canned beans, such as white, navy, or kidney beans, rinsed and drained
1 cup tomato juice
½ cup vegetable stock
Handful fresh basil leaves, rinsed
Himalayan pink salt
Freshly ground black pepper

Directions:

In a large pot over medium-high heat, heat the coconut oil. Add the onion, garlic, sweet potato, zucchini, eggplant, and carrot. Sauté for 3 minutes.
Stir in the beans, tomato juice, and vegetable stock. Bring to a boil. Reduce the heat to simmer and cook for 10 minutes.
Stir in the basil, season with salt and pepper, and serve.

Nutrition:

Calories: 168
Total fat: 7g
Total carbohydrates: 25g
Fiber: 6g
Sugar: 11g
Protein: 4g

26. Pesto Soba Noodles

Preparation Time: 5 minutes

Cooking Time: 15 minutes

Servings: 2

Ingredients:

3 tablespoons extra-virgin olive oil
1 bunch fresh basil leaves, rinsed
1 bunch fresh parsley, rinsed
1 bunch fresh cilantro, rinsed
3½ ounces soba buckwheat noodles, cooked according to package directions
Himalayan pink salt
Freshly ground black pepper

Directions:

In a blender, combine the olive oil, basil, parsley, and cilantro. Blend until smooth.
In a large bowl, combine the cooked noodles and sauce. Toss to coat, season with salt and pepper, and serve.

Nutrition:

Calories: 355
Total fat: 21g
Total carbohydrates: 36g
Fiber: 1g
Sugar: 0g
Protein: 9g

27. Quinoa Burrito Bowl

Preparation Time: 10 minutes

Cooking Time: 10 minutes

Servings: 4

Ingredients:

1 cup quinoa, rinsed well
Boiling filtered water
1 can of black beans, washed and rinsed
4 scallions, white parts only, rinsed and sliced
4 garlic cloves, minced
1 teaspoon ground cumin
1 teaspoon red pepper flakes
Juice of 2 limes
2 avocados, peeled, pitted, and sliced
Handful fresh cilantro, rinsed and chopped

Directions:

In a small saucepan over medium heat, combine the quinoa with enough boiling water to shield and then simmer for 8 to 10 minutes, until the water has absorbed. Drain, rinse and set aside.

Meanwhile, in another small saucepan over low heat, stir together the black beans, scallions, garlic, cumin, red pepper flakes, and lime juice. Simmer for 10 minutes to warm.

In a large bowl, stir collected the quinoa and warmed beans. Top with the avocado and cilantro and serve.

Nutrition:

Calories: 420
Total fat: 9g
Carbohydrates: 70g
Fiber: 18g
Sugar: 2g
Protein: 10g

28. Millet Pilaf

Preparation Time: 10 minutes

Cooking Time: 15 minutes

Servings: 4

Ingredients:

1 cup millet
2 tomatoes, rinsed, seeded, and chopped
1¾ cups of filtered water
2 tablespoons extra-virgin olive oil
¼ cup chopped dried apricot
Zest of 1 lemon
Juice of 1 lemon
½ cup fresh parsley, rinsed and chopped
Himalayan pink salt
Freshly ground black pepper

Directions:

In an electric pressure cooker, combine the millet, tomatoes, and water. Lock the lid into place, select manual and high pressure, and cook for 7 minutes.

When the beep sounds, quick release the pressure by pressing Cancel and twisting the steam valve to the Venting position. Carefully remove the lid.

Stir in the olive oil, apricot, lemon zest, lemon juice, and parsley. Taste, season with salt and pepper, and serve.

Nutrition:

Calories: 270
Total fat: 8g
Total carbohydrates: 42g
Fiber: 5g
Sugar: 3g
Protein: 6g

29. Basil and Olive Pizza

Preparation Time: 10 minutes

Cooking Time: 30 minutes

Servings: 4

Ingredients:

FOR THE PIZZA SAUCE

1 (15-ounce) can tomatoes
1 tablespoon extra-virgin olive oil
½ cup fresh basil leaves, rinsed
2 garlic cloves, chopped
1 teaspoon onion powder
¼ teaspoon dried oregano
¼ teaspoon dried sage
¼ teaspoon dried rosemary
¼ teaspoon red chili flakes (optional)
1 teaspoon Himalayan pink salt
Pinch freshly ground black pepper

FOR THE PIZZAS

4 spelt flour pita slices of bread
4 ounces' vegan mozzarella, shredded
1 cup mixed veggies of your choice (tomatoes, eggplant, onion, green pepper, mushroom, etc.), rinsed and finely sliced
⅔ cup pitted olives, chopped
1 tablespoon extra-virgin olive oil
5 fresh basil leaves, rinsed and torn

Directions:

TO MAKE THE PIZZA SAUCE

In a blender, blend the tomatoes, olive oil, basil, garlic, onion powder, oregano, sage, rosemary, chili flakes, salt, and pepper on low until the basil and garlic are in very small pieces.

Transfer to a pot over middle heat and simmer for about 20 minutes, until the sauce reduces slightly and thickens.

TO MAKE THE PIZZAS

Preheat the oven to 500°F. Line a baking sheet with parchment paper and set aside. Spread the pizza sauce evenly over the pitas. Top with the vegan mozzarella and scatter the sliced veggies and olives on top.

Bake for 8 minutes, or until golden on top. Drizzle the pizzas with the olive oil and scatter the basil leaves over them. Freeze leftovers in an airtight container for up to three weeks.

Nutrition:

Calories: 400
Total fat: 10g
Total carbohydrates: 64g
Fiber: 5g
Sugar: 2g
Protein: 10g

30. Black Bean Chili

Preparation Time: 15 minutes

Cooking Time: 20 minutes

Servings: 4

Ingredients:

1 tablespoon coconut oil
1 small onion, rinsed and diced
6 mushrooms, cleaned and sliced
2 tablespoons ground coriander
2 tablespoons paprika
2 tablespoons ground cumin
1 tablespoon ground cinnamon
1 tablespoon ground nutmeg
1 tablespoon chili powder
1 (15-ounce) can tomatoes
1 can of black beans, washed and rinsed
1 (15.5-ounce) can kidney beans, rinsed and drained
5 cherry tomatoes, rinsed
2 tablespoons tomato purée
1 tablespoon raw honey or agave nectar
½ cup red wine or grape juice

3 squares dark chocolate, or 1 heaping tablespoon cocoa powder
7 ounces uncooked brown rice
4 tablespoons coconut yogurt, for serving (optional)
4 fresh cilantro sprigs, for serving (optional)

Directions:

In a great pan over average heat, heat the coconut oil. Include the onion and mushrooms, and sauté for 5 minutes. Stir in the coriander, paprika, cumin, cinnamon, nutmeg, and chili powder.

Add the canned tomatoes with their juices, black beans, kidney beans, cherry tomatoes, and tomato purée. Mix to combine and carry to a simmer. Cook for 5 minutes.

Stir in the honey, wine, and chocolate. Turn the heat to little and simmer for 10 minutes. While the chili cooks, cook the rice according to the package directions. Rinse and drain. Serve the chili above the rice, garnished with yogurt (if using), and cilantro (if using).

Nutrition:

Calories: 580g - Total fat: 5g
Total carbohydrates: 102g
Fiber: 18g - Sugar: 14g - Protein: 19g

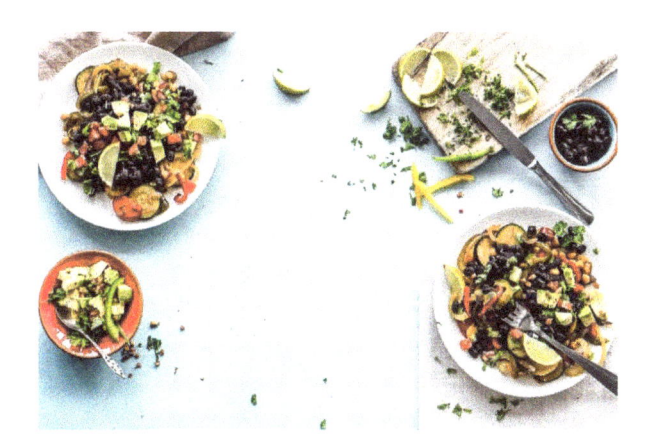

31. Mixed Lentils

Preparation Time: 15 minutes

Cooking Time: 30 minutes

Servings: 4

Ingredients:

2 tablespoons coconut oil
1 onion, rinsed and diced
2 carrots, rinsed and diced
2 celery stalks, rinsed and diced
1 sweet potato, rinsed and diced
1 cup dried red lentils
1 cup dried puy lentils
5 cups vegetable stock
Himalayan pink salt
Freshly ground black pepper

Directions:

In a large pot over medium heat, heat the coconut oil. Include the onion and fry for 3 minutes, or until it has softened. Supplement the carrots, celery, and sweet potato, and cook for 2 minutes.

Add the red and puy lentils and vegetable stock. Carry to a boil and lower the heat to simmer. Cook this for 25 minutes, or until the lentils are soft. Season with salt and pepper and serve.

Nutrition:

Calories: 330
Total fat: 10g
Total carbohydrates: 49g
Fiber: 20g
Sugar: 8g
Protein: 17g

32. Zucchini-Broccoli Stir-Fry

Preparation Time: 15 minutes

Cooking Time: 15 minutes

Servings: 4

Ingredients:

2 tablespoons coconut oil
2 tablespoons sesame oil
1 (2-inch) piece fresh ginger, peeled and finely chopped
4 garlic cloves, minced
2 onions, rinsed and chopped
1 head broccoli, rinsed and broken into florets
1 zucchini, rinsed and cut into long, fettuccine-like strips
3 scallions, white parts only, rinsed and chopped
1 tablespoon fresh basil leaves, rinsed and chopped
1-ounce coconut aminos

Directions:

In a wok or large skillet over medium heat, heat the coconut and sesame oils. Mix the ginger and garlic and sauté for 5 minutes, until fragrant.
Add the onion and broccoli, and cook for 3 minutes, until the onion softens slightly.
Add the zucchini, scallions, and basil. Stir to combine and heat for 4 minutes, until the vegetables are tender.
Remove the wok from the heat, sprinkle in the coconut aminos, and serve.

Nutrition:

Calories: 180 - Total fat: 14g
Total carbohydrates: 13g
Fiber: 3g - Sugar: 4g
Protein: 3g

33. Tomato Spelt Pasta

Preparation Time: 15 minutes

Cooking Time: 20 minutes

Servings: 4

Ingredients:

3 tablespoons extra-virgin olive oil
2 garlic cloves, crushed
1 onion, rinsed and diced
1 eggplant, rinsed and diced
2 zucchinis, rinsed and diced
3 tomatoes, rinsed and diced
⅔ cup sun-dried tomatoes
2 teaspoons dried basil
1 teaspoon dried oregano
1 cup vegetable stock
1 tablespoon red wine vinegar
Himalayan pink salt
Freshly ground black pepper
7 ounces spelt pasta
Boiling filtered water

Directions:

In a great pan over average heat, heat the olive oil. Add the garlic, onion, and eggplant, and sauté for 8 minutes.
Add the zucchini, tomatoes, sun-dried tomatoes, basil, and oregano. Cook for 8 minutes, stirring.
Stir in the vegetable stock and vinegar, and season with salt and pepper. Let simmer for a few minutes.
Meanwhile, in a separate, saucepan over medium heat, combine the pasta with enough boiling water to cover and cook for about 10 minutes, until soft. Drain.
Serve the pasta with the sauce.

Nutrition:

Calories: 460 - Total fat: 12g
Carbohydrates: 75g - Fiber: 10g
Sugar: 11g - Protein: 17g

34. Green Tomatoes Crisps

Preparation Time: 14 minutes

Cooking Time: 16 minutes

Servings: 3

Ingredients:

¼ cup coconut flour
A pinch of salt
A pinch of pepper
4 green tomatoes
1 cup applesauce
½ cup almond flour
¼ cup olive oil

Directions:

First is to mix the coconut flour, salt, and pepper in a bowl. Mix the tomatoes. Toss until well coated.
In another bowl, pour applesauce. Add almond flour. Mix until well combined. Heat the oil. Dip the tomatoes into the applesauce mixture and the almond mixture. Fry tomatoes in batches until golden brown. Serve.

Nutrition:

Calories 113
Total Fat 4.2 g
Saturated Fat 0.8 g
Cholesterol 0 mg
Sodium 861 mg
Total Carbs 22.5 g
Fiber 6.3 g
Sugar 2.3 g
Protein 9.2 g

35. Fruit Salad in Cider

Preparation Time: 11 minutes

Cooking Time: 16 minutes

Servings: 3

Ingredients:

For the salad:

1 piece, small apple, cubed
1 piece, small apricot, cubed
¼ piece, small grapefruit pulp, shredded into bite-sized pieces
¼ cup, loosely packed jicama, cubed

For cider sauce:

2 tbsp. apple cider vinegar, warmed in the microwave oven
A dash of cinnamon powder

Directions:

Combine apple cider vinegar and cinnamon powder in a small bowl. Mix well.
Place salad ingredients in a large bowl; pour in cider sauce. Toss well to combine; spoon equal portions into plates. Serve immediately.

Nutrition:

Calories 123
Total Fat 14.2 g
Saturated Fat 0.7 g
Cholesterol 0 mg
Sodium 661 mg
Total Carbs 22.5 g
Fiber 6.3 g
Sugar 2.9 g
Protein 9.2 g

36. Roasted Vegetables

Preparation Time: 14 minutes

Cooking Time: 17 minutes

Servings: 3

Ingredients:

4 Tbsp. olive oil, reserve some for greasing
2 heads, large garlic, tops sliced off
2 large eggplants/aubergine, tops removed, cubed
2 large shallots, peeled, quartered
1 large carrot, peeled, cubed
1 large parsnip, peeled, cubed
1 small green bell pepper, deseeded, ribbed, cubed
1 small red bell pepper, deseeded, ribbed, cubed
½ pound Brussels sprouts, halved, do not remove cores
1 sprig, large thyme, leaves picked
Sea salt, coarse-grained

For garnish:

1 large lemon, halved, ½ squeezed, ½ sliced into smaller wedges
⅛ cup fennel bulb, minced

Directions:

Preheat the oven to 425°F or 220°C for at least 5 minutes before using.

Line deep roasting pan with aluminium foil; lightly grease with oil. Tumble in bell peppers, Brussels sprouts, carrots, eggplants, garlic, parsnips, rosemary leaves, shallots, and thyme. Add a pinch of sea salt; drizzle in remaining oil and lemon juice. Toss well to combine.

Cover roasting pan with a sheet of aluminium foil. Place this on the middle rack of the oven. Bake for 20 to 30 minutes. Remove aluminium foil. Roast, for another 5 to 10 minutes, or until some vegetables brown at the edges. Remove roasting pan from the oven. Cool slightly before ladling equal portions into plates.

Garnish with fennel and a wedge of lemon. Squeeze lemon juice on top of the dish before eating.

Nutrition:

Calories 163 - Total Fat 4.2 g
Saturated Fat 0.8 g - Cholesterol 0 mg
Sodium 861 mg - Total Carbs 22.5 g
Fiber 6.3 g - Sugar 2.3 g - Protein 9.2 g

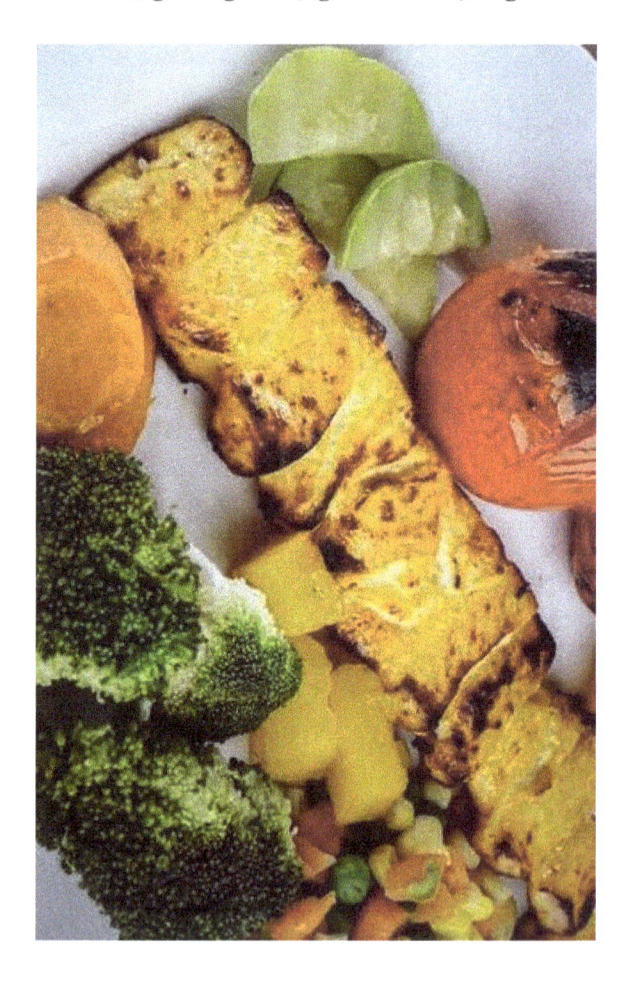

37. Sweet and Sour Onions

Preparation Time: 10 minutes

Cooking Time: 11 minutes

Servings: 4

Ingredients:

4 large onions, halved
2 garlic cloves, crushed
3 cups vegetable stock
1 ½ tablespoon balsamic vinegar
½ teaspoon Dijon mustard
1 tablespoon sugar

Directions:

Combine onions and garlic in a pan. Fry for 3 minutes, or till softened.

Pour stock, vinegar, Dijon mustard, and sugar. Bring to a boil.

Reduce heat. Cover and let the combination simmer for 10 minutes.

Get rid of from heat. Continue stirring until the liquid is reduced and the onions are brown. Serve.

Nutrition:

Calories 203
Total Fat 41.2 g
Saturated Fat 0.8 g
Cholesterol 0 mg
Sodium 861 mg
Total Carbs 29.5 g
Fiber 16.3 g
Sugar 29.3 g
Protein 19.2 g

38. Sautéed Apples and Onions

Preparation Time: 14 minutes

Cooking Time: 16 minutes

Servings: 3

Ingredients:

2 cups dry cider
1 large onion, halved
2 cups vegetable stock
4 apples, sliced into wedges
A pinch of salt
A pinch of pepper

Directions:

Combine cider and onion in a saucepan. Bring to a boil until the onions are cooked and liquid is almost gone.

Pour the stock and the apples. Season with salt and pepper. Stir occasionally. Cook for about 10 minutes or until the apples are tender but not mushy. Serve.

Nutrition:

Calories 343
Total Fat 51.2 g
Saturated Fat 0.8 g
Cholesterol 0 mg
Sodium 861 mg
Total Carbs 22.5 g
Fiber 6.3 g
Sugar 2.3 g
Protein 9.2 g

39. Zucchini Noodles with Portabella Mushrooms

Preparation Time: 14 minutes

Cooking Time: 16 minutes

Servings: 3

Ingredients:

1 zucchini, processed into spaghetti-like noodles
3 garlic cloves, minced
2 white onions, thinly sliced
1 thumb-sized ginger, julienned
1 lb. chicken thighs
1 lb. portabella mushrooms, sliced into thick slivers
2 cups chicken stock
3 cups of water
A pinch of sea salt, add more if needed
A pinch of black pepper, add more if needed
2 tsp. sesame oil
4 tbsp. coconut oil, divided
¼ cup fresh chives, minced, for garnish

Directions:

Pour 2 tablespoons of coconut oil into a large saucepan. Fry mushroom slivers in batches for 5 minutes or until seared brown. Set aside. Transfer these to a plate.
Sauté the onion, garlic, and ginger for 3 minutes or until tender. Add in chicken thighs, cooked mushrooms, chicken stock, water, salt, and pepper stir mixture well. Bring to a boil.
Decrease gradually the heat and allow simmering for 20 minutes or until the chicken is forking tender. Tip in sesame oil. Serve by placing an equal amount of zucchini noodles into bowls. Ladle soup and garnish with chives.

Nutrition:

Calories 163
Total Fat 4.2 g
Saturated Fat 0.8 g
Cholesterol 0 mg
Sodium 861 mg
Total Carbs 22.5 g
Fiber 6.3 g
Sugar 2.3 g
Protein 9.2 g

40. Grilled Tempeh with Pineapple

Preparation Time: 12 minutes

Cooking Time: 16 minutes

Servings: 3

Ingredients:

10 oz. tempeh, sliced
1 red bell pepper, quartered
1/4 pineapple, sliced into rings
6 oz. green beans
1 tbsp. coconut aminos
2 1/2 tbsp. orange juice, freshly squeeze
1 1/2 tbsp. lemon juice, freshly squeezed
1 tbsp. extra virgin olive oil
1/4 cup hoisin sauce

Directions:

Blend the olive oil, orange and lemon juices, coconut aminos or soy sauce, and hoisin sauce in a bowl. Add the diced tempeh and set aside.
Heat up the grill or place a grill pan over medium-high flame. Once hot, lift the marinated tempeh from the bowl with a pair of tongs and transfer them to the grill or pan. Grill for 2 to 3 minutes, or until browned all over.
Grill the sliced pineapples alongside the tempeh, then transfer them directly onto the serving platter.

Place the grilled tempeh beside the grilled pineapple and cover with aluminium foil to keep warm.

Meanwhile, place the green beans and bell peppers in a bowl and add just enough of the marinade to coat.

Prepare the grill pan and add the vegetables. Grill until fork tender and slightly charred. Transfer the grilled vegetables to the serving platter and arrange artfully with the tempeh and pineapple. Serve at once.

Nutrition:

Calories 163 - Total Fat 4.2 g
Saturated Fat 0.8 g - Cholesterol 0 mg
Sodium 861 mg - Total Carbs 22.5 g
Fiber 6.3 g - Sugar 2.3 g - Protein 9.2 g

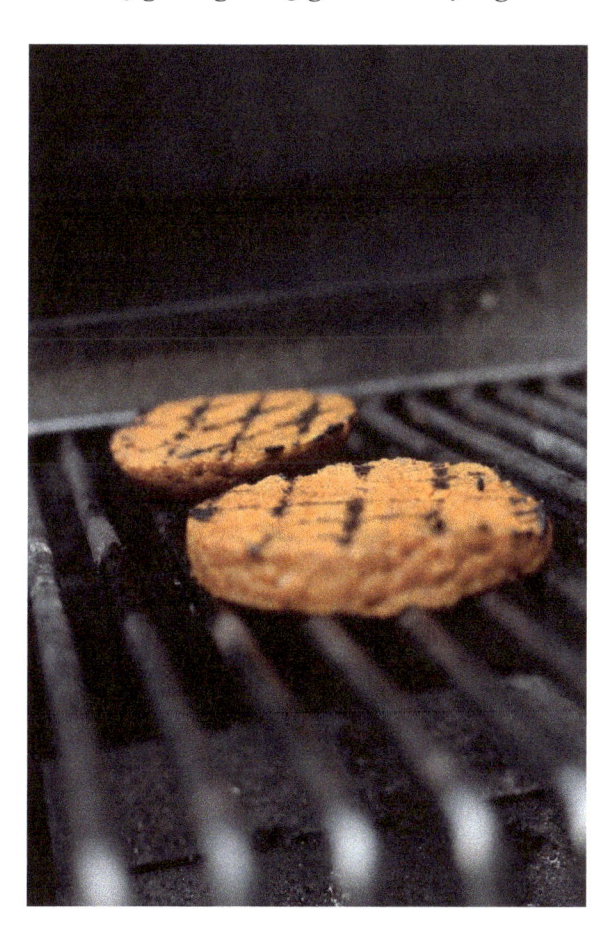

41. Courgettes in Cider Sauce

Preparation Time: 13 minutes

Cooking Time: 17 minutes

Servings: 3

Ingredients:

2 cups baby courgettes
3 tablespoons vegetable stock
2 tablespoons apple cider vinegar
1 tablespoon light brown sugar
4 spring onions, finely sliced
1 piece of fresh ginger root, grated
1 teaspoon of corn flour
2 teaspoons of water

Directions:

Bring a pan with salted water to a boil. Add courgettes. Bring to a boil for 5 minutes. Meanwhile, in a pan, combine vegetable stock, apple cider vinegar, brown sugar, onions, ginger root, lemon juice and rind, and orange juice and rind. Take to a boil. Lower the heat and allow simmering for 3 minutes.

Mix the corn flour with water. Stir well. Pour into the sauce. Continue stirring until the sauce thickens.

Drain courgettes. Transfer to the serving dish. Spoon over the sauce. Toss to coat courgettes. Serve.

Nutrition:

Calories 173 - Total Fat 9.2 g
Saturated Fat 0.8 g
Cholesterol 0 mg
Sodium 861 mg
Total Carbs 22.5 g
Fiber 6.3 g - Sugar 2.3 g
Protein 9.2 g

42. Baked Mixed Mushrooms

Preparation Time: 8 minutes

Cooking Time: 20 minutes

Servings: 3

Ingredients:

2 cups mixed wild mushrooms
1 cup chestnut mushrooms
2 cups dried porcini
2 shallots
4 garlic cloves
3 cups raw pecans
½ bunch fresh thyme
1 bunch flat-leaf parsley
2 tablespoons olive oil
2 fresh bay leaves
1 ½ cups stale bread

Directions:

Remove skin and finely chop garlic and shallots. Roughly chop the wild mushrooms and chestnut mushrooms. Pick the leaves of the thyme and tear the bread into small pieces. Put inside the pressure cooker.
Place the pecans and roughly chop the nuts. Pick the parsley leaves and roughly chop. Place the porcini in a bowl then add 300ml of boiling water. Set aside until needed.
Heat oil in the pressure cooker. Add the garlic and shallots. Cook for 3 minutes while stirring occasionally.
Drain porcini and reserve the liquid. Add the porcini into the pressure cooker together with the wild mushrooms and chestnut mushrooms. Add the bay leaves and thyme. Position the lid and lock in place. Put to high heat and bring to high pressure. Adjust heat to stabilize. Cook for 10 minutes. Adjust taste if necessary.
Transfer the mushroom mixture into a bowl and set aside to cool completely.
Once the mushrooms are completely cool, add the bread, pecans, a pinch of black pepper and sea salt, and half of the reserved liquid into the bowl. Mix well. Add more reserved liquid if the mixture seems dry. Add more than half of the parsley into the bowl and stir. Transfer the mixture into a 20cm x 25cm lightly greased baking dish and cover with tin foil.
Bake in the oven for 35 minutes. Then, get rid of the foil and cook for another 10 minutes. Once done, sprinkle the remaining parsley on top and serve with bread or crackers. Serve.

Nutrition:

Calories 343
Total Fat 4.2 g
Saturated Fat 0.8 g
Cholesterol 0 mg
Sodium 861 mg
Total Carbs 22.5 g
Fiber 6.3 g
Sugar 2.3 g
Protein 9.2 g

43. Spiced Okra

Preparation Time: 14 minutes

Cooking Time: 16 minutes

Servings: 3

Ingredients:

2 cups okra
¼ teaspoon stevia
1 teaspoon chilli powder
½ teaspoon ground turmeric
1 tablespoon ground coriander
2 tablespoons fresh coriander, chopped
1 tablespoon ground cumin
¼ teaspoon salt
1 tablespoon desiccated coconut
3 tablespoons vegetable oil
½ teaspoon black mustard seeds
½ teaspoon cumin seeds
Fresh tomatoes, to garnish

Directions:

Trim the okra. Wash and dry.
Combine stevia, chilli powder, turmeric, ground coriander, fresh coriander, cumin, salt, and desiccated coconut in a bowl.
Heat the oil in a pan. Cook mustard and cumin seeds for 3 minutes. Stir continuously.
Add okra. Tip in the spice mixture. Cook on low heat for 8 minutes.
Transfer to a serving dish. Garnish with fresh tomatoes.

Nutrition:

Calories 163 - Total Fat 4.2 g
Saturated Fat 0.8 g
Cholesterol 0 mg
Sodium 861 mg - Total Carbs 22.5 g
Fiber 6.3 g - Sugar 2.3 g - Protein 9.2 g

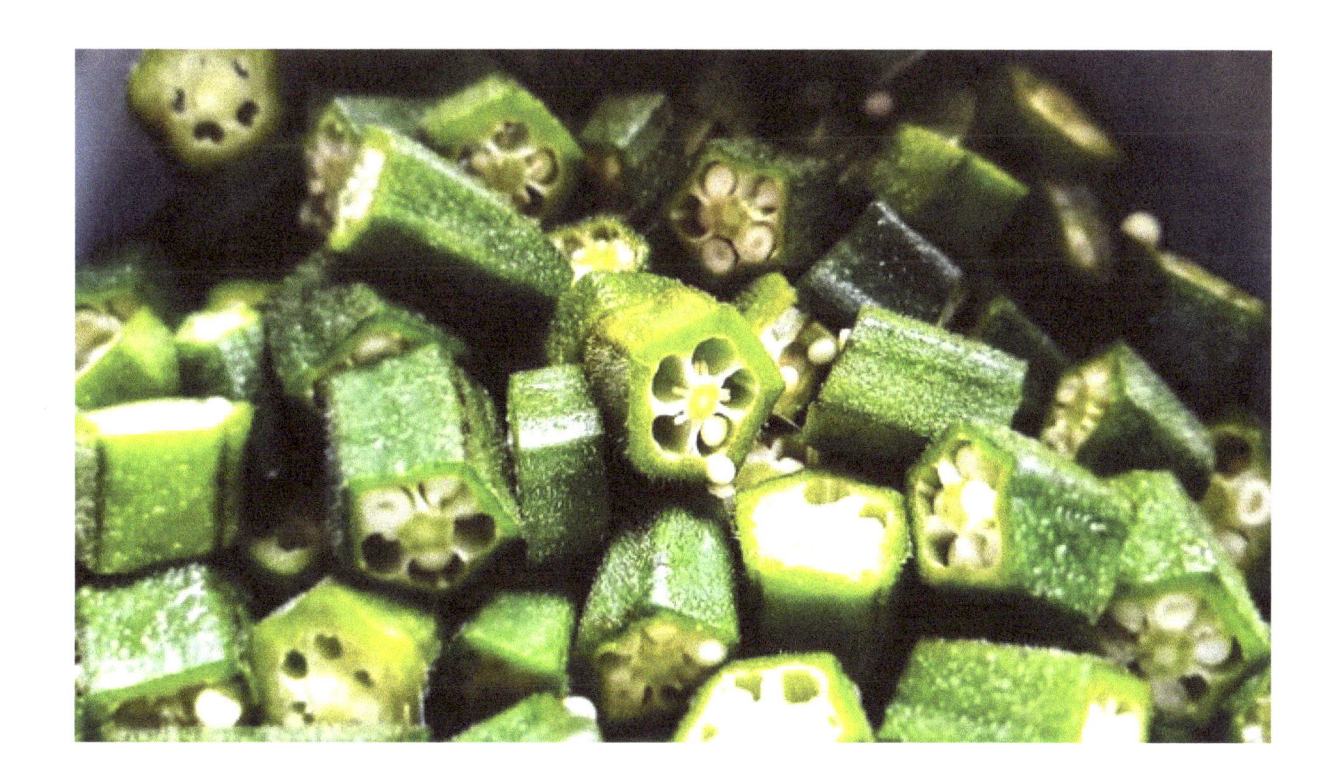

Sauces

1. Alkaline Salsa Mexicana

Preparation Time: 14 minutes

Cooking Time: 16 minutes

Servings: 3

Ingredients:

Cayenne pepper, one (1) pinch
Spring onions, two (2)
Tomatoes (big), three (3)
Cilantro (a handful)
Juice of lime, one (1)
Organic or sea salt (one pinch)
Chilies (green), two (2)
Garlic, two (2) cloves

Directions:

Chop garlic cloves in tiny pieces, cut the chilies in small pieces, cut the onions in rings, and put the tomatoes in small cubes. There are two ways you can about it, depend on how you prefer your salsa (either smooth or chunky).
For a smooth salsa; add all the ingredients in a mixing pan and mix well.
Empty the mix in a food processor and blast for a few seconds.
Add salt and pepper to taste.
Serve.
However, for a chunky salsa; add all ingredients together in a mixing bowl and mix properly.
Add salt and pepper to taste.
Serve.

Nutrition:

Calories: 5
Carbohydrates: 1g

2. Tofu Salad Dressing

Preparation Time: 14 minutes

Cooking Time: 16 minutes

Servings: 3

Ingredients:

Stevia powder, one (1) teaspoon
Tofu, 100g
Alkaline water, Five (5) tablespoons
Random spices and herbs of your choice
Sea salt, ½ teaspoon

Directions:

Include all elements in a food processor and process until it is fine to consistency.
Enjoy it with salad.

Nutrition:

Calories: 80 - Carbohydrates: 1g
Fat: 9g - Protein: 1g

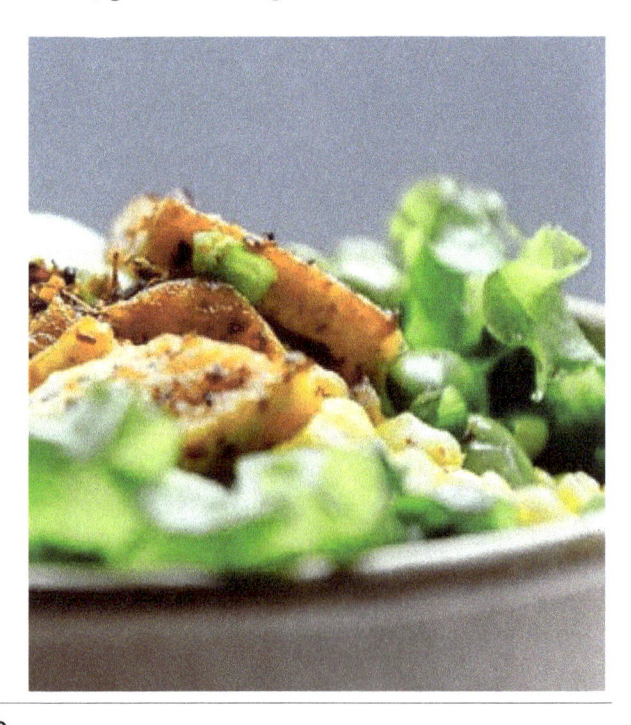

3. Millet Spread

Preparation Time: 14 minutes

Cooking Time: 16 minutes

Servings: 3

Ingredients:

Pepper, one (1) pinch
White onion (big), one (1)
Millet, one (1) cup
Any garden herb of your choice, one (1) teaspoon
Virgin olive oil (cold-pressed extra), one (1) tablespoon
Alkaline water, two (2) cups
Organic/sea salt, one (1) pinch
Yeast-free vegetable stock, one (1) teaspoon

Directions:

Get a small pot over medium heat, add water, the vegetable stock, and millet and boil for ten minutes, and put the pot aside for some minutes.
In a different pan, add oil and stir fry the roughly chopped onion.
Once that is done, add the stir-fried onion to the millet.
Mix properly, then add salt and pepper to taste.
Place it in a mixer and blend for 40 seconds. Serve.

Nutrition:

Calories: 25
Carbohydrates: 5 g

4. Alkaline Eggplant Dip

Preparation Time: 14 minutes

Cooking Time: 16 minutes

Servings: 3

Ingredients:

Garlic, two (2) cloves
Lemon juice (fresh), five (5) tablespoons
Parsley (a handful)
Cayenne pepper (a pinch)
Organic salt or sea salt (a pinch)
Eggplant (700g)
Sesame paste, six (6) tablespoons

Directions:

Firstly, it is necessary to preheat the oven to around 400 degrees Fahrenheit.
Wash the eggplants and use a fork to prick several places.
Place in the oven on a grid and heat for between thirty to forty minutes.
While this is going, chop the parsley and garlic and set aside.
Take off the eggplant from the oven after forty minutes and allow it to cool.
Once it's cooled, peel the eggplants and scoop out the pulp.
Chop the pulp finely on a chopping board and empty it in a mixing bowl.
In the mixing bowl, sprinkle the lemon juice and mash with a spoon until it becomes smooth.
Finally, add garlic, the parsley, and the sesame paste.
Season with pepper and salt to taste. Serve.

Nutrition:

Calories: 30 - Carbohydrates: 2 g
Fat: 3 g - Protein: 1g

5. Coriander Spread

Preparation Time: 14 minutes

Cooking Time: 16 minutes

Servings: 3

Ingredients:

Chili (green), 1-2
Ginger (fresh), ½ inch
Lime juice (fresh), two (2) tablespoons
Coconut flakes (freshly grated), one (1) cup
Coriander leaves (fresh), three (3) cups
Alkaline water, four (4) tablespoons
Organic or sea salt, one pinch

Directions:

Chop the ginger, chili, and coriander leaves. Include all elements in a blender machine and blend until the mix is smooth to consistency.
When that is done, you can add some organic or sea salt and season to taste.
Lastly, it is recommended that you put the mix in the fridge for about an hour.
Serve.

Nutrition:

Calories: 22
Carbohydrates: 2 g
Fat: 43 g

6. Polo Salad Dressing

Preparation Time: 14 minutes

Cooking Time: 16 minutes

Servings: 3

Ingredients:

Dates, two (2)
Juice of lemon, (½ lemon)
Alkaline water, ½ cup
Cayenne pepper and sea salt, one (1) dash
Extra virgin oil (cold-pressed), 1/3 cup
Miso, one (1) tablespoon

Directions:

Include all elements in a blender machine and blast until the mix is smooth to consistency.
You can add additional salt and pepper if desired.
Serve

Nutrition:

Calories: 71
Carbohydrates: 8g
Fat: 3 g
Protein: 2g

7. Citrus Alkaline Salad Dressing

Preparation Time: 14 minutes

Cooking Time: 16 minutes

Servings: 3

Ingredients:

Garlic powder, one (1) teaspoon
Rosemary (dried), ¼ teaspoon
Cumin (ground), ½ teaspoon
Oregano (ground), ½ teaspoon
Basil (dried), one (1) teaspoon
Olive oil (cold-pressed), ¾ cup
Cayenne pepper and sea salt, one (1) dash
Fresh lime or lemon juice, 1/3 cup

Directions:

Add all the ingredients in a mixer and blast until the mix is smooth to consistency.
You can season with pepper and salt if desired.
Serve.

Nutrition:

Calories: 43 - Carbohydrates: 3 g - Fat: 3 g

8. Avocado Spinach Dip

Preparation Time: 14 minutes

Cooking Time: 16 minutes

Servings: 3

Ingredients:

Dill, one (1) cup
Avocado, one (1)
Garlic, one (1) clove
Parsley, one (1) cup
Spinach (fresh), 150g
Tahini, one (1) tablespoon
Chili, one (1)
Pepper and sea salt to taste

Directions:

Include all elements in a blender machine
Blend until the mix turns creamy and smooth to consistency.
You can consist of pepper and salt to taste.
Serve.

Nutrition:

Calories: 46
Carbohydrates: 3g
Fat: 3g
Protein: 2g

9. Alkaline Vegetable Spread

Preparation Time: 14 minutes

Cooking Time: 16 minutes

Servings: 3

Ingredients:

Pepper, one (1) pinch
Tomato, one (1)
Avocado, one (1)
Yeast-free vegetable stock, one (1) teaspoon
Bean sprouts, ½ cup
Celery stalk, one (1)
Alfalfa sprouts, ½ cup
Sunflower seeds, one (1) handful
Organic salt or sea salt, one (1) pinch
Any garden herb of your choice, one (1) teaspoon
Extra virgin oil (cold-pressed), one (1) tablespoon
Cucumber ½

Directions:

Depending on how you like your spread, you can either blend it or not. Since we want this spread to be chunky, we won't Blend.
So, chop the alfalfa sprouts, cucumber, tomato, celery, and bean sprout into tiny pieces.
Get a mixing bowl and toss all the chopped ingredients into it.
Add sunflower seeds and mix properly.
Mash the avocado and add in a separate bowl, along with the olive oil, vegetable stock, lemon juice, salt and pepper, and herbs.
Stir until it forms a creamy paste.
Finally, mix the mashed avocado cream with the vegetables.
Stir consistently until all ingredients are mixed properly.
Refrigerate for about an hour.
Serve.

Nutrition:

Calories: 12
Carbohydrates: 1 g
Fat: 7 g

10. Alkaline Sunflower Sauce

Preparation Time: 14 minutes

Cooking Time: 16 minutes

Servings: 3

Ingredients:

Tomato, one (1)
Sunflower seeds, 200g
Red pepper, one (1)
Garlic, one (1) clove
Extra virgin olive oil (cold-pressed), one (teaspoon)
Pepper (a pinch)
Organic salt or sea salt (a pinch)
Any herb of your choice

Directions:

Note: Before you start this process, you should soak the sunflower seeds for about four (4) hours before commencement.
Add all ingredients in a blender and blast till the mix turns into a smooth cream.
Add your favourite herbs, pepper, and salt to taste.
Serve.

Nutrition:

Calories: 200
Protein: 7g

11. Almond-Red Bell Pepper Dip

Preparation Time: 14 minutes

Cooking Time: 16 minutes

Servings: 3

Ingredients:

Garlic, 2-3 cloves
Sea salt, one (1) pinch
Cayenne pepper, one (1) pinch
Extra virgin olive oil (cold-pressed), one (1) tablespoon
Almonds, 60g
Red bell pepper, 280g

Directions:

First of all, cook garlic and pepper until they are soft.
Add all ingredients in a mixer and blend until the mix becomes smooth and creamy.
Finally, add pepper and salt to taste.
Serve.

Nutrition:

Calories: 51
Carbohydrates: 10g
Fat: 1g
Protein: 2g

12. Hummus

Preparation Time: 14 minutes

Cooking Time: 16 minutes

Servings: 3

Ingredients:

Olive oil (cold pressed), one (1) tablespoon
Fresh Lemon juice, two (2) tablespoons
Chili, one (1)
Pepper and sea salt to taste
Tahini, one (1) tablespoon
Garlic (finely chopped), two (2) cloves
Chickpeas (home-cooked), 300g-400g
Vegetable broth (yeast-free), 50ml

Directions:

Blend all the ingredients until it becomes creamy and smooth.
Add pepper and salt to taste.
Serve.

Nutrition:

Calories: 70 - Carbohydrates: 4g
Fat: 5g - Protein: 2 g

Sweet Barbecue Sauce

Preparation Time: 14 minutes

Cooking Time: 16 minutes

Servings: 3

Ingredients:

6 quartered plum tomatoes
1/4 cup of chopped white onions
1/4 cup of date sugar
2 teaspoons of pure sea salt
2 teaspoons agave syrup
1/4 teaspoon cayenne
2 teaspoons of onion powder
1/2 teaspoon ground ginger
1/8 teaspoon cloves

Directions:

Add all ingredients, excluding date sugar, to a blender and blend them thoroughly. Pour mixture into a saucepan and add a date sugar. Cook over average heat, stirring occasionally to prevent sticking until boiling. Reduce heat to a simmer. Cover the saucepan with a lid and cook for 15 minutes, stirring from time to time.

Use an immersion blender to blend the sauce until it is smooth. Remain to cook at low heat until the sauce thickens for about 10 minutes. Allow mixture to cool before using it. Serve and enjoy your sweet barbecue sauce!

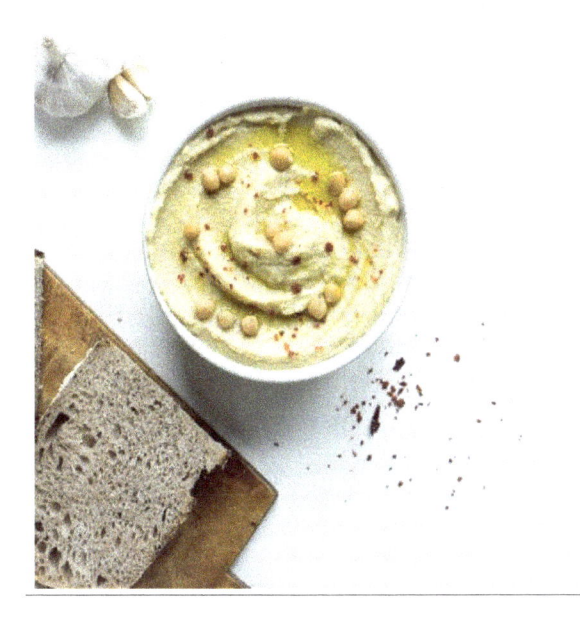

Nutrition:

Calories: 30
Carbohydrates: 4 g
Fat: 1 g

13. Avocado Sauce

Preparation Time: 14 minutes

Cooking Time: 16 minutes

Servings: 3

Ingredients:

1 ripe avocado
1 pinch of basil
½ teaspoon of oregano
1/2 teaspoon of onion powder
2 teaspoons of minced onion
1/2 teaspoon of pure sea salt

Directions:

Cut the avocado in half, peel it and remove the seed. Slice it into small pieces and throw into a food processor. Add all other ingredients and blend for 2 to 3 minutes until smooth. Serve and enjoy your avocado sauce!

Nutrition:

Calories: 14
Carbohydrates: 2 g
Protein: 1g

14. Fragrant Tomato Sauce

Preparation Time: 14 minutes

Cooking Time: 16 minutes

Servings: 3

Ingredients:

5 Roma tomatoes
1 pinch of basil
1 teaspoon of oregano
1 teaspoon of onion powder
2 teaspoon of minced onion
2 teaspoon agave syrup
1 teaspoon of pure sea salt
2 tablespoons of grape seed oil

Directions:

Make an X cut on the lowermost of the Roma tomatoes and place them into a pot of hot water for just 1 minute. Take away the tomatoes from the water using a spoon and shock them, placing them in cold water for 30 seconds. Take them out and immediately peel with your fingers or a knife. Put all the ingredients into a mixer or a food processor and blend for 1 minute until smooth. Serve and enjoy your fragrant tomato sauce.

Nutrition:

Calories: 20
Carbohydrates: 2 g
Protein: 1g

15. Guacamole

Preparation Time: 14 minutes

Cooking Time: 16 minutes

Servings: 3

Ingredients:

1 minced Roma tomato
2 avocados
1/2 cup of chopped cilantro
1/2 cup of minced red onion
1/2 teaspoon of cayenne powder
1/2 teaspoon of onion powder
1/2 teaspoon of pure sea salt
Juice from ½ lime

Directions:

Cut the avocados in half, peel, and remove the seeds. Slice into tiny pieces and put them in a medium bowl. Add all other ingredients, excluding the Roma tomato, to the bowl. Using a masher, mix together until becomes smooth. Add the minced Roma tomatoes to the mixture and mix well.
Serve and enjoy your delicious guacamole!

Nutrition:

Calories: 12
Fat: 1 g

16. Garlic Sauce

Preparation Time: 14 minutes

Cooking Time: 16 minutes

Servings: 3

Ingredients:

1/4 cup of diced shallots
1 tablespoon of onion powder
1/4 teaspoon of dill
1/2 teaspoon of ginger
1/2 teaspoon of pure sea salt
1 cup of grapeseed oil

Directions:

Find a glass jar with a lid. Put all ingredients for the sauce in the jar and shake them well. Place the sauce mixture in the refrigerator for at least 1 hour. Serve and enjoy your "garlic" sauce!

Nutrition:

Calories: 48

Carbohydrates: 2 g
Fat: 4 g

17. Pesto Saucy Cream Recipe

Preparation Time: 14 minutes

Cooking Time: 16 minutes

Servings: 3

Ingredients:

1 small avocado (Hass)
1 cup walnuts
3 tablespoons sour orange or lime
1/8 teaspoon basil
1/4 teaspoon onion powder
1/4 teaspoon cayenne pepper
1 teaspoon spring water

Directions:

Make a slit with a knife lengthwise around the avocado. Split open the avocado into two. Then using your heavy knife carefully, hit down the avocado seed, turn and pull out the seed. Scoop out the avocado meat and remove the skin. Then, add all of the ingredients to your blender and blend until all of the ingredients are thoroughly mixed and becomes smooth.

Nutrition:

Calories: 65 - Carbohydrates: 4 g
Fat: 5 g - Protein: 3 g

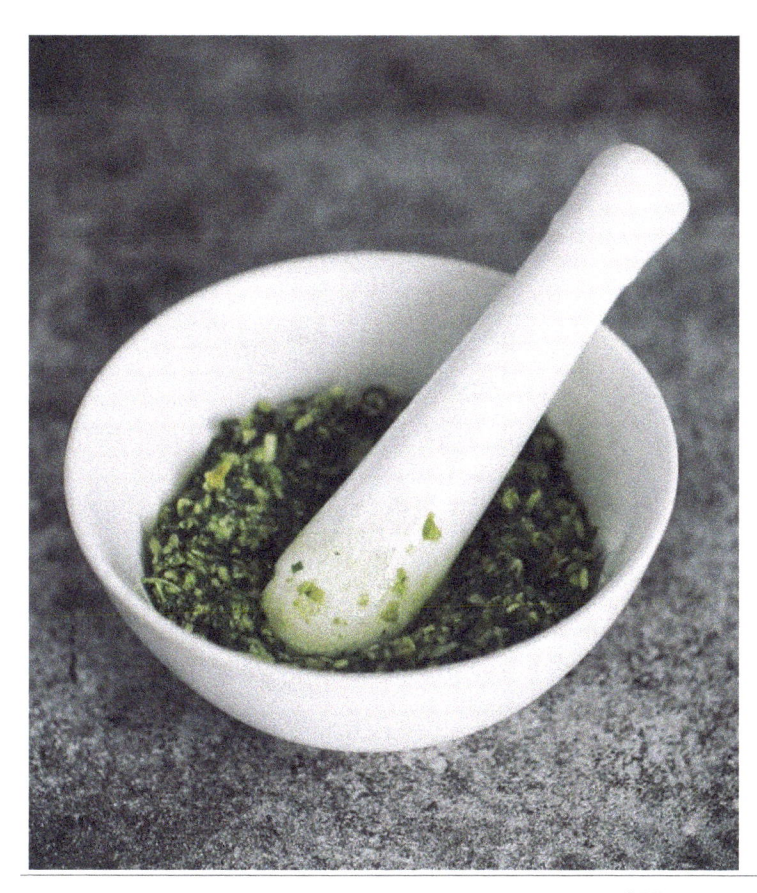

Special Ingredients

1. Homemade Hemp Seed Milk

Preparation Time: 15 minutes

Cooking Time: 2 hours

Servings: 2 cups

Ingredients:

2 tablespoons of hemp seeds
2 tablespoons of agave syrup
1/8 teaspoon of pure sea salt
2 cups of spring water
Fruits (optional)*

Directions:

Place all ingredients, except fruits, into the blender.
Blend them for two minutes.
Add fruits and repeatedly blend for 30 to 50 seconds.
Leave milk in a refrigerator until cold.
Enjoy your homemade hemp seed milk!

Nutrition:

Calories: 83
Carbohydrates: 1.3 g
Protein: 4.7 g
Fat: 7.3 g

2. Spicy Infused Oil

Preparation Time: 5 minutes

Cooking Time: 24 hours

Servings: 1 cup

Ingredients:

1 tablespoon of crushed cayenne pepper
3/4 cup of grapeseed oil

Directions:

Fill a glass jar with a lid or a squeeze bottle with grapeseed oil.
Add crushed cayenne pepper to the jar/bottle.
Shake it and let the oil infuse for at least 24 hours.
Add it to a dish and enjoy your spicy infused oil!

Nutrition:

Calories: 120
Fat: 14 g

3. Italian Infused Oil

Preparation Time: 5 minutes

Cooking Time: 24 hours

Servings: 1 cup

Ingredients:

1 teaspoon of oregano
1 teaspoon of basil
1 pinch of pure sea salt
3/4 cup of grapeseed oil

Directions:

Fill a glass jar with a lid or a squeeze bottle with grapeseed oil.
Mix seasoning together and add them to the jar/bottle.
Shake it and let the oil infuse for at least 24 hours.
Add it to a dish and enjoy your Italian infused oil!

Nutrition:

Calories: 120
Fat: 14 g

4. Garlic Infused Oil

Preparation Time: 5 minutes

Cooking Time: 24 hours

Servings: 1 cup

Ingredients:

1/2 teaspoon of dill
1/2 teaspoon of ginger powder
1 tablespoon of onion powder
1/2 teaspoon of pure sea salt
3/4 cup of grapeseed oil

Directions:

Fill a glass jar with a lid or a squeeze bottle with Grape Seed Oil.
Add the seasonings to the jar/bottle.
Shake it and let the oil infuse for at least 24 hours.
Add it to a dish and enjoy your "Garlic" Infused Oil!

Nutrition:

Calories: 130
Fat: 14 g

5. Papaya Seed Mango Dressing

Preparation Time: 5 minutes

Cooking Time: 10 minutes

Servings: 1/2 cups

Ingredients:

1 cup of chopped mango
1 teaspoon of ground papaya seeds
1 teaspoon of basil
1 teaspoon of onion powder
1 teaspoon of agave syrup
2 tablespoons of lime juice
1/4 cup of grapeseed oil
1/4 teaspoon of pure sea salt

Directions:

Prepare and place all ingredients into the blender.
Blend for one minute until smooth.
Add it to a salad and enjoy your papaya seed mango dressing!

Nutrition:

Calories: 120
Fat: 14 g

6. Tomato Ginger Dressing

Preparation Time: 5 minutes

Cooking Time: 10 minutes

Servings: 1/2 cups

Ingredients:

2 chopped plum tomatoes
1 teaspoon of minced ginger*
1 tablespoon of agave syrup
2 tablespoons of chopped onion
2 tablespoons of sesame seeds
1 tablespoon of lime juice

Directions:

Prepare and place all ingredients into the blender.
Blend for one minute until smooth.
Add it to a salad and enjoy your tomato ginger dressing!

Nutrition:

Calories: 40.3
Fat: 4.1 g
Fiber: 0.1 g

7. Dill Cucumber Dressing

Preparation Time: 5 minutes

Cooking Time: 10 minutes

Servings: 1/2 cups

Ingredients:

1 teaspoon of fresh dill*
1 cup of quartered cucumbers
1/2 teaspoon of onion powder
2 teaspoons of agave syrup
1 tablespoon of lime juice
1/4 cup of Avocado oil

Directions:

Prepare and place all ingredients into the blender.
Blend for one minute until smooth.
Add it to a salad and enjoy your dill cucumber dressing!

Nutrition:

Calories: 60
Carbohydrates: 3 g
Fat: 5

8. Homemade Walnut Milk

Preparation Time: 15 minutes

Cooking Time: Minimum 8 hours

Servings: 4 cups

Ingredients:

1 cup of raw walnuts
1/8 teaspoon of pure sea salt
3 cups of spring water + extra for soaking

Directions:

Put raw walnuts in a small pot and cover them with three inches of water.
Soak the walnuts for at least eight hours.
Drain and rinse the walnuts with cold water.
Add the soaked walnuts, pure sea salt, and three cups of spring water to a blender.
Mix well until smooth.
Strain it if you need to.
Enjoy your homemade walnut milk!

Nutrition:

Calories: 200 - Carbohydrate: 3.89 gr
Sugar: 1 g - Fiber: 2 g - Protein: 5 g - Fat: 20

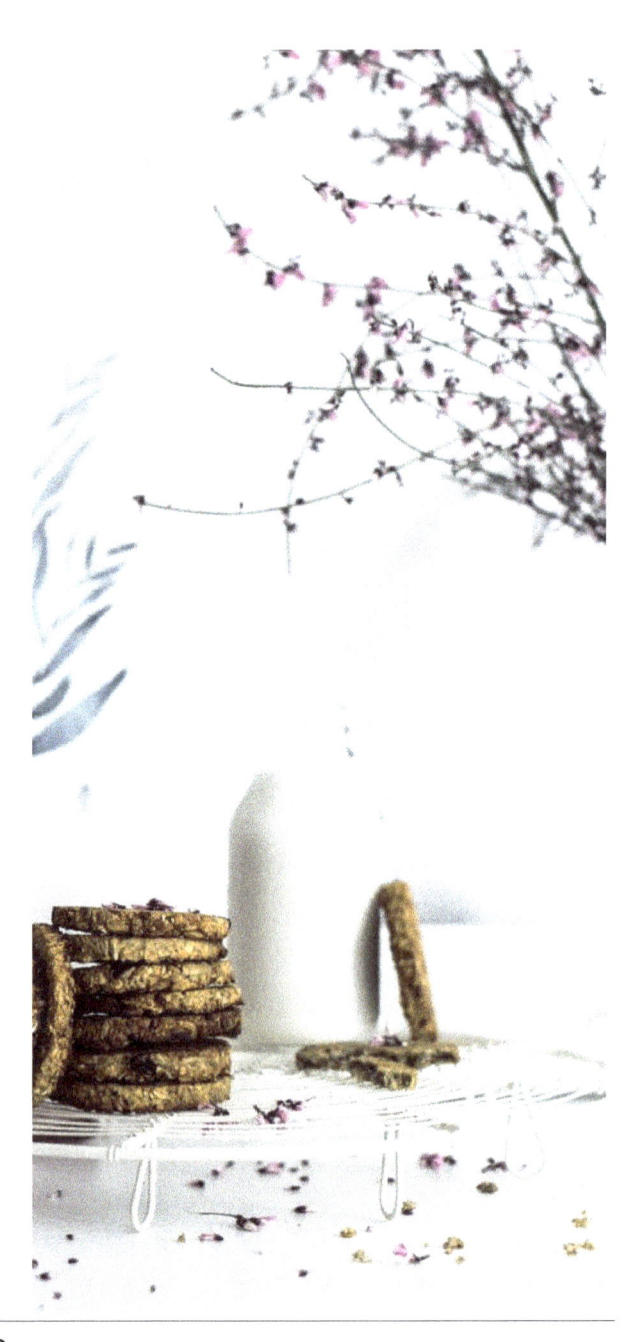

9. Aquafaba

Preparation Time: 15 minutes

Cooking Time: 2 Hours 30 Minutes

Servings: 2-4 Cups

Ingredients:

1 bag of garbanzo beans
1 teaspoon of pure sea salt
6 cups of spring water + extra for soaking

Directions:

Place garbanzo beans in a large pot, add spring water and pure sea salt. Bring to a rolling boil.

Remove from the heat and leave to soak kindly for 30 to 40 minutes.

Strain garbanzo beans and add 6 cups of spring water.

Boil for 1 hour and 30 minutes on medium heat.

Strain the garbanzo beans. This strained water is Aquafaba.

Pour Aquafaba into a glass jar with a lid and place it into the refrigerator.

After cooling, Aquafaba becomes thicker. If it is too liquid, repeatedly boil for 10-20 minutes.

Useful tips:

Aquafaba is a good alternative for an egg:
2 tablespoons of Aquafaba = 1 egg white
3 tablespoons of Aquafaba = 1 egg.

Nutrition:

Calories: 46 - Carbs: 8 g
Fiber: 2 g - Protein: 3 g

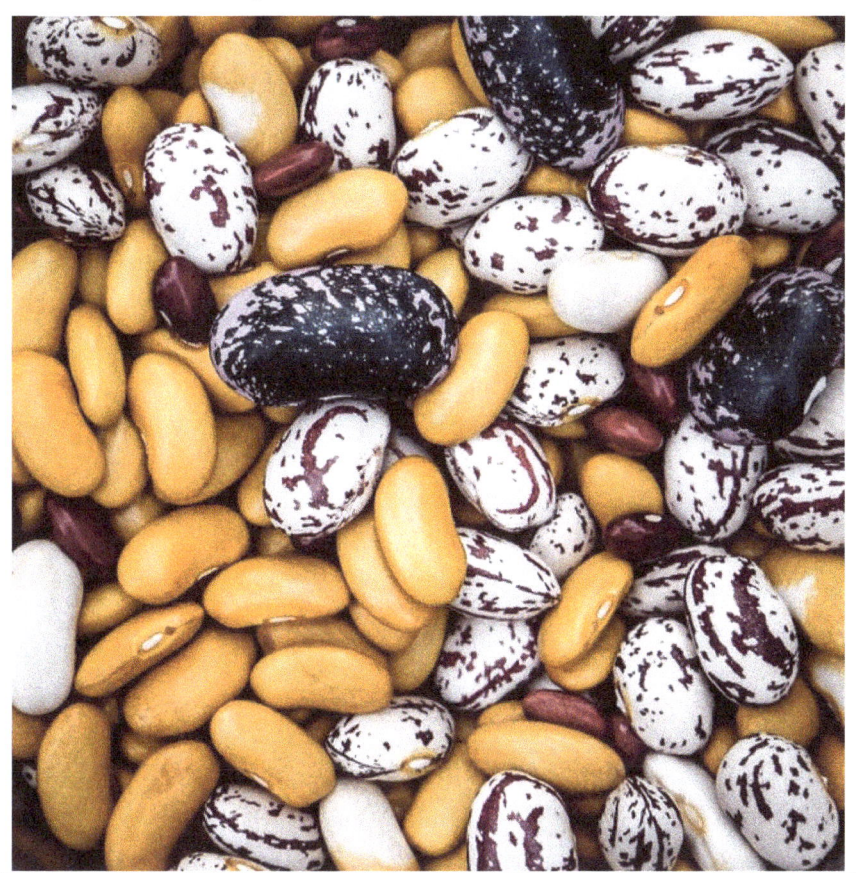

Snacks & Bread

1. Spinach and Sesame Crackers

Preparation Time: 5 minutes

Cooking Time: 15 minutes

Servings: 4

Ingredients:

2 tablespoons white sesame seeds
1 cup fresh spinach, washed
1 2/3 cups of all-purpose flour
1/2 cup of water
1/2 teaspoon baking powder
1 teaspoon olive oil
1 teaspoon of salt

Directions:

Transfer the spinach to a blender with a half cup of water and blend until smooth.
Add 2 tablespoons white sesame seeds, ½ teaspoon baking powder, 1 2/3 cups all-purpose flour, and 1 teaspoon salt to a bowl and stir well until combined. Add in 1 teaspoon olive oil and spinach water. Mix again and knead by using your hands until you obtain a smooth dough.
If the made dough is too gluey, then add more flour.
Using your parchment paper lightly roll out the dough as thin as possible. Cut into squares with a pizza cutter.
Bake into a preheated oven at 400° for about 15to 20 minutes. Once done, let cool and then serve.

Nutrition:

223 calories
3g fat - 41g total carbohydrates
6g protein

2. Mini Nacho Pizzas

Preparation Time: 5 minutes

Cooking Time: 10 minutes

Servings: 4

Ingredients:

1/4 cup refried beans, vegan
2 tablespoons tomato, diced
2 English muffins, split in half
1/4 cup onion, sliced
1/3 cup vegan cheese, shredded
1 small jalapeno, sliced
1/3 cup roasted tomato salsa
1/2 avocado, diced and tossed in lemon juice

Directions:

Add the refried beans/salsa onto the muffin bread. Sprinkle with shredded vegan cheese followed by the veggie toppings.
Transfer to a baking sheet and place in a preheated oven at 350 to 400 F on a top rack. Put into the oven for 10 minutes and then broil for 2minutes, so that the top becomes bubbly.
Take out from the oven and let them cool at room temperature.
Top with avocado. Enjoy!

Nutrition:

133 calories
4.2g fat
719g total carbohydrates
6g protein

3. Pizza Sticks

Preparation Time: 10 minutes

Cooking Time: 30 minutes

Servings: 16 sticks

Ingredients:

5 tablespoons tomato sauce
Few pinches of dried basil
1 block extra firm tofu
2 tablespoon + 2 teaspoon nutritional yeast

Directions:

Cape the tofu in a paper tissue and put a cutting board on top, place something heavy on top and drain for about 10 to 15 minutes. In the meantime, line your baking sheet with parchment paper. Cut the tofu into 16 equal pieces and place them on a baking sheet. Spread each pizza stick with a teaspoon of marinara sauce.
Sprinkle each stick with a half teaspoon of yeast, followed by basil on top.
Bake into a preheated oven at 425 F for about 28 to 30 minutes. Serve and enjoy!

Nutrition:

33 calories - 1.7g fat
2g total carbs - 3g protein

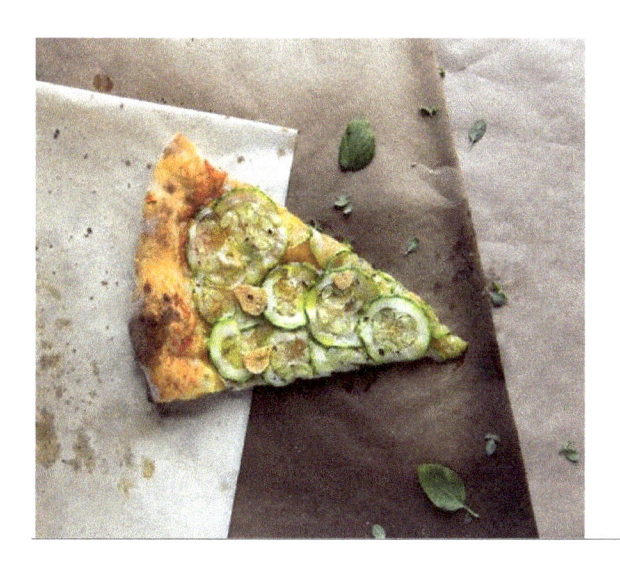

4. Raw Broccoli Poppers

Preparation Time: 2 minutes

Cooking Time: 8 minutes

Servings: 4

Ingredients:

1/8 cup of water
1/8 teaspoon of fine sea salt
4 cups broccoli florets, washed and cut into 1-inch pieces
1/4 teaspoon turmeric powder
1 cup unsalted cashews, soaked overnight or at least 3-4 hours and drained
1/4 teaspoon onion powder
1 red bell pepper, seeded and
2 heaping tablespoons nutritional
2 tablespoons lemon juice

Directions:

Transfer the drained cashews to a high-speed blender and pulse for about 30 seconds. Add in the chopped pepper and pulse again for 30 seconds.
Add some 2 tablespoons of lemon juice, 1/8 cup of water, 2 heaping tablespoons of nutritional yeast, ¼ teaspoon of onion powder, 1/8 teaspoon of fine sea salt, and 1/4 teaspoon of turmeric powder. Pulse for about 45 seconds until smooth.
Handover the broccoli into a bowl and add in chopped cheesy cashew mixture. Toss well until coated.
Transfer the pieces of broccoli to the trays of a yeast dehydrator.
Follow the dehydrator's instructions and dehydrate for about 8 minutes at 125 F or until crunchy.

Nutrition:

408 calories, 32g fat - 22g Carbohydrates
15g protein

5. Blueberry Cauliflower

Preparation Time: 2 minutes

Cooking Time: 5 minutes

Servings: 1

Ingredients:

¼ cup of frozen strawberries
2 teaspoons maple syrup
¾ cup unsweetened cashew milk
1 teaspoon vanilla extract
½ cup of plain cashew yogurt
5 tablespoons powdered peanut butter
¾ cup of frozen wild blueberries
½ cup of cauliflower florets, coarsely chopped

Directions:

Add all the smoothie ingredients to a high-speed blender.
Blitz to combine until smooth.
Pour into a chilled glass and serve.

Nutrition:

340 calories
11g fat
48g total carbohydrates
16g protein

6. Candied Ginger

Preparation Time: 10 minutes

Cooking Time: 40 minutes

Servings: 3 to 5

Ingredients:

2 1/2 cups salted pistachios, shelled
1 1/4 teaspoons powdered ginger
3 tablespoons pure maple syrup

Directions:

Add 1 1/4 teaspoons powdered ginger to a bowl with pistachios. Stir well until combined. There should be no lumps.
Drizzle with 3 tablespoons of maple syrup and stir well.
Transfer to a baking sheet lined with parchment paper and spread evenly.
Cook into a preheated oven at 275 F for about 20 minutes.
Take out from the oven, stir, and cook for further 10 to 15 minutes.
Let it cool for about a few minutes until crispy. Enjoy!

Nutrition:

378 calories
27.6g fat
26g total carbohydrates
13g protein

7. Chia Crackers

Preparation Time: 20 minutes

Cooking Time: 1 hour

Servings: 24-26 crackers

Ingredients:

1/2 cup of pecans, chopped
1/2 cup of chia seeds
1/2 teaspoon cayenne pepper
1 cup of water
1/4 cup of nutritional yeast
1/2 cup of pumpkin seeds
1/4 cup of ground flax
Salt and pepper, to taste

Directions:

Mix around 1/2 cup chia seeds and 1 cup water. Keep it aside.
Take another bowl and combine all the remaining ingredients. Combine well and stir in the chia water mixture until you obtained dough.
Transfer the dough onto a baking sheet and rollout (¼" thick).
Transfer into a preheated oven at 325°F and

bake for about half an hour.

Take out from the oven, flip over the dough, and cut it into desired cracker shape/squares.

Spread and back again for a further half an hour, or until crispy and browned.

Once done, take out from the oven and let them cool at room temperature. Enjoy!

Nutrition:

41 calories

3.1g fat

2g total carbohydrates

2g protein

8. Orange- Spiced Pumpkin Hummus

Preparation Time: 2 minutes

Cooking Time: 5 minutes

Servings: 4 cups

Ingredients:

1 tablespoon maple syrup

1/2 teaspoon salt

1 can (16oz.) garbanzo beans,

1/8 teaspoon ginger or nutmeg

1 cup of canned pumpkin

1/8 teaspoon cinnamon

1/4 cup of tahini

1 tablespoon fresh orange juice

A pinch of orange zest, for garnish

1 tablespoon apple cider vinegar

Directions:

Mix all the ingredients to a food processor blender and blend until slightly chunky. Serve right away and enjoy it!

Nutrition:

291 calories

22.9g fat

15g total carbohydrates

12g protein

9. Cinnamon Maple Sweet Potato Bites

Preparation Time: 5 minutes

Cooking Time: 25 minutes

Servings: 3 to 4

Ingredients:

½ teaspoon corn-starch

1 teaspoon cinnamon

4 medium sweet potatoes, then peeled, and cut into bite-size cubes

2 to 3 tablespoons maple syrup

3 tablespoons butter, melted

Directions:

Transfer the potato cubes to a Ziploc bag and add in 3 tablespoons of melted butter. Seal and shake well until the potato cubes are coated with butter.

Add in the remaining ingredients and shake again.

Transfer the potato cubes to a parchment-lined baking sheet. Cubes shouldn't be stacked on one another.

Sprinkle with cinnamon, if needed, and bake in a preheated oven at 425°F for about 25 to 30 minutes, stirring once during cooking.

Once done, take them out and stand at room temperature. Enjoy!

Nutrition:

436 calories

17.4g fat

71.8g total carbohydrates

4.1g protein

10. Cheesy Kale Chips

Preparation Time: 3 minutes

Cooking Time: 12 minutes

Servings: 4

Ingredients:

3 tablespoons nutritional yeast
1 head curly kale, washed, ribs
3/4 teaspoon garlic powder
1 tablespoon olive oil
1 teaspoon onion powder
Salt, to taste

Directions:

Line cookie sheets with parchment paper. Drain the kale leaves and spread on a paper removed and leaves torn into a chip-towel. Then, kindly transfer the leaves to a bowl and sized pieces. Add in 1 teaspoon of onion powder, 3 tablespoons of nutritional yeast, 1 tablespoon of olive oil, and ¾ teaspoon of garlic powder. Mix with your hands.
Spread the kale onto prepared cookie sheets. They shouldn't touch each other.
Bake into a preheated oven for about 350 F for about 10 to 12 minutes.
Once crisp, take out from the oven, and sprinkle with a bit of salt. Serve and enjoy!

Nutrition:

71 calories
4g fat
5g total carbohydrates
4g protein

11. Lemon Roasted Bell Pepper

Preparation Time: 10 minutes

Cooking Time: 5 minutes

Servings: 4

Ingredients:

4 bell peppers
1 teaspoon olive oil
1 tablespoon mango juice
1/4 teaspoon garlic, minced
1 teaspoons oregano
1 pinch of salt
1 pinch of pepper

Directions:

Start heating the Air Fryer to 390 degrees F.
Place some bell pepper in the air fryer.
Drizzle it with the olive oil and air fry for 5 minutes.
Take a serving plate and transfer it.
Take a small bowl and add garlic, oregano, mango juice, salt, and pepper.
Mix them well and drizzle the mixture over the peppers.
Serve and enjoy!

Nutrition:

Calories: 59 kcal
Carbohydrates: 6 g
Fat: 5 g
Protein: 4 g

12. Subtle Roasted Mushrooms

Preparation Time: 10 minutes

Cooking Time: 5 minutes

Servings: 4

Ingredients:

2 teaspoons mixed Sebi Friendly herbs
1 tablespoon olive oil
1/2 teaspoon garlic powder
2 pounds' mushrooms
2 tablespoons date sugar

Directions:

Wash mushrooms and turn dry in a plate of mixed greens spinner.
Quarter and put them in a safe spot.
Put garlic, oil, and spices in the dish of your oar type air fryer.
Warmth for 2 minutes.
Stir it.
Add some mushrooms and cook 25 minutes.
Then include vermouth and cook for 5 minutes more.
Serve and enjoy!

Nutrition:

Calories: 94 - Carbohydrates: 3 g
Fat: 8 g - Protein: 2 g

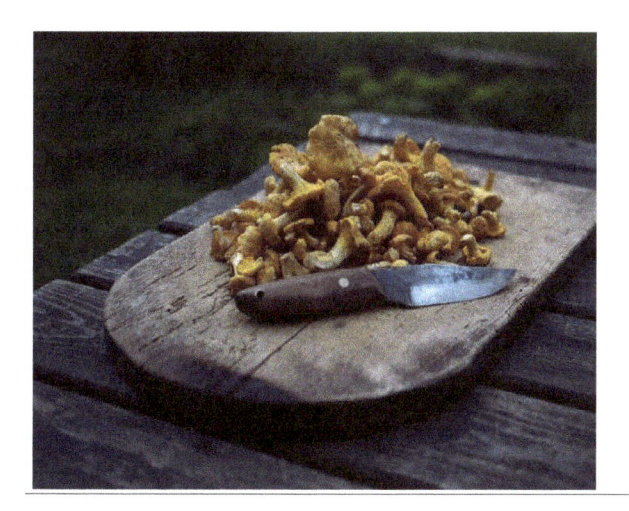

13. Fancy Spelt Bread

Preparation Time: 10 minutes

Cooking Time: 5 minutes

Servings: 4

Ingredients:

1 cup spring water
1/2 cup of coconut milk
3 tablespoons avocado oil
1 teaspoon baking soda
1 tablespoon agave nectar
4 and 1/2 cups spelt flour
1 and 1/2 teaspoon salt

Directions:

Preheat your Air Fryer to 355 degrees F.
Take a big bowl and add baking soda, salt, flour whisk well.
Add 3/4 cup of water, plus coconut milk, oil, and mix well.
Sprinkle your working surface with flour, add dough to the flour.
Roll well.
Knead for about three minutes, adding small amounts of flour until dough is a nice ball.
Place parchment paper in your cooking basket.
Lightly grease your pan and put the dough inside.
Transfer into Air Fryer and bake for 30-45 minutes until done.
Remove then insert a stick to check for doneness.
If done already serve and enjoy, if not, let it cook for a few minutes more.

Nutrition:

Calories: 203 kcal
Carbohydrates: 37 g
Fat: 4g
Protein: 7 g

14. Crispy Crunchy Hummus

Preparation Time: 10 minutes

Cooking Time: 10-15 minutes

Servings: 4

Ingredients:

1/2 a red onion
2 tablespoons fresh coriander
1/4 cup of cherry tomatoes
1/2 a red bell pepper
1 tablespoon dulse flakes
Juice of lime
Salt to taste
3 tablespoons olive oil
2 tablespoons tahini
1 cup of warm chickpeas

Directions:

Prepare your Air Fryer cooking basket
Add chickpeas to your cooking container and cook for 10-15 minutes, making a point to continue blending them every once in a while until they are altogether warmed
Add warmed chickpeas to a bowl and include tahini, salt, lime
Utilize a fork to pound chickpeas and fixings in glue until smooth
Include hacked onion, cherry tomatoes, ringer pepper, dulse drops, and olive oil
Blend well until consolidated
Serve hummus with a couple of cuts of spelt bread

Nutrition:

Calories: 95 kcal
Carbohydrates: 5 g
Fat: 5 g
Protein: 5 g

15. Chick Pea and Kale Dish

Preparation Time: 10 minutes

Cooking Time: 25-30 minutes

Servings: 4

Ingredients:

2 cups chickpea flour
1/2 cup green bell pepper, diced
1/2 cup onions, minced
1 tablespoon oregano
1 tablespoon salt
1 teaspoon cayenne
4 cups spring water
2 tablespoons grapeseed oil

Directions:

Boil spring water in a large pot.
Lower heat into medium and whisk in chickpea flour.
Add some minced onions, diced green bell pepper, seasoning to the pot and cook for 10 minutes.
Cover dish using a baking sheet, grease with oil.
Pour batter into the sheet and spread with a spatula.
Cover with another sheet.
Transfer to a fridge and chill, for 20 minutes.
Remove from the freezer and cut the batter into fry shapes.
Preheat the Air Fryer to 385 degrees F.
Transfer fries into the cooking basket, lightly greased, and cover with parchment.
Bake for about 15 minutes, flip and bake for 10 minutes more until golden brown.
Serve and enjoy!

Nutrition:

Calories: 271 kcal
Carbohydrates: 28 g - Fat: 15 g
Protein: 9 g

16. Zucchini Chips

Preparation Time: 10 minutes

Cooking Time: 12-15 minutes

Servings: 4

Ingredients:

Salt to taste
Grapeseed oil as needed
6 zucchinis

Directions:

Preheat the Air Fryer to 330 F.
Wash zucchini, slice zucchini into thin strips.
Put slices in a bowl and add oil, salt, and toss.
Spread over the cooking basket, fry for 12-15 minutes.
Serve and enjoy!

Nutrition:

Calories: 92 - Carbohydrates: 6 g
Fat: 7 g - Protein: 2 g

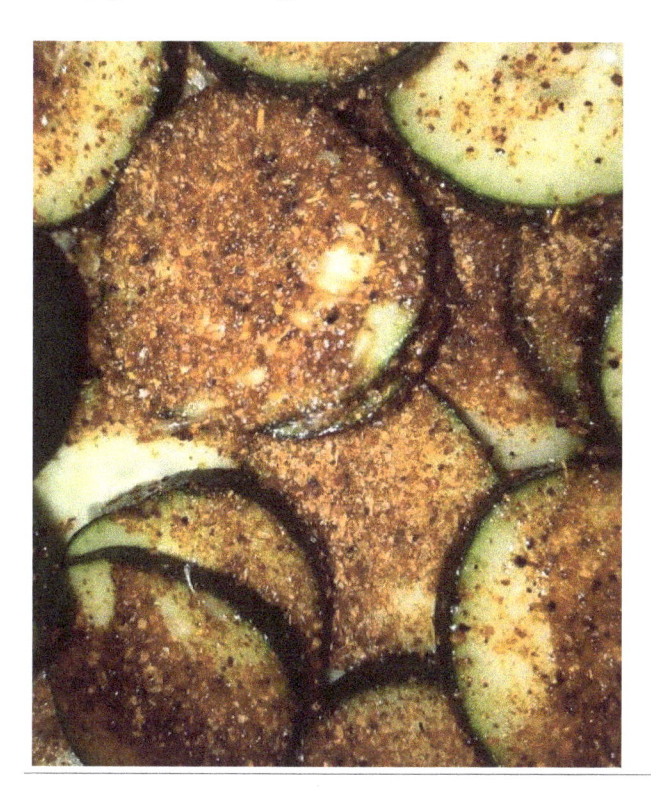

17. Classic Blueberry Spelt Muffins

Preparation Time: 10 minutes

Cooking Time: 12-15 minutes

Servings: 4

Ingredients:

1/4 sea salt
1/3 cup of maple syrup
1 teaspoon baking powder
1/2 cup of sea moss
3/4 cup of spelt flour
3/4 cup of Kamut flour
1 cup of hemp milk
1 cup of blueberries

Directions:

Preheat Air Fryer to 380 degrees F.
Take your muffin tins and gently grease them.
Take a bowl and add flour, syrup, salt, baking powder, seamless, and mix well.
Add milk and mix well.
Fold in blueberries.
Pour into muffin tins.
Transfer to the cooking basket, bake for 20-25 minutes until nicely baked.
Serve and enjoy!

Nutrition:

Calories: 217 kcal,
Carbohydrates: 32 g
Fat: 9 g
Protein: 4 g

18. Genuine Healthy Crackers

Preparation Time: 10 minutes

Cooking Time: 12-15 minutes

Servings: 4

Ingredients:

1/2 cup of Rye flour
1 cup of spelt flour
2 teaspoons sesame seed
1 teaspoon agave syrup
1 teaspoon salt
2 tablespoons grapeseed oil
3/4 cup of spring water

Directions:

Preheat the Air Fryer to 330 degrees F.
Take a medium bowl and add all ingredients, mix well.
Make dough ball.
Prepare a place for rolling out the dough, cover with a piece of parchment.
Lightly grease the paper with grape seed oil, place dough.
Roll out, dough with a rolling pin, add more flour if needed.
Take a shape cutter and cut dough into squares.
Place squares in the Air Fryer cooking basket.
Brush with more oil.
Sprinkle salt.
Bake for 10-15 minutes until golden.
Let it cool, serve, and enjoy!

Nutrition:

Calories: 226 kcal
Carbohydrates: 41 g
Fat: 3 g
Protein: 11 g

19. Dr. Sebi's Tortilla Chips

Preparation Time: 10 minutes

Cooking Time: 8-12 minutes

Servings: 4

Ingredients:

2 cups of spelt flour
1 teaspoon of salt
1/2 cup of spring water
1/3 cup of grapeseed oil

Directions:

Preheat your Air Fryer into 320 degrees F.
Take the food processor then add salt, flour, and process well for 15 seconds.
Gradually add grapeseed oil until mixed.
Keep mixing until you have a nice dough.
Formulate work surface and cover in a piece of parchment, sprinkle flour.
Knead the dough for 1-2 minutes.
Grease cooking basket with oil.
Transfer dough on the cooking basket, brush oil and sprinkle salt.
Cut dough into 8 triangles.
Bake for about 8-12 minutes until golden brown.
Serve and enjoy once done!

Nutrition:

Calories: 288 - Carbohydrates: 18 g
Fat: 17 g - Protein: 16 g

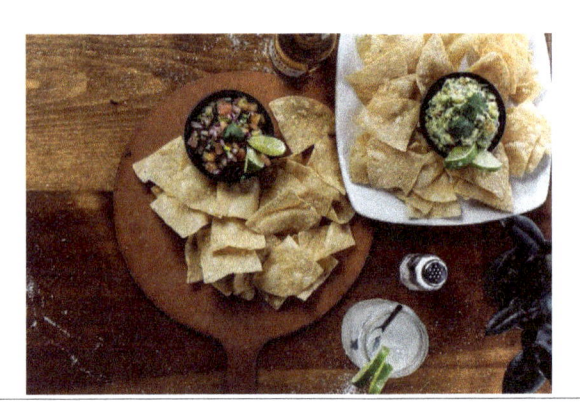

20. Pumpkin Spice Crackers

Preparation Time: 10 minutes

Cooking Time: 60 minutes

Servings: 06

Ingredients:

⅓ cup of coconut flour
2 tablespoons pumpkin pie spice
¾ cup of sunflower seeds
¾ cup of flaxseed
⅓ cup of sesame seeds
1 tablespoon ground psyllium husk powder
1 teaspoon of sea salt
3 tablespoons coconut oil, melted
1⅓ cups of alkaline water

Directions:

Set your oven to 300 degrees F.
Combine all dry ingredients in a bowl.
Add water and oil to the mixture and mix well.
Let the dough stay for 2 to 3 minutes.
Spread the dough evenly on a cookie sheet lined with parchment paper.
Bake for 30 minutes.
Reduce the oven heat to low and bake for another 30 minutes.
Crack the bread into bite-size pieces.
Serve

Nutrition:

Calories 248
Total Fat 15.7 g
Saturated Fat 2.7 g
Cholesterol 75 mg
Sodium 94 mg
Total Carbs 0.4 g
Fiber 0g
Sugar 0 g
Protein 24.9 g

21. Spicy Roasted Nuts

Preparation Time: 10 minutes

Cooking Time: 15 minutes

Servings: 4

Ingredients:

8 oz. pecans or almonds or walnuts
1 teaspoon of sea salt
1 tablespoon of olive oil or coconut oil
1 teaspoon of ground cumin
1 teaspoon of paprika powder or chili powder

Directions:

Add all the ingredients to a skillet.
Roast the nuts until golden brown.
Serve and enjoy.

Nutrition:

Calories 287
Total Fat 29.5 g
Saturated Fat 3 g
Cholesterol 0 mg
Total Carbs 5.9 g
Sugar 1.4g
Fiber 4.3 g
Sodium 388 mg
Protein 4.2 g

22. Wheat Crackers

Preparation Time: 10 minutes

Cooking Time: 20 minutes

Servings: 4

Ingredients:

1 3/4 cups almond flour
1 1/2 cups coconut flour
3/4 teaspoon of sea salt
1/3 cup of vegetable oil
1 cup of alkaline water
Sea salt for sprinkling

Directions:

Set your oven to 350 degrees F.
Mix coconut flour, almond flour, and salt in a bowl.
Stir in vegetable oil and water. Mix well until smooth.
Spread this dough on a floured surface into a thin sheet.
Cut small squares out of this sheet.
Arrange the dough squares on a baking sheet lined with parchment paper.
For about 20 minutes, bake until it turns light golden.
Serve.

Nutrition:

Calories 64
Total Fat 9.2 g
Saturated Fat 2.4 g
Cholesterol 110 mg
Sodium 276 mg
Total Carbs 9.2 g
Fiber 0.9 g
Sugar 1.4 g
Protein 1.5 g

23. Potato Chips

Preparation Time: 10 minutes

Cooking Time: 20 minutes

Servings: 4

Ingredients:

1 tablespoon vegetable oil
1 potato, sliced paper-thin
Sea salt, to taste

Directions:

Toss potato with oil and sea salt.
Spread the slices in a baking dish in a single layer.
Cook in a microwave for 5 minutes until golden brown.
Serve.

Nutrition:

Calories 80
Total Fat 3.5 g
Saturated Fat 0.1 g
Cholesterol 320 mg
Sodium 350 mg
Total Carbs 11.6 g
Fiber 0.7 g
Sugar 0.7 g
Protein 1.2 g

24. Zucchini Pepper Chips

Preparation Time: 10 minutes

Cooking Time: 15 minutes

Servings: 04

Ingredients:

1 2/3 cups vegetable oil
1 teaspoon garlic powder
1 teaspoon onion powder
1/2 teaspoon black pepper
3 tablespoons crushed red pepper flakes
2 zucchinis, thinly sliced

Directions:

Mix oil with all the spices in a bowl.
Add zucchini slices and mix well.
Transfer the mixture to a Ziplock bag and seal it.
Refrigerate for 10 minutes.
Spread the zucchini slices on a greased baking sheet.
Bake for 15 minutes
Serve.

Nutrition:

Calories 172
Total Fat 11.1 g
Saturated Fat 5.8 g
Cholesterol 610 mg
Sodium 749 mg
Total Carbs 19.9 g
Fiber 0.2 g
Sugar 0.2 g
Protein 13.5 g

25. Apple Chips

Preparation Time: 5 minutes

Cooking Time: 45 minutes

Servings: 4

Ingredients:

2 Golden Delicious apples, cored and thinly sliced
1 1/2 teaspoons white sugar
1/2 teaspoon ground cinnamon

Directions:

Set your oven to 225 degrees F.
Place apple slices on a baking sheet.
Sprinkle sugar and cinnamon over apple slices.
Bake for 45 minutes.
Serve

Nutrition:

Calories 127
Total Fat 3.5 g
Saturated Fat 0.5 g
Cholesterol 162 mg
Sodium 142 mg
Total Carbs 33.6g
Fiber 0.4 g
Sugar 0.5 g
Protein 4.5 g

26. Kale Crisps

Preparation Time: 10 minutes

Cooking Time: 10 minutes

Servings: 04

Ingredients:

1 bunch kale, remove the stems, leaves torn into even pieces
1 tablespoon of olive oil
1 teaspoon of sea salt

Directions:

Set your oven to 350 degrees F. Layer a baking sheet with parchment paper.
Spread the kale leaves on a paper towel to absorb all the moisture.
Toss the leaves with sea salt and olive oil.
Kindly spread them on the baking sheet and bake for 10 minutes.
Serve.

Nutrition:

Calories 113 - Total Fat 7.5 g
Saturated Fat 1.1 g - Cholesterol 20 mg
Sodium 97 mg - Total Carbs 1.4 g
Fiber 0 g - Sugar 0 g - Protein 1.1g

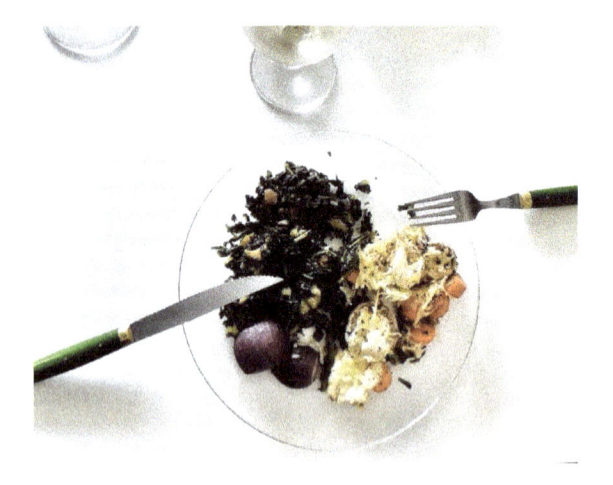

27. Carrot Chips

Preparation Time: 5 minutes

Cooking Time: 12 minutes

Servings: 4

Ingredients:

4 carrots, washed, peeled and sliced
2 teaspoons of extra-virgin olive oil
1/4 teaspoon of sea salt

Directions:

Set your oven to 350 degrees F.
Toss carrots with salt and olive oil.
Spread the slices into two baking sheets in a single layer.
Bake for 6 minutes on the upper and lower rack of the oven.
Switch the baking racks and bake for another 6 minutes.
Serve.

Nutrition:

Calories 153
Total Fat 7.5 g
Saturated Fat 1.1 g
Cholesterol 20 mg
Sodium 97 mg
Total Carbs 20.4 g
Fiber 0 g
Sugar 0 g
Protein 3.1g

28. Pita Chips

Preparation Time: 5 minutes

Cooking Time: 12 minutes

Servings: 4

Ingredients:

12 pita bread pockets, sliced into triangles
1/2 cup olive oil
1/2 teaspoon ground black pepper
1 teaspoon of garlic salt
1/2 teaspoon dried basil
1 teaspoon dried chervil

Directions:

Set your oven to 400 degrees F.
Toss pita with all the remaining ingredients in a bowl.
Spread the seasoned triangles on a baking sheet.
Bake for 7 minutes until golden brown.
Serve with your favourite hummus.

Nutrition:

Calories 201
Total Fat 5.5 g
Saturated Fat 2.1 g
Cholesterol 10 mg
Sodium 597 mg
Total Carbs 2.4 g
Fiber 0 g
Sugar 0 g
Protein 3.1g

29. Sweet Potato Chips

Preparation Time: 5 minutes

Cooking Time: 5 minutes

Servings: 4

Ingredients:

1 sweet potato, thinly sliced
2 teaspoons olive oil, or as needed
Coarse sea salt, to taste

Directions:

Toss sweet potato with oil and salt.
Spread the slices in a baking dish in a single layer.
Cook in a microwave for 5 minutes until golden brown.
Serve.

Nutrition:

Calories 213
Total Fat 8.5 g
Saturated Fat 3.1 g
Cholesterol 120 mg
Sodium 497 mg
Total Carbs 21.4 g
Fiber 0 g
Sugar 0 g
Protein 0.1g

Desserts

1. Chocolate Crunch Bars

Preparation Time: 5 minutes

Cooking Time: 5 minutes

Servings: 4

Ingredients:

1 1/2 cups sugar-free chocolate chips
1 cup almond butter
Stevia to taste
1/4 cup coconut oil
3 cups pecans, chopped

Directions:

Layer an 8-inch baking pan with parchment paper.
Mix chocolate chips with butter, coconut oil, and sweetener in a bowl.
Melt it by heating in a microwave for 2 to 3 minutes until well mixed.
Stir in nuts and seeds. Mix gently.
Pour this batter carefully into the baking pan and spread evenly.
Refrigerate for 2 to 3 hours.
Slice and serve.

Nutrition:

Calories 316
Total Fat 30.9 g
Saturated Fat 8.1 g
Cholesterol 0 mg
Total Carbs 8.3 g
Sugar 1.8 g
Fiber 3.8 g
Sodium 8 mg
Protein 6.4 g

2. Homemade Protein Bar

Preparation Time: 5 minutes

Cooking Time: 10 minutes

Servings: 4

Ingredients:

1 cup nut butter
4 tablespoons coconut oil
2 scoops vanilla protein
Stevia, to taste
½ teaspoon of sea salt

Optional Ingredients:

1 teaspoon cinnamon

Directions:

Mix coconut oil with butter, protein, stevia, and salt in a dish.
Stir in cinnamon and chocolate chip.
Press the mixture firmly and freeze until firm.
Cut the crust into small bars.
Serve and enjoy.

Nutrition:

Calories 179
Total Fat 15.7 g
Saturated Fat 8 g
Cholesterol 0 mg
Total Carbs 4.8 g
Sugar 3.6 g
Fiber 0.8 g
Sodium 43 mg
Protein 5.6 g

3. Shortbread Cookies

Preparation Time: 10 minutes

Cooking Time: 70 minutes

Servings: 6

Ingredients:

2 1/2 cups almond flour
6 tablespoons nut butter
1/2 cup erythritol
1 teaspoon vanilla essence

Directions:

Preheat your oven to 350 degrees F.
Layer a cookie sheet with parchment paper.
Beat butter with erythritol until fluffy.
Stir in vanilla essence and almond flour. Mix well until becomes crumbly.
Spoon out a tablespoon of cookie dough onto the cookie sheet.
Add more dough to make as many cookies.
Bake for 15 minutes until brown.
Serve.

Nutrition:

Calories 288
Total Fat 25.3 g
Saturated Fat 6.7 g
Cholesterol 23 mg
Total Carbs 9.6 g
Sugar 0.1 g
Fiber 3.8 g
Sodium 74 mg
Potassium 3 mg
Protein 7.6 g

4. Coconut Chip Cookies

Preparation Time: 10 minutes

Cooking Time: 15 minutes

Servings: 4

Ingredients:

1 cup almond flour
½ cup cacao nibs
½ cup coconut flakes, unsweetened
1/3 cup erythritol
½ cup almond butter
¼ cup nut butter, melted
¼ cup almond milk
Stevia, to taste
¼ teaspoon of sea salt

Directions:

Preheat your oven to 350 degrees F.
Layer a cookie sheet with parchment paper.
Add and then combine all the dry ingredients in a glass bowl.
Whisk in butter, almond milk, vanilla essence, stevia, and almond butter.
Beat well, then stir in the dry mixture. Mix well.
Spoon out a tablespoon of cookie dough on the cookie sheet.
Add more dough to make as many as 16 cookies.
Flatten each cookie using your fingers.
Bake for 25 minutes until golden brown.
Let them sit for 15 minutes.
Serve.

Nutrition:

Calories 192 - Total Fat 17.44 g
Saturated Fat 11.5 g - Cholesterol 125 mg
Total Carbs 2.2 g
Sugar 1.4 g - Fiber 2.1 g - Sodium 135 mg
Protein 4.7 g

5. Peanut Butter Bars

Preparation Time: 10 minutes

Cooking time: 10 minutes

Servings: 6

Ingredients:

3/4 cup almond flour
2 oz. almond butter
1/4 cup Swerve
1/2 cup peanut butter
1/2 teaspoon vanilla

Directions:

Combine all the ingredients for bars.
Transfer this mixture to a 6-inch small pan.
Press it firmly.
Refrigerate for 30 minutes.
Slice and serve.

Nutrition:

Calories 214
Total Fat 19 g
Saturated Fat 5.8 g
Cholesterol 15 mg
Total Carbs 6.5 g
Sugar 1.9 g
Fiber 2.1 g
Sodium 123 mg
Protein 6.5 g

6. Zucchini Bread Pancakes

Preparation Time: 15 minutes

Cooking Time: 35 minutes

Servings: 3

Ingredients:

Grape seed oil, 1 tbsp.
Chopped walnuts, .5 c
Walnut milk, 2 c
Shredded zucchini, 1 c
Mashed burro banana, .25 c
Date sugar, 2 tbsp.
Kamut flour or spelt, 2 c

Directions:

Place the date sugar and flour into a bowl. Whisk together.
Add in the mashed banana and walnut milk. Stir until combined. Remember to scrape the bowl to get all the dry mixture. Add in walnuts and zucchini. Stir well until combined.
Place the grape seed oil onto a griddle and warm.
Pour .25 cup batter on the hot griddle. Leave it along until bubbles begin forming on to surface. Carefully turn over the pancake and cook another four minutes until cooked through.
Place the pancakes onto a serving plate and enjoy with some agave syrup.

Nutrition:

Calories: 246
Carbohydrates: 49.2 g
Fiber: 4.6 g
Protein: 7.8 g

7. Berry Sorbet

Preparation Time: 10 minutes

Cooking Time: 20 minutes

Servings: 6

Ingredients:

Water, 2 c
Blend strawberries, 2 c
Spelt flour, 1.5 tsp.
Date sugar, .5 c

Directions:

Add the water into a large pot and let the water begin to warm. Add the flour and date sugar and stir until dissolved. Allow this mixture to start boiling and continue to cook for around ten minutes. It should have started to thicken. Take off the heat and set to the side to cool.

Once the syrup has cooled off, add in the strawberries, and stir well to combine.

Pour into a container that is freezer safe and put it into the freezer until frozen.

Take sorbet out of the freezer, cut into chunks, and put it either into a blender or a food processor. Hit the pulse button until the mixture is creamy.

Pour this into the same freezer-safe container and put it back into the freezer for four hours.

Nutrition:

Calories: 99
Carbohydrates: 8 g

8. Quinoa Porridge

Preparation Time: 5 minutes

Cooking Time: 15 minutes

Servings: 04

Ingredients:

Zest of one lime
Coconut milk, .5 c
Cloves, .5 tsp.
Ground ginger, 1.5 tsp.
Spring water, 2 c
Quinoa, 1 c
Grated apple, 1

Directions:

Cook the quinoa. Follow the instructions on the package. When the quinoa has been cooked, drain well. Place it back into the pot and stir in spices.

Add coconut milk and stir well to combine. Grate the apple now and stir well.

Divide equally into bowls and add the lime zest on top. Sprinkle with nuts and seeds of choice.

Nutrition:

Calories: 180
Fat: 3 g
Carbohydrates: 40 g
Protein: 10 g

9. Apple Quinoa

Preparation Time: 15 minutes

Cooking Time: 30 minutes

Servings: 04

Ingredients:

Coconut oil, 1 tbsp.
Ginger
Key lime .5
Apple, 1
Quinoa, .5 c
Optional toppings:
Seeds
Nuts
Berries

Directions:

Fix the quinoa according to the instructions on the package. When you are getting close to the end of the cooking time, grate in the apple and cook for 30 seconds.
Zest the lime into the quinoa and squeeze the juice in. Stir in the coconut oil.
Divide evenly into bowls and sprinkle with some ginger.
You can add in some berries, nuts, and seeds right before you eat.

Nutrition:

Calories: 146
Fiber: 2.3 g
Fat: 8.3 g

10. Kamut Porridge

Preparation Time: 10 minutes

Cooking Time: 25 minutes

Servings: 04

Ingredients:

Agave syrup, 4 tbsp.
Coconut oil, 1 tbsp.
Sea salt, .5 tsp.
Coconut milk, 3.75 c
Kamut berries, 1 c
Optional toppings
Berries
Coconut chips
Ground nutmeg
Ground cloves

Directions:

You need to "crack" the Kamut berries. You can try this by placing the berries into a food processor and pulsing until you have 1.25 cups of Kamut.
Place the cracked Kamut in a pot with salt and coconut milk. Give it a good stir in order to combine everything. Allow this mixture to come to a full rolling boil and then turn the heat down until the mixture is simmering. Stir every now and then until the Kamut has thickened to your likeness. This normally takes about ten minutes.
Take off heat, stir in agave syrup and coconut oil.
Garnish with toppings of choice and enjoy.

Nutrition:

Calories: 114
Protein: 5 g
Carbohydrates: 24g
Fiber: 4 g

11. Hot Kamut with Peaches, Walnuts, and Coconut

Preparation Time: 10 minutes

Cooking Time: 35 minutes

Servings: 04

Ingredients:

Toasted coconut, 4 tbsp.
Toasted and chopped walnuts, .5 c
Chopped dried peaches, 8
Coconut milk, 3 c
Kamut cereal, 1 c

Directions:

Mix the coconut milk into a saucepan and allow it to warm up. When it begins simmering, add in the Kamut. Let this cook about 15 minutes, while stirring every now and then.
When done, divide evenly into bowls and top with the toasted coconut, walnuts, and peaches.
You could even go one more and add some fresh berries.

Nutrition:

Calories: 156
Protein: 5.8 g
Carbohydrates: 25 g
Fiber: 6 g

12. Overnight "Oats"

Preparation Time: 5 minutes

Cooking Time: 0 minutes

Servings: 04

Ingredients:

Berry of choice, .5 c
Walnut butter, .5 tbsp.
Burro banana, .5
Ginger, .5 tsp.
Coconut milk, .5 c
Hemp seeds, .5 c

Directions:

Put the hemp seeds, salt, and coconut milk into a glass jar. Mix well.
Place the lid on the jar then put it in the refrigerator to sit overnight.
The next morning, add the ginger, berries, and banana. Stir well and enjoy it.

Nutrition:

Calories: 139
Fat: 4.1 g
Protein: 9 g
Sugar: 7 g

13. Blueberry Cupcakes

Preparation Time: 15 minutes
Cooking Time: 40 minutes
Servings: 04
Ingredients:

Grape seed oil
Sea salt, .5 tsp.
Sea moss gel, .25 c
Agave, .3 c
Blueberries, .5 c
Teff flour, .75 c
Spelt flour, .75 c
Coconut milk, 1 c

Directions:

Warm your oven to 365. Place paper liners into a muffin tin.
Place sea moss gel, sea salt, agave, flour, and milk in a large bowl. Mix well to combine.
Gently fold in blueberries.
Gently pour batter into paper liners. Place in oven and bake 30 minutes.
They are done if they have turned a nice golden colour, and they spring back when you touch them.

Nutrition:

Calories: 85
Fat: 0.7 g
Carbohydrates: 12 g
Protein: 1.4 g
Fiber: 5 g

14. Brazil Nut Cheese

Preparation Time: 2 hours
Cooking Time: 0 minutes
Servings: 04
Ingredients:

Grape seed oil, 2 tsp.
Water, 1.5 c
Hemp milk, 1.5 c
Cayenne, .5 tsp.
Onion powder, 1 tsp.
Juice of .5 lime
Sea salt, 2 tsp.
Brazil nuts, 1 lb.
Onion powder, 1 tsp.

Directions:

You will need to start the process by soaking the Brazil nuts in some water. You just put the nuts into a bowl and make sure the water covers them. Soak no less than two hours or overnight. Overnight would be best.
Now you need to put everything except water into a food processor or blender.
Add just 5 cups water and blend for two minutes.
Continue adding the 5 cups of water and blending until you have the consistency you want.
Scrape into an airtight container and enjoy.

Nutrition:

Calories: 187.
Protein: 4.1 g
Fat: 19 g
Carbs: 3.3 g
Fiber: 2.1 g

15. Baked Stuffed Pears

Preparation Time: 15 minutes

Cooking Time: 35 minutes

Servings: 04

Ingredients:

Agave syrup, 4 tbsp.
Cloves, .25 tsp.
Chopped walnuts, 4 tbsp.
Currants, 1 c
Pears, 4

Directions:

Make sure your oven has been warmed to 375.

Slice the pears in two lengthwise and remove the core. To get the pear to lay flat, you can slice a small piece off the backside.

Place the agave syrup, currants, walnuts, and cloves in a small bowl and mix well. Set this to the side to be used later.

Put the pears on a cookie sheet that has parchment paper on it. Make sure the cored sides are facing up. Sprinkle each pear half with about .5 tablespoon of the chopped walnut mixture.

Place into the oven and cook for 25 to 30 minutes. Pears should be tender.

Nutrition:

Calories: 103.9
Fiber: 3.1 g
Carbohydrates: 22 g

16. Butternut Squash Pie

Preparation Time: 25 minutes

Cooking Time: 35 minutes

Servings: 04

Ingredients:

For the crust:

Cold water
Agave, splash
Sea salt, a pinch
Grape seed oil, .5 c
Coconut flour, .5 c
Spelt Flour, 1 c

For the filling:

Butternut squash, peeled, chopped
Water
Allspice, to taste
Agave syrup, to taste
Hemp milk, 1 c
Sea moss, 4 tbsp.

Directions:

You will need to warm your oven to 350.
For the crust:
Place the grape seed oil and water into the refrigerator to get it cold. This will take about one hour.

Place all ingredients into a large bowl. Now you need to add in the cold water a little bit in small amounts until a dough forms. Place this onto a surface that has been sprinkled with some coconut flour. Knead for a few minutes and roll the dough as thin as you can get it. Carefully, pick it up and place it inside a pie plate.

Place the butternut squash into a Dutch oven and pour in enough water to cover. Bring this to a full rolling boil. Let this cook until the squash has become soft.

Completely drain and place into a bowl.

Using a potato masher, mash the squash. Add in some allspice and agave to taste. Add in the sea moss and hemp milk. Using a hand mixer, blend well. Pour into the pie crust. Place into an oven and bake for about one hour.

Nutrition:

Calories: 245
Carbohydrates: 50 g
Fat: 10 g

17. Cheesecake

Ingredients:

Sea salt, .25 tsp.
Sea moss gel, 1 tbsp.
Lime juice, 2 tbsp.
Dates, 5 to 6
Agave, .25 c
Hemp or walnut milk, 1.5 c
Brazil nuts, 2 c

Crust:

Sea salt, .25 tsp.
Agave, .25 c
Coconut flakes, 1.5 c
Dates, 1.5 c

Topping:

Blackberries
Blueberries
Sliced raspberries
Sliced strawberry
Sliced mango

Directions:

Mix all of the crust ingredients into your food processor and blend it for about 20 seconds. Spread your crust out into a Springform pan that has been covered with parchment. Place the mango slices along the side of the pan and then place it in the freezer as you prepare everything else.

Add everything for the cheesecake to your blender and mix it until it creates a smooth mixture.

Get rid of the Springform pan from the freezer and pour the filling in. Wrap in foil and let it sit for three to four hours. Carefully remove from the pan, and then place the rest of the toppings over the top. All of the leftovers should be kept in the freezer.

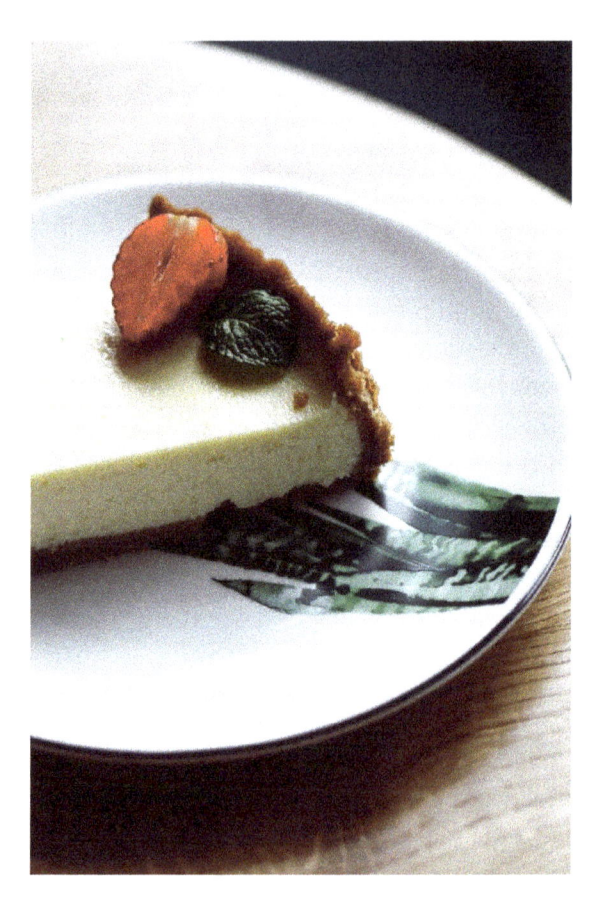

18. Coconut Chia Cream Pot

Preparation Time: 5 minutes

Cooking Time: 5 minutes

Servings: 04

Ingredients:

Date, one (1)
Coconut milk (organic), one (1) cup
Coconut yogurt, one (1) cup
Vanilla extract, ½ teaspoon
Chia seeds, ¼ cup
Sesame seeds, one (1) teaspoon
Flaxseed (ground), one (1) tablespoon or flax meal, one (1) tablespoon

Toppings:

Fig, one (1)
Blueberries, one (1) handful
Mixed nuts (brazil nuts, almonds, pistachios, macadamia, etc.)
Cinnamon (ground), one teaspoon

Directions:

First, blend the date with coconut milk (the idea is to sweeten the coconut milk).
Get a mixing bowl and add the coconut milk with the vanilla, sesame seeds, chia seeds, and flax meal.
Refrigerate for between twenty to thirty minutes or wait till the chia expands.
To serve, pour a layer of coconut yogurt in a small glass, then add the chia mix, followed by pouring another layer of the coconut yogurt.
It's alkaline, creamy, and delicious.

Nutrition:

Calories: 310
Carbohydrates: 39 g
Protein: 4 g
Fiber: 8.1 g

19. Chocolate Avocado Mousse

Preparation Time: 10 minutes

Cooking Time: 5 minutes

Servings: 04

Ingredients:

Coconut water, 2/3 cup
Hass avocado, ½
Raw cacao, 2 teaspoons
Vanilla, 1 teaspoon
Dates, three (3)
Sea salt, one (1) teaspoon
Dark chocolate shavings

Directions:

Blend all ingredients.
Blast until it becomes thick and smooth, as you wish.
Put in a fridge and allow it to get firm.

Nutrition:

Calories: 181.8
Fat: 151. g
Protein: 12 g

20. Chia Vanilla Coconut Pudding

Preparation Time: 5 minutes

Cooking Time: 5 minutes

Servings: 2

Ingredients:

Coconut oil, 2 tablespoons
Raw cashew, ½ cup
Coconut water, ½ cup
Cinnamon, 1 teaspoon
Dates (pitted), 3
Vanilla, 2 teaspoons
Coconut flakes (unsweetened), 1 teaspoon
Salt (Himalayan or Celtic Grey)
Chia seeds, 6 tablespoons
Cinnamon or pomegranate seeds for garnish (optional)

Directions:

Get a blender, add all the ingredients (minus the pomegranate and chia seeds), and blend for about forty to sixty seconds.
Reduce the blender speed to the lowest and add the chia seeds.
Pour the content into an airtight container and put it in a refrigerator for five to six hours.
To serve, you can garnish with the cinnamon powder of pomegranate seeds.

Nutrition:

Calories: 201
Fat: 10 g
Sodium: 32.8 mg

21. Sweet Tahini Dip with Ginger Cinnamon Fruit

Preparation Time: 10 minutes

Cooking Time: 5 minutes

Servings: 2

Ingredients:

Cinnamon, one (1) teaspoon
Green apple, one (1)
Pear, one (1)
Fresh ginger, two (2) or three (3)
Celtic sea salt, one (1) teaspoon

Ingredients for sweet Tahini:

Almond butter (raw), three (3) teaspoons
Tahini (one big scoop), three (3) teaspoons
Coconut oil, two (2) teaspoons
Cayenne (optional), ¼ teaspoons
Wheat-free tamari, two (2) teaspoons
Liquid coconut nectar, one (1) teaspoon

Directions:

Get a clean mixing bowl.
Grate the ginger, add cinnamon, sea salt, and mix in the bowl.
Dice apple and pear into little cubes, turn into the bowl, and mix.
Get a mixing bowl and mix all the ingredients.
Then, add the sprinkle, the sweet Tahini, and dip all over the ginger cinnamon fruit.
Serve.

Nutrition:

Calories: 109
Fat: 10.8 g
Sodium: 258 mg

22. Coconut Butter and Chopped Berries with Mint

Preparation Time: 5 minutes

Cooking Time: 5 minutes

Servings: 04

Ingredients:

Chopped mint, one (1) tablespoon
Coconut butter (melted), two (2) tablespoons
Mixed berries (strawberries, blueberries, and raspberries)

Directions:

Get a small bowl and add the berries.
Drizzle the melted coconut butter and sprinkle the mint.
Serve.

Nutrition:

Calories: 159
Fat: 12 g
Carbohydrates: 18 g

23. Alkaline Raw Pumpkin Pie

Preparation Time: 5 minutes

Cooking Time: 5 minutes

Servings: 04

Ingredients:

Ingredients for pie crust:

Cinnamon, one (1) teaspoon
Dates/Turkish apricots, one (1) cup
Raw almonds, one (1) cup
Coconut flakes (unsweetened), one (1) cup

Ingredients for pie filling:

Dates, six (6)
Cinnamon, ½ teaspoon
Nutmeg, ½ teaspoon
Pecans (soaked overnight), one (1) cup
Organic pumpkin Blends (12 oz.), 1 ¼ cup
Nutmeg, ½ teaspoon
Sea salt (Himalayan or Celtic Sea Salt), ¼ teaspoon
Vanilla, 1 teaspoon
Gluten-free tamari

Directions:

Directions for pie crust:

Get a food processor and blend all the pie crust ingredients at the same time.
Make sure the mixture turns oily and sticky before you stop mixing.
Put the mixture in a pie pan and mold against the sides and floor, to make it stick properly.

Directions for the pie filling:

Mix ingredients together in a blender.
Add the mixture to fill in the pie crust.
Pour some cinnamon on top.
Refrigerate until it's cold and then mold.

Nutrition:

Calories 135
Calories from Fat 41.4.
Total Fat 4.6 g
Cholesterol 11.3 mg

24. Strawberry Sorbet

Preparation Time: 5 minutes

Cooking Time: 4 hours

Servings: 4

Ingredients:

2 cups of strawberries*
1 1/2 teaspoons of spelt flour
1/2 cup of date sugar
2 cups of spring water

Directions:

Add date sugar, spring water, and spelt flour to a medium pot and boil on low heat for about ten minutes. The mixture should thicken, like syrup.
Remove the pot from the heat and allow it to cool.
After cooling, add Blend Strawberry and mix gently.
Put the mixture in a container and freeze.
Cut it into pieces, put the sorbet into a processor, and blend until smooth.
Put everything back in the container and leave in the refrigerator for at least four hours.
Serve and enjoy your Strawberry Sorbet!

Nutrition:

Calories: 198
Carbohydrates: 28 g

25. Blueberry Muffins

Preparation Time: 5 minutes

Cooking Time: 1 Hour

Servings: 3

Ingredients:

1/2 cup of blueberries
3/4 cup of teff flour
3/4 cup of spelt flour
1/3 cup of agave syrup
1/2 teaspoon of pure sea salt
1 cup of coconut milk
1/4 cup of sea moss gel (optional, check information)
Grape Seed Oil

Directions:

Preheat your oven to 365 degrees Fahrenheit.
Grease or line 6 standard muffin cups.
Add Teff, Spelt flour, Pure Sea Salt, Coconut Milk, Sea Moss Gel, and Agave Syrup to a large bowl. Mix them together.
Add Blueberries to the mixture and mix well.
Divide muffin batter among the 6 muffin cups.
Bake for 30 minutes until golden brown.
Serve and enjoy your Blueberry Muffins!

Nutrition:

Calories: 65
Fat: 0.7 g
Carbohydrates: 12 g
Protein: 1.4 g
Fiber: 5 g

26. Banana Strawberry Ice Cream

Preparation Time: 5 minutes

Cooking Time: 4 hours

Servings: 5

Ingredients:

1 cup of strawberry*
5 quartered baby bananas*
1/2 avocado, chopped
1 tablespoon of agave syrup
1/4 cup of homemade walnut milk

Directions:

Mix ingredients into the blender and blend them well.
Taste. If it is too thick, add extra milk or agave syrup if you want it sweeter.
Put in a container with a lid and allow to freeze for at least 5 to 6 hours.
Serve it and enjoy your banana strawberry ice cream!

Nutrition:

Calories: 200 - Fat: 0.5 g
Carbohydrates: 44 g

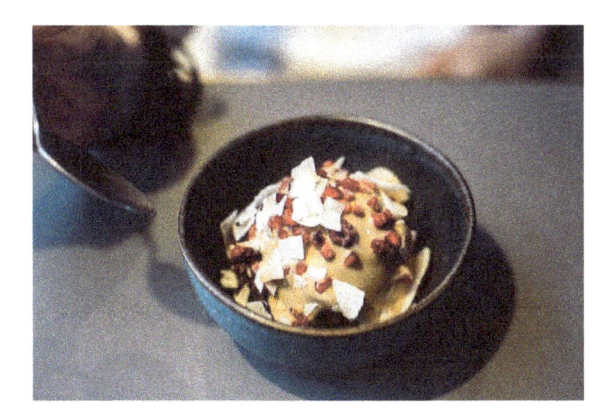

27. Homemade Whipped Cream

Preparation Time: 5 minutes

Cooking Time: 10 minutes

Servings: 1 Cup

Ingredients:

1 cup of Aquafaba
1/4 cup of agave syrup

Directions:

Add agave syrup and Aquafaba into a bowl. Mix at high speed around 5 minutes with a stand mixer or 10 to 15 minutes with a hand mixer.
Serve and enjoy your homemade whipped cream!

Nutrition:

Calories: 21
Fat: 0g
Sodium: 0.3g
Carbohydrates: 5.3g
Fiber: 0g
Sugars: 4.7g
Protein: 0g

28. "Chocolate" Pudding

Preparation Time: 5 minutes

Cooking Time: 20 minutes

Servings: 4

Ingredients:

1 to 2 cups of black sapote
1/4 cup of agave syrup
1/2 cup of soaked Brazil nuts (overnight or for at least 3 hours)
1 tablespoon of hemp seeds
1/2 cup of spring water

Directions:

Cut 1 to 2 cups of black sapote in half. Remove all seeds. You should have 1 full cup of de-seeded fruit.

Mix all ingredients into a blender and blend until smooth.

Serve and enjoy your "chocolate" pudding!

Nutrition:

Calories: 134
Fat: 0.5 g
Carbohydrates: 15 g
Protein: 2.5 g
Fiber: 10 g

29. Banana Nut Muffins

Preparation Time: 5 minutes

Cooking Time: 1 Hour

Servings: 6

Ingredients:

Dry ingredients:

1 1/2 cups of spelt or teff flour
1/2 teaspoon of pure sea salt
3/4 cup of date syrup

Wet ingredients:

2 medium blended burro bananas
¼ cup of grape seed oil
¾ cup of homemade walnut milk (see recipe)*
1 tablespoon of key lime juice

Filling ingredients:

½ cup of chopped walnuts (plus extra for decorating)
1 chopped burro banana

Directions:

Preheat your oven to 400 degrees Fahrenheit.

Take a muffin tray and grease 12 cups or line with cupcake liners.

Put all dry ingredients in a large bowl and mix them thoroughly.

Add all wet ingredients to a separate, smaller bowl and mix well with blended bananas.

Mix ingredients from the two bowls in one large container. Be careful not to over mix.

Add the filling ingredients and fold in gently.

Pour muffin batter into the 12 prepared muffin cups and garnish with a couple of Walnuts.

Bake it for 22 to 26 minutes until golden brown.

Allow cooling for 10 minutes.

Serve and enjoy your banana nut muffins!

Nutrition:

Calories: 150
Fat: 10 g
Carbohydrates: 30 g
Protein: 2.4 g
Fiber: 2 g

30. Mango Nut Cheesecake

Cooking Time: 4 Hour 30 Minutes

Servings: 8 Servings

Ingredients:

Filling:

2 cups of Brazil nuts
5 to 6 dates
1 tablespoon of sea moss gel (check information)
1/4 cup of agave syrup
1/4 teaspoon of pure sea salt
2 tablespoons of lime juice
1 1/2 cups of homemade walnut milk (see recipe)*

Crust:

1 1/2 cups of quartered dates
1/4 cup of agave syrup
1 1/2 cups of coconut flakes
1/4 teaspoon of pure sea salt

Toppings:

Sliced mango
Sliced strawberries

Directions:

Put all crust ingredients in a food processor and blend for 30 seconds.
With parchment paper, cover a baking form and spread out the blended crust ingredients.
Put sliced mango across the crust and freeze for 10 minutes.
Mix all filling ingredients using a blender until it becomes smooth.
Pour the filling above the crust, cover with foil or parchment paper, and let it stand for about 3 to 4 hours in the refrigerator.
Take out from the baking form and garnish with toppings.
Serve and enjoy your mango nut cheesecake!

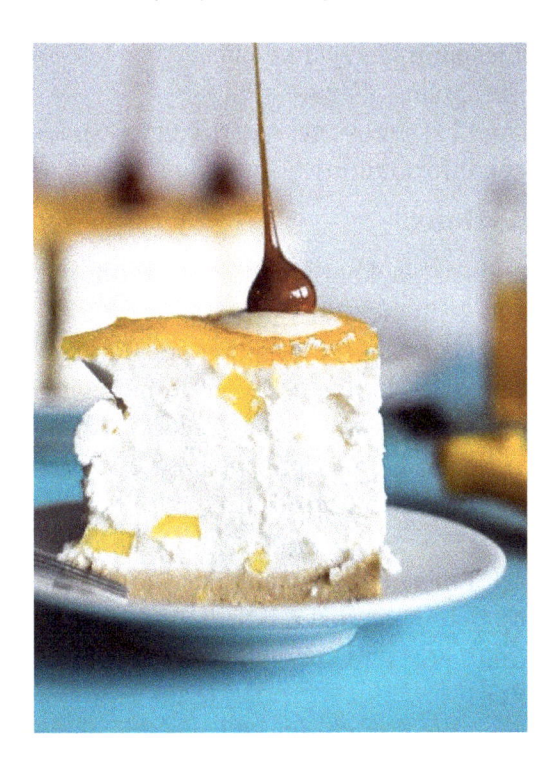

31. Blackberry Jam

Preparation Time: 5 minutes

Cooking Time: 4 hours 30 minutes

Servings: 1 cup

Ingredients:

3/4 cup of blackberries
1 tablespoon of key lime juice
3 tablespoons of agave syrup
¼ cup of sea moss gel + extra 2 tablespoons (check information)

Directions:

Put rinsed blackberries into a medium pot and cook on medium heat.
Stir blackberries until liquid appears.
Once berries soften, use your immersion blender to chop up any large pieces. If you don't have a blender put the mixture in a food processor, mix it well, then return to the pot.
Add sea moss gel, key lime juice, and agave syrup to the blended mixture. Boil on medium heat and stir well until it becomes thick.
Remove from the heat and leave it to cool for 10 minutes.
Serve it with bread pieces or the Flatbread (see recipe).
Enjoy your blackberry jam!

Nutrition:

Calories: 43
Fat: 0.5 g
Carbohydrates: 13 g

32. Blackberry Bars

Preparation Time: 5 minutes

Cooking Time: 1 hour 20 minutes

Servings: 4

Ingredients:

3 burro bananas or 4 baby bananas
1 cup of spelt flour
2 cups of quinoa flakes
1/4 cup of agave syrup
1/4 teaspoon of pure sea salt
1/2 cup of grape seed oil
1 cup of prepared blackberry jam

Directions:

Preheat your oven to 350 degrees Fahrenheit.
Remove the skin of the bananas and mash with a fork in a large bowl.
Combine agave syrup and grape seed oil with the blend and mix well.
Add spelt flour and quinoa flakes. Knead the dough until it becomes sticky to your fingers.
Cover a 9x9-inch baking pan with parchment paper.
Take 2/3 of the dough and smooth it out over the parchment pan with your fingers.
Spread blackberry jam over the dough.
Crumble the remaining dough and sprinkle on the top.
Bake for 20 minutes.
Remove from the oven and let it cool for at 10 to 15 minutes.
Cut into small pieces.
Serve and enjoy your blackberry bars!

Nutrition:

Calories: 43 - Fat: 0.5 g
Carbohydrates: 10 g
Protein: 1.4 g
Fiber: 5 g

Smoothies

1. Raisins – Plume Smoothie (RPS)

Preparation Time: 10 minutes

Cooking Time: 0 minutes

Servings: 1

Ingredients:

1 teaspoon raisins
2 sweet cherry
1 skinned black plume
1 cup Dr. Sebi's stomach calming herbal tea/cuachalalate back powder
¼ coconut water

Directions:

Flash 1 teaspoon of raisins in warm water for 5 seconds and drain the water completely.
Rinse, cube sweet cherry and skinned black plum
Get 1 cup of water boiled; put ¾ Dr. Sebi's stomach calming herbal tea for 10 – 15minutes.
If you are unable to get Dr. Sebi's stomach calming herbal tea, you can alternatively cook 1 teaspoon of powdered cuachalalate with 1 cup of water for 5 – 10 minutes, remove the extract and allow it to cool.
Pour all the ARPS items inside a blender and blend till you achieve a homogenous smoothie.
It is now okay for you to enjoy the inevitable detox smoothie.

Nutrition:

Calories: 150
Fat: 1.2 g
Carbohydrates: 79 g
Protein: 3.1 g

2. Nori Clove Smoothies (NCS)

Preparation Time: 10 minutes

Cooking Time: 0 minutes

Servings: 1

Ingredients:

¼ cup fresh nori
1 cup cubed banana
1 teaspoon diced onion or ¼ teaspoon powdered onion
½ teaspoon clove
1 cup Dr. Sebi's energy booster
1 tablespoon agave syrup

Directions:

Rinse ANCS Items with clean water.
Finely chop the onion to take one teaspoon and cut fresh nori.
Boil 1½ teaspoon with 2 cups of water, remove the particle, allow to cool, measure 1 cup of the tea extract.
Pour all the items inside a blender with the tea extract and blend to achieve homogenous smoothies.
Transfer into a clean cup and have a nice time with a lovely body detox and energizer.

Nutrition:

Calories: 78
Fat: 2.3 g
Carbohydrates: 5 g
Protein: 6 g

3. Brazil Lettuce Smoothies (BLS)

Preparation Time: 10 minutes

Cooking Time: 0 minutes

Servings: 1

Ingredients:

1 cup raspberries
½ handful Romaine lettuce
½ cup homemade walnut milk
2 Brazil nuts
½ large grape with seed
1 cup soft jelly coconut water
Date Sugar to Taste

Directions:

In a clean bowl rinse the fruits with clean water.
Chop the Romaine lettuce and cubed raspberries and add other items into the blender and blend to achieve homogenous smoothies.
Serve your delicious medicinal detox.

Nutrition:

Calories: 168
Fat: 4.5 g
Carbohydrates: 31.3 g
Sugar: 19.2 g
Protein: 3.6 g

4. Apple – Banana Smoothie (ABS)

Preparation Time: 10 minutes

Cooking Time: 0 minutes

Servings: 1

Ingredients:

1 cup cubed apple
½ burro banana
½ cup cubed mango
½ cup cubed watermelon
½ teaspoon powdered onion
3 tablespoon Key lime juice
Date sugar to taste (If you like)

Directions:

In a clean bowl rinse the fruits with clean water.
Add cubed banana, apple, mango, watermelon, and add other items into the blender and blend to achieve homogenous smoothies.
Serve your delicious medicinal detox.
Alternatively, you can add one tablespoon of finely dices raw red onion if the powdered onion is not available.

Nutrition:

Calories: 99
Fat: 0.3g
Carbohydrates: 23 grams
Protein: 1.1 g

5. Ginger – Pear Smoothie (GPS)

Preparation Time: 10 minutes

Cooking Time: 0 minutes

Servings: 1

Ingredients:

1 big pear with seed and cured
½ avocado
¼ handful watercress
½ sour orange
½ cup of ginger tea
½ cup of coconut water
¼ cup of spring water
2 tablespoons agave syrup
Date sugar to satisfaction

Directions:

Firstly, boil 1 cup of ginger tea, cover the cup and allow it cool to room temperature.
Pour all the AGPS Items into your clean blender and homogenize them to smooth fluid.
You have just prepared yourself a wonderful detox Romaine smoothie.

Nutrition:

Calories: 101.
Protein: 1 g
Carbs: 27 g
Fiber: 6 g

6. Cantaloupe – Amaranth Smoothie (CAS)

Preparation Time: 10 minutes

Cooking Time: 0 minutes

Servings: 1

Ingredients:

½ cup of cubed cantaloupe
¼ handful green amaranth
½ cup homemade hemp milk
¼ teaspoon Dr. Sebi's bromide plus powder
1 cup of coconut water
1 teaspoon agave syrup

Directions:

You will have to rinse all the ACAS items with clean water.
Chop green amaranth, cubed cantaloupe, transfer all into a blender and blend to achieve a homogenous smoothie.
Pour into a clean cup; add Agave syrup and homemade hemp milk.
Stir them together and drink.

Nutrition:

Calories: 55
Fiber: 1.5 g
Carbohydrates: 8 mg

7. Garbanzo Squash Smoothie (GSS)

Preparation Time: 10 minutes

Cooking Time: 0 minutes

Servings: 1

Ingredients:

1 large cubed apple
1 fresh tomato
1 tablespoon finely chopped fresh onion or ¼ teaspoon powdered onion
¼ cup boiled garbanzo bean
½ cup of coconut milk
¼ cubed Mexican squash chayote
1 cup energy booster tea

Directions:

You will need to rinse the AGSS items with clean water.
Boil 1½ Dr. Sebi's energy booster tea with 2 cups of clean water. Filter the extract, measure 1 cup, and allow it to cool.
Cook Garbanzo beans, drain the water and allow it to cool.
Pour all the AGSS items into a high-speed blender and blend to achieve a homogenous smoothie.
You may add date sugar.
Serve your amazing smoothie and drink.

Nutrition:

Calories: 82.
Carbs: 22 g
Protein: 2 g
Fiber: 7 g

8. Strawberry – Orange Smoothies (SOS)

Preparation Time: 10 minutes

Cooking Time: 0 minutes

Servings: 1

Ingredients:

1 cup of diced strawberries
1 removed back of Seville orange
¼ cup cubed cucumber
¼ cup Romaine lettuce
½ kelp
½ burro banana
1 cup soft jelly coconut water
½ cup of water
Date sugar.

Directions:

Use clean water to rinse all the vegetable items of ASOS into a clean bowl.
Chop Romaine lettuce; dice strawberry, cucumber, and banana; remove the back of Seville orange and divide into four.
Transfer all the ASOS items inside a clean blender and blend to achieve a homogenous smoothie.
Pour into a clean big cup and fortify your body with a palatable detox.

Nutrition:

Calories 298
Calories from Fat 9.
Fat 1g
Cholesterol 2mg
Sodium 73mg
Potassium 998mg
Carbohydrates 68g
Fiber 7g
Sugar 50g

9. Tamarind – Pear Smoothie (TPS)

Preparation Time: 10 minutes

Cooking Time: 0 minutes

Servings: 1

Ingredients:

½ burro banana
½ cup of watermelon
1 raspberry
1 prickly pear
1 grape with seed
3 tamarinds
½ medium cucumber
1 cup of coconut water
½ cup Distilled water

Directions:

Use clean water to rinse all the ATPS items. Remove the pod of tamarinds and collect the edible part around the seed into a container. If you must use the seeds, then you have to boil the seed for 15 minutes and add to the tamarind edible part in the container.
Cube all other vegetable fruits and transfer all the items into a high-speed blender and blend to achieve a homogenous smoothie.

Nutrition:

Calories: 199
Carbohydrates: 47 g
Fat: 1g
Protein: 6g

10. Currant Elderberry Smoothie (CES)

Preparation Time: 10 minutes

Cooking Time: 0 minutes

Servings: 1

Ingredients:

¼ cup cubed elderberry
1 sour cherry
2 currants
1 cubed burro banana
1 fig
1 cup 4 bay leaves tea
1 cup energy booster tea
Date sugar to your satisfaction

Directions:

Use clean water to rinse all the ACES items. Initially boil ¾ teaspoon of energy Booster Tea with 2 cups of water on a heat source and allow boiling for 10 minutes.
Add 4 bay leaves and boil together for another 4 minutes.
Drain the tea extract into a clean big cup and allow it to cool.
Transfer all the items into a high-speed blender and blend till you achieve a homogenous smoothie.
Pour the palatable medicinal smoothie into a clean cup and drink.

Nutrition:

Calories: 63
Fat: 0.22g
Sodium: 1.1mg
Carbohydrates: 15.5g
Fiber: 4.8g
Sugars: 8.25g
Protein: 1.6g

11. Sweet Dream Strawberry Smoothie

Preparation Time: 15 minutes

Cooking Time: 0

Servings: 1

Ingredients:

5 strawberries
3 dates – pits eliminated
2 burro bananas or small bananas
Spring water for 32 fluid ounce of smoothie

Directions:

Strip off the skin of the bananas.
Wash the dates and strawberries.
Include bananas, dates, and strawberries to a blender container.
Include a couple of water and blend.
Keep on including adequate water to persuade up to be 32 oz. of smoothie.

Nutrition:

Calories: 282 - Fat: 11g
Carbohydrates: 4g - Protein: 7g

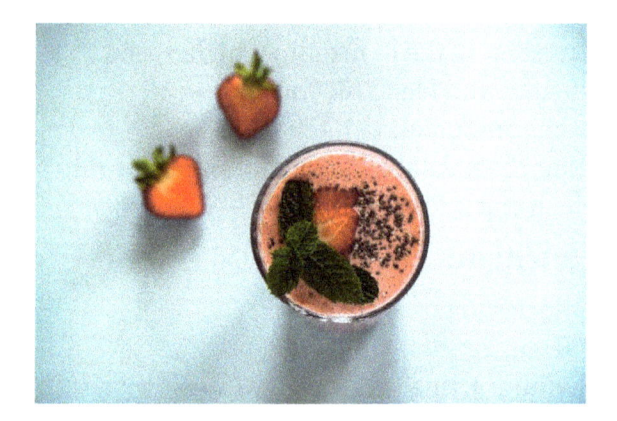

12. Alkaline Green Ginger and Banana Cleansing Smoothie

Preparation Time: 15 minutes

Cooking Time: 0

Servings: 1

Ingredients:

One handful of kale
One banana, frozen
Two cups of hemp seed milk
One inch of ginger, finely minced
Half cup of chopped strawberries, frozen
1 tablespoon of agave or your preferred sweetener

Directions:

Mix all the ingredients in a blender and mix on high speed.
Allow it to blend evenly.
Pour into a pitcher with a few decorative straws and voila, you are one happy camper. Enjoy!

Nutrition:

Calories: 350
Fat: 4g
Carbohydrates: 52g
Protein: 16g

13. Orange Mixed Detox Smoothie

Preparation Time: 15 minutes

Cooking Time: 0

Servings: 1

Ingredients:

One cup of veggies (amaranth, dandelion, lettuce or watercress)
Half avocado
One cup of tender-jelly coconut water
One Seville orange
Juice of one key lime
One tablespoon of bromide plus powder

Directions:

Peel and cut the Seville orange in chunks. Mix all the ingredients collectively in a high-speed blender until done.

Nutrition:

Calories: 71
Fat: 1g
Carbohydrates: 12g
Protein: 2g

14. Cucumber Toxin Flush Smoothie

Preparation Time: 15 minutes

Cooking Time: 0

Servings: 1

Ingredients:

1 cucumber
1 key lime
1 cup of watermelon (seeded), cubed

Directions:

Mix all the above ingredients in a high-speed blender.
Considering that watermelon and cucumbers are largely water, you may not want to add any extra, however, you can do so if you want.
Juice the key lime and add it to your smoothie.
Enjoy!

Nutrition:

Calories: 219
Fat: 4g
Carbohydrates: 48g
Protein: 5g

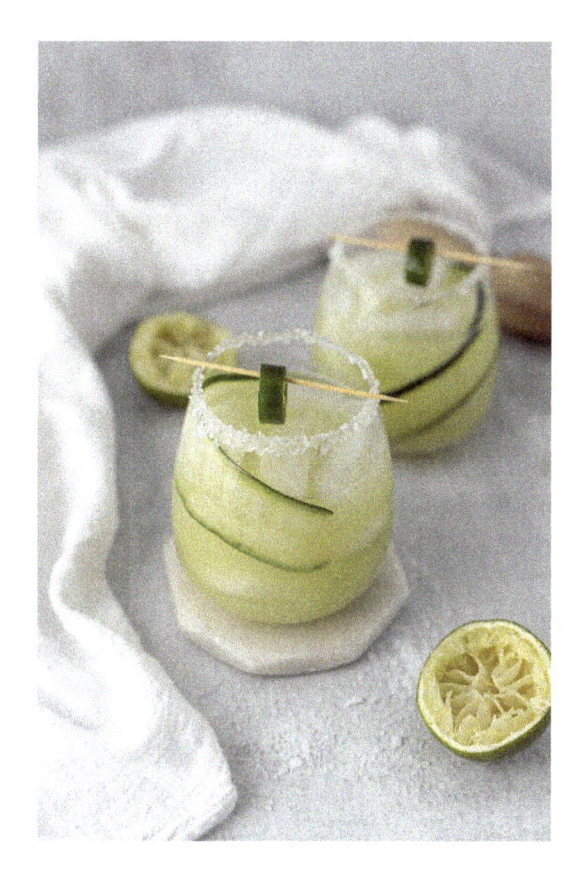

15. Apple Blueberry Smoothie

Preparation Time: 15 minutes

Cooking Time: 0

Servings: 1

Ingredients:

Half apple
One date
Half cup of blueberries
Half cup of sparkling callaloo
One tablespoon of hemp seeds
One tablespoon of sesame seeds
Two cups of sparkling soft-jelly coconut water
Half tablespoon of bromide plus powder

Directions:

Mix all of the ingredients in a high-speed blender and enjoy!

Nutrition:

Calories: 167.4
Fat: 6.4g
Carbohydrates: 22.5g
Protein: 6.7g

16. Detox Berry Smoothie

Preparation Time: 15 minutes

Cooking Time: 0

Servings: 1

Ingredients:

Spring water
1/4 avocado, pitted
One medium burro banana
One Seville orange
Two cups of fresh lettuce
One tablespoon of hemp seeds
One cup of berries (blueberries or an aggregate of blueberries, strawberries, and raspberries)

Directions:

Add the spring water to your blender.
Put the fruits and veggies right inside the blender.
Blend all ingredients until smooth.

Nutrition:

Calories: 202.4
Fat: 4.5g
Carbohydrates: 32.9g
Protein: 13.3g

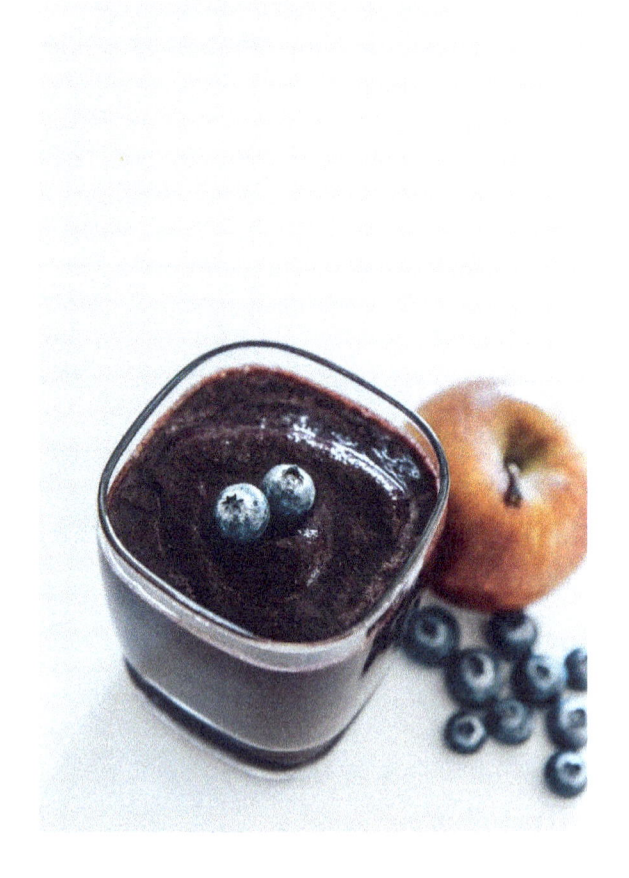

17. Papaya Detox Smoothie

Preparation Time: 15 minutes

Cooking Time: 0

Servings: 1

Ingredients:

Two cups papaya
One tablespoon of papaya seeds
Juice of a Lime
One cup of filtered water

Directions:

Chop the papaya into square portions and scoop out a tablespoon of clean and raw papaya seeds.
Mix all of the ingredients right into a high-speed blender for 1 minute until the whole thing is blended.
Pour into a tumbler and enjoy this tasty drink your liver will love.
Enjoy!

Nutrition:

Calories: 197
Fat: 0.7g
Carbohydrates: 49.4g
Protein: 5.4g

Directions:

Put all the ingredients collectively in a blender.
Blend all the ingredients evenly.
Enjoy this delicious smoothie.

Nutrition:

Calories: 133
Fat: 4g
Carbohydrates: 24g
Protein: 3g

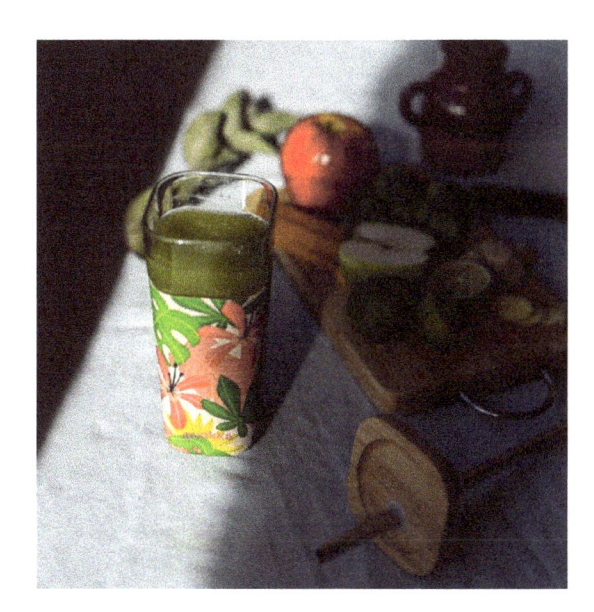

18. Apple and Amaranth Detoxifying Smoothie

Preparation Time: 15 minutes

Cooking Time: 0

Servings: 1

Ingredients:

1/4 avocado
1 key lime
Two apples, chopped
Two cups of water
Two cups of amaranth veggie

19. Avocado Mixed Smoothie

Preparation Time: 15 minutes

Cooking Time: 0

Servings: 1

Ingredients:

One cup of water
One ounce of blueberries
One pear, chopped
1/4 avocado, pitted
1/4 cup cooked quinoa

Directions:

Mix all ingredients in a high-speed blender and enjoy!

Nutrition:

Calories: 187
Fat: 21g
Carbohydrates: 29g
Protein: 11g

20. Peach Berry Smoothie

Preparation Time: 15 minutes

Cooking Time: 0

Servings: 1

Ingredients:

Half cup of frozen peaches
Half cup of frozen blueberries
Half cup of frozen cherries
Half cup of frozen strawberries
One tablespoon of sea moss gel
One tablespoon of hemp seeds
One tablespoon of coconut water
One tablespoon of agave

Directions:

Blend all ingredients for one minute. If the combination is too thick, add extra ¼ cup of coconut water and blend for another 20 secs.
Enjoy your peach berry smoothie!

Nutrition:

Calories: 170 - Fat: 0g
Carbohydrates: 43g - Protein: 0g

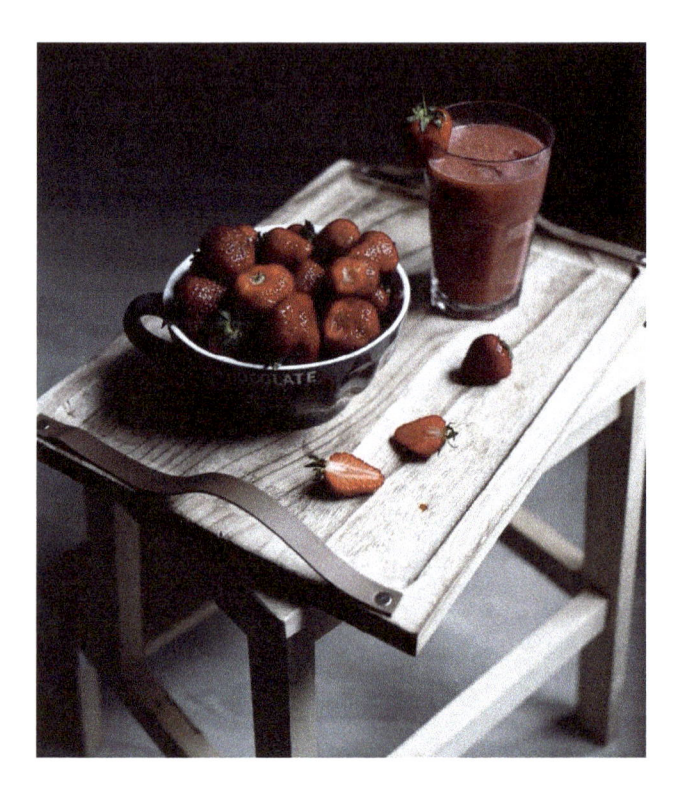

21. Irish Sea Moss Smoothie

Preparation Time: 15 minutes

Cooking Time: 0

Servings: 1

Ingredients:

2 oz. of whole wild sea moss, soaked
2 cups of spring water

Directions:

To prepare Irish sea moss smoothie, use two whole and wild sea moss.
Carefully wash away any sand and debris.
Do a final wash and chop up longer ones to safeguard your blender's blade.
Add your sea moss and two cups of spring water to blend in the blender.
Put in a jar and refrigerate. This smoothie can last for many weeks.
Enjoy your delicious smoothie.

Nutrition:

Calories: 220
Fat: 3g
Carbohydrates: 45g
Protein: 2g

22. Cucumber Mixed Detox Smoothie

Preparation Time: 15 minutes

Cooking Time: 0

Servings: 1

Ingredients:

Half cucumber, chopped
One inch of ginger
One pinch of pure sea salt
Two grapefruits, squeezed
Two lemons, squeezed
One avocado, chopped
Half cup of filtered or spring water
One pinch cayenne pepper

Directions:

Blend all ingredients. Sip and experience this tasty nutritious smoothie!

Nutrition:

Calories: 48 - Fat: 0g
Carbohydrates: 12g - Protein: 1g

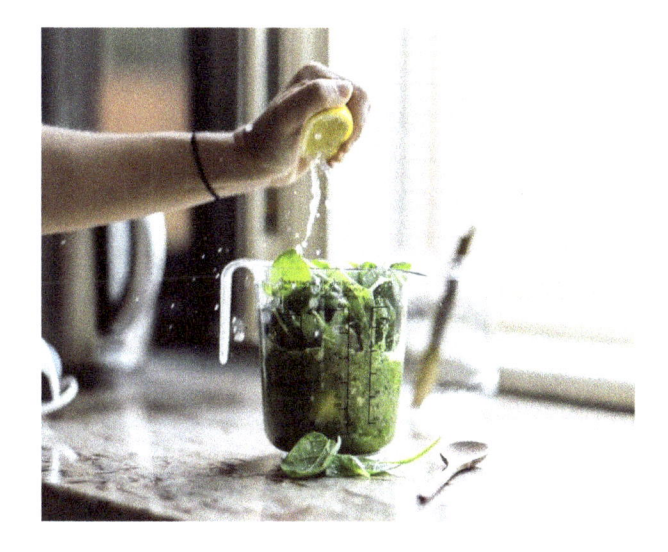

23. Strawberry Banana Smoothie

Preparation Time: 15 minutes

Cooking Time: 0

Servings: 1-2

Ingredients:

2 cups hemp milk
4 banana
8 oz. strawberry
¾ cup dates
1 tbsp. agave

Directions:

To make this delicious smoothie, you need to place the strawberries and date in a high-speed blender.
Blend them for a minute or two or until they are slightly broken down.
After that, add the banana along with the hemp milk and agave.
Blend them for 2 to 3 minutes or until combined well.
Enjoy.

Nutrition:

Calories: 148
Fat: 2g
Carbohydrates: 21g
Protein: 1g

24. Green Monster Smoothie

Preparation Time: 15 minutes

Cooking Time: 0

Servings: 1

Ingredients:

½ of 1 avocado, diced
½ of 1 mango, diced
2 to 3 dates, pitted
1 tbsp. soursop pulp
1 bunch of rainbow Kale, leaves torn
½ cup of coconut water

Directions:

To make this smoothie, place all the ingredients in a high-speed blender and blend it for 2 to 3 minutes or until everything comes together and smooth.
Move the mixture to a serving glass and serve it with ice cubes if you desire to take it cold.

Nutrition:

Calories: 179.4
Fat: 2.3g
Carbohydrates: 36.8g
Protein: 6.8g

25. Apple Smoothie

Preparation Time: 15 minutes

Cooking Time: 0

Servings: 2

Ingredients:

2 cups of apple juice, fresh
2 cups ice cube
1 tbsp. sea moss
1 clove, grounded
1 tbsp. ginger, grounded

Directions:

To start with, place all the ingredients needed to make the smoothie in a high-speed blender. Blend all ingredients wait for 2 to 3 minutes or until you get a smooth mixture. Serve and enjoy.

Nutrition:

Calories: 431.5
Fat: 10.8g
Carbohydrates: 53.1g
Protein: 38.4g

26. Weight Loss Apple Cucumber Smoothie

Preparation Time: 15 minutes

Cooking Time: 0

Servings: 1

Ingredients:

One large to medium size of sliced cucumber
One large cubed apple
One large sliced bell pepper
Six seeded dates (rinsed)
Six large strawberries
Five sliced tomatoes (rinsed)
Half to one cupful of water

Directions:

Combine the whole recipes and blend very well until smooth. Wow! The first-day breakfast is settled, enjoy.

Nutrition:

65 calories
Carb 57 g
Protein 2 g
Fat 4 g

27. Toxins Removal Smoothie

Preparation Time: 15 minutes

Cooking Time: 0

Servings: 1

Ingredients:

One seeded and sliced small to large-sized watermelon
One large key lime (removes the juice and discards the seed
One large cucumber (sliced)

Directions:

Transfer the lime juice into the blender.
Add the remaining recipes and blend very well to obtain a smooth mixture.
Wow! This means you have successfully completed the second-day smoothie. Enjoy.

Nutrition:

45 calories
Carb 35 g
Protein 6 g
Fat 4 g

28. Multiple Berries Smoothie

Preparation Time: 15 minutes

Cooking Time: 0

Servings: 1

Ingredients:

A quarter cupful of blueberries
A quarter cupful of strawberries
A quarter cupful of raspberries
One large banana (peeled and sliced)
Agave syrup as desired
A half cupful of water

Directions:

Transfer the water into the blender.
Add the remaining recipes and blend until smooth.
I really love this smoothie because it is very sweet without adding sugar and the colour is also inviting.

Nutrition:

Calories: 210
Carbohydrates: 55 g
Sodium: 20 mg

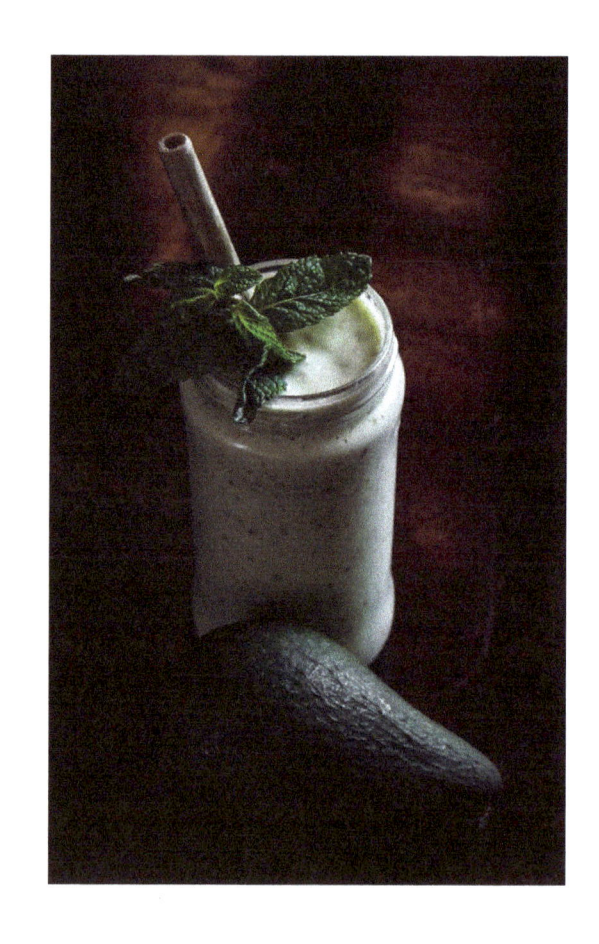

29. Dandelion Avocado Smoothie

Preparation Time: 15 minutes

Cooking Time: 0

Servings: 1

Ingredients:

One cup of dandelion
One orange (juiced)
Coconut water
One avocado
One key lime (juice)

Directions:

In a high-speed blend all ingredients until smooth.

Nutrition:

Calories: 160 - Fat: 15 grams
Carbohydrates: 9 grams
Protein: 2 grams

30. Amaranth Greens and Avocado Smoothie

Preparation Time: 15 minutes

Cooking Time: 0

Servings: 1

Ingredients:

One key lime (juice)
Two sliced apples (seeded)
Half avocado
Two cups of amaranth greens
Two cups of watercress
One cup of water

Directions:

Add the whole recipes together and transfer them into the blender. Blend thoroughly until smooth.

Nutrition:

Calories: 160
Fat: 15 grams
Carbohydrates: 9 grams
Protein: 2 grams

Conclusion

Thank you for making it to the end of Dr. Sebi's book of recipes. Dr. Sebi's eating regimen is an antacid dinner plan, which is generally a veggie lover diet. The eating regimen depends on plants that control human-made weight control plans and cross breed nourishments as well. The eating regimen likewise guarantees that there are least degrees of corrosive in the nourishments you devour and the bodily fluid in one's body.

He additionally accepts that when individuals follow the two strategies, they make a domain, basic, not perfect for the endurance of maladies in the human body.

What inspired the specialist to receive the eating regimen is his starting point back in Honduras. The inspiration driving Dr. Sebi's eating routine focuses back to Alfredo Darrington Bowman (Dr. Sebi). He is a local Honduran, known as an intracellular specialist, botanist, and common healer.

Eating food is an everyday schedule that people should experience. The idea of substances and nourishments that we devour ordinary can bring about a lifetime utilization propensity on the off chance that it isn't directed. Before hopping into the basic way of life, you have to contemplate it. It will assist you with abstaining from making void vows to self.

This eating routine diminishes body contaminants and supports general prosperity. It will make you take a more secure, better way to deal with food.

It will likewise raise the odds of different infections. On the chance that you need to shed pounds, it can spur you to do it effectively and dependably. This is identified with improved quality and versatility that everybody requires.

Dr. Sebi's eating regimen is an altogether new way to deal with food. Thusly, it may be difficult to become acclimated to it, particularly toward the beginning.

It is prudent to attempt Dr. Sebi's Directions for 30 days if you don't completely receive another dietary system. Connect with for a month and see the upgrades. Following a month, you should change to this eating regimen altogether.

Dr. Sebi's diet advances eating entire, natural, plant-based food. Numerous people have used to cause a noteworthy change in their wellbeing. They are perfect in moving from acidic to soluble. You can similarly utilize them for occasionally keeping up your body framework and improving your wellbeing.

Not exclusively will you eat scrumptious suppers, you will likewise be helping yourself and your family to feel much improved and improve in general wellbeing just by eating affirmed Doctor Sebi's food. How incredible is that?

Now there is just one thing for you to do: Take action!

I hope you enjoyed reading this book. If you are looking to follow a more plant-based eating pattern, Dr. Sebi's diet has many healthy diets that are more flexible and sustainable.

I wish you great success in your journey for good health!

CPSIA information can be obtained
at www.ICGtesting.com
Printed in the USA
BVHW051109250221
601118BV00010B/680